PREFACE

In this study guide, which should be utilized in conjunction with *Schwartz, et al.: Principles of Surgery*, Second Edition, 1974, I have attempted to transform general surgical information and principles into questions, as a means of testing one's absorption and comprehension of the subject matter in surgery. The organized format should prove a valuable study aid to medical students, surgical residents, practicing surgeons and other physicians interested in the clinical application of these facts.

The reader is advised to read his textbook completely, as this guide is not meant to be a substitute for the educational benefits which are derived from an excellent textbook.

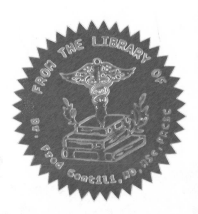

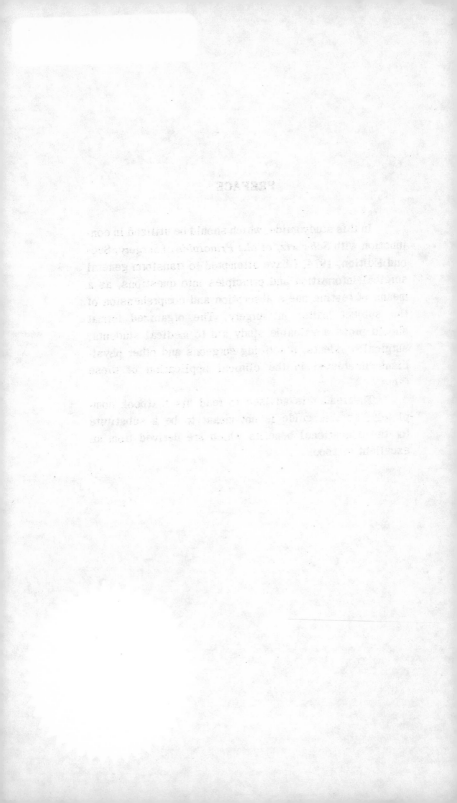

Medical Examination Review Book

Volume 5A

TEXTBOOK STUDY GUIDE
OF
SURGERY

Second Edition

1,894 MULTIPLE CHOICE QUESTIONS
AND REFERENCED ANSWERS

By

ALFRED N. BUTNER, M.D.
Clinical Instructor
Department of Surgery
Stanford University
School of Medicine

and

Staff Surgeon
Sunnyvale Medical Clinic
Sunnyvale, California
El Camino Hospital
Mountainview, California

MEDICAL EXAMINATION PUBLISHING COMPANY, INC.
65-36 Fresh Meadow Lane
Flushing, New York 11365

MEDICAL EXAMINATION REVIEW BOOK
TEXTBOOK STUDY GUIDE OF SURGERY
Volume 5A - Second Edition

TABLE OF CONTENTS

SECTION

I   PHYSICAL AND METABOLIC RESPONSE TO TIS-
SUE DESTRUCTION AND TRANSPLANTATION
Questions 1-584   7

II   PHYSIOLOGIC MONITORING
Questions 585-603 71

III   DISEASES OF THE INTEGUMENT
Questions 604-650 74

IV   HEAD AND NECK SURGERY
Questions 651-686 80

V   THORACIC AND CARDIOVASCULAR SURGERY
Questions 687-940 84

VI   SURGICAL HYPERTENSION
Questions 941-966 113

VII   GASTROINTESTINAL SURGERY
Questions 967-1231 116

VIII MECHANISMS OF ABDOMINAL PROTECTION
AND SUPPORT
Questions 1232-1306 146

IX   ENDOCRINE AXIS
Questions 1307-1424 156

X   PEDIATRIC SURGERY
Questions 1425-1445 168

XI   UROLOGIC SURGERY
Questions 1446-1475 171

XII   GYNECOLOGIC SURGERY
Questions 1476-1517 175

Table of Contents (Continued)

SECTION

XIII   NEUROLOGIC SURGERY
Questions 1518-1572 180

XIV   ACQUIRED AND CONGENITAL MUSCULO-
SKELETAL DISORDERS: RECONSTRUCTION
AND REHABILITATION
Questions 1573-1894 186

ANSWER KEY 220

ANSWER THE FOLLOWING QUESTIONS BY USING THE KEY
OUTLINED BELOW:
A. If both statement and reason are correct and related cause and effect
B. If both statement and reason are correct but not related cause and
    effect
C. If statement is true but reason is false
D. If statement is false but reason is true
E. If both statement and reason are false

1.   ACTH secretion in response to trauma will not occur if the injured area is
     deinnervated BECAUSE the release of ACTH is dependent upon venous re-
     turn of humeral agents from the traumatized area.
                                        Ref. p. 1

2.   A paraplegic patient would not be expected to produce 17-OHCS in response
     to surgery below the level of the cord lesion BECAUSE ACTH blood levels
     are at a maximum and cannot be stimulated beyond that point.
                                        Ref. p. 2

SELECT THE MOST APPROPRIATE ANSWER(S):

3.   HYPOVOLEMIA MAY ACT AS A PRIMARY STIMULUS FOR ALL, EXCEPT:
     A. Aldosterone secretion
     B. Antidiuretic hormone secretion
     C. Thyroid stimulating hormone
     D. Epinephrine and norepinephrine release
     E. Cortisol secretion   Ref. p. 2

4.   HYPOVOLEMIA STIMULATES WHICH OF THE FOLLOWING PRESSURE
     SENSITIVE SYSTEMS TO PRODUCE RENIN?:
     A. Aortic arch
     B. Carotid sinus
     C. Juxtaglomerular apparatus
     D. Hypothalamic volume sensors
     E. Hypothalamic pressure sensors   Ref. p. 2

5.   IN A PARAPLEGIC PATIENT WITH A SEVERE BURN BELOW THE LEVEL
     OF THE CORD LESION, THE STIMULUS WHICH BRINGS ABOUT ACTH
     RELEASE FIRST WOULD MOST LIKELY BE:
     A. Local burn destruction   D. Infection
     B. Hypovolemia   E. All of the above
     C. Acidosis   Ref. p. 3

6.   WHICH OF THE FOLLOWING STATES IS AN EXAMPLE OF THIRD SPACE
     SEQUESTRATION?:
     A. Burn edema
     B. Large collections of blood secondary to fractured femur
     C. Ileus of small bowel with accumulated intraluminal fluids
     D. All of the above   Ref. p. 3

7.   WHICH OF THE FOLLOWING IS NOT RELEASED BY BACTERIAL
     ENDOTOXIN?:
     A. ACTH
     B. Epinephrine + Norepinephrine
     C. ADH
     D. Renin
     E. None of the above   Ref. p. 3

SECTION I - PHYSICAL AND METABOLIC RESPONSE TO TISSUE DESTRUCTION AND TRANSPLANTATION

8. ACIDOSIS MAY BE PRODUCED BY:
    A. Prolonged shock
    B. Respiratory hyperpnea
    C. Open heart surgical procedures with extracorporeal circulation
    D. Prolonged Levine tube suction
    E. Cirrhosis   Ref. p. 3

9. IN ENDOTOXIN RELEASE IN AN ANIMAL WITH A SECTIONED CORD, WHICH WOULD BE PRODUCED?:
    A. ACTH
    B. Adrenal medullary epinephrine
    C. Both   Ref. p. 3

10. BACTERIAL ENDOTOXIN GIVEN INTRAVENOUSLY IN AN ANIMAL WHOSE SPINAL CORD IS SECTIONED AT C7 EXHIBITS WHICH OF THE FOLLOW-ING FINDINGS?:
    A. Elevation in ACTH level, elevation in 17-OHCS level, elevation in epinephrine secretion
    B. No change in ACTH level, elevation in 17-OHCS level, no change in epinephrine secretion
    C. Elevation in ACTH level, no change in 17-OHCS level, no change in epinephrine secretion
    D. Elevation in ACTH level, elevation in 17-OHCS level, no change in epinephrine secretion   Ref. p. 3

11. WHAT EFFECT DOES EMOTIONAL TRAUMA USUALLY HAVE ON THE BODY'S ENDOCRINE RESPONSE TO TRAUMA?:
    A. Synergistic
    B. Antagonistic
    C. No effect   Ref. p. 4

12. ANOXIA MAY BE A "PRIMARY TRAUMA" IN OUR SPACE AGE, OR SECONDARY TO CHEST TRAUMA, AND RESULTS IN STIMULATION OF WHICH OF THE FOLLOWING?:
    A. ADH   D. Growth hormone
    B. Catecholamine   E. Renin
    C. 17-OHCS   Ref. p. 4

13. WHICH OF THE FOLLOWING IS STIMULATED BY HYPOGLYCEMIA?:
    A. ACTH   D. Norepinephrine
    B. GH   E. All of the above
    C. Epinephrine   Ref. p. 4

    ANSWER THE FOLLOWING QUESTIONS BY USING THE KEY OUTLINED BELOW:
    A. If both statement and reason are correct and related cause and effect
    B. If both statement and reason are correct but not related cause and effect
    C. If statement is true but reason is false
    D. If statement is false but reason is true
    E. If both statement and reason are false

14. An increased release of catecholamine is noted in the presence of hypo-glycemia BECAUSE it directly stimulates the hypothalamus.
                                        Ref. p. 4

15. ACTH release in anesthetized animals undergoing operative trauma is de-creased BECAUSE with hypothermia the effects of anesthesia are abolished.
                                        Ref. p. 5

16. An anencephalic patient is able to release ACTH from its anterior pituitary
in response to trauma BECAUSE the primary site of stimulation is the
medulla.   Ref. p. 5

MATCH THE FOLLOWING HYPOTHALAMIC CENTERS AND THEIR
ENDOCRINE SECRETIONS. EACH LETTERED ANSWER MAY BE USED
ONLY ONCE:

17. ___ Anterior supraoptic nucleus   A. LH, FSH
18. ___ Posterior supraoptic nucleus   B. CRF (corticotropin releas-
19. ___ Paraventricular nucleus   ing factor) TSH
20. ___ Tuberal nucleus   C. Epinephrine, norepinephrine
21. ___ Median eminence   D. ADH
22. ___ Posterior hypothalamus   E. Control over gonadotropic
                                              hormones
                                           F. Oxytocin
                                           Ref. p. 6

ANSWER THE FOLLOWING QUESTION BY USING THE KEY
OUTLINED BELOW:
A. If both statement and reason are correct and related cause and effect
B. If both statement and reason are correct and not related cause and effect
C. If statement is true but reason is false
D. If statement is false but reason is true
E. If both statement and reason are false

23. Exogenous corticosteroids for a prolonged period will induce disuse adrenal
atrophy AND an unresponsive gland to ACTH stimulation induced by operative trauma.   Ref. p. 7

ANSWER THE FOLLOWING STATEMENT T(RUE) OR F(ALSE):

24. Unrecognized adrenal insufficiency at operation will most likely result in
death in the operative or early postoperative period.
                                                      Ref. p. 8

SELECT THE MOST APPROPRIATE ANSWER:

25. THE MOST COMMON FORM OF UNRECOGNIZED ADRENAL INSUFFI-
CIENCY IN MALES IS:
A. Adrenogenital syndrome
B. Iatrogenic corticosteroid medication withdrawal
C. Waterhouse-Friderichsen syndrome
D. Addison's disease   Ref. p. 8

SELECT THE MOST APPROPRIATE ANSWER:

26. CORTISOL IS DEACTIVATED BY GLUCURONIC ACID OR SULFURIC ACID
CONJUGATION IN_____, AND THEREFORE, ABNORMAL ELEVA-
TIONS OF STEROID WOULD BE PRESENT IF DAMAGE TO THE ORGAN(S)
WOULD OCCUR:
A. Liver
B. Kidney
C. Both liver and kidney   Ref. p. 9

27. IN A PARAPLEGIC PATIENT, WHICH OF THE FOLLOWING WOULD NOT
STIMULATE CORTICOSTEROID PRODUCTION?:
A. Infection   D. Hypoglycemia
B. Trauma - operative   E. Hemorrhage
C. Excitatory anesthetic agent   Ref. p. 9

SECTION I - PHYSICAL AND METABOLIC RESPONSE TO TISSUE
                    DESTRUCTION AND TRANSPLANTATION

FILL IN THE APPROPRIATE ANSWERS. EACH LETTERED ITEM
MAY BE USED MORE THAN ONCE: (Questions 28-31)

A. Elevated
B. Decreased
C. Unchanged

In Nembutal anesthesia, the 17-OHCS are 28) _____ and the epinephrine,
norepinephrine secretions are 29) _____ while in ether anesthesia,
17-OHCS are 30) _____ and epinephrine, norepinephrine secretions are
31) _____ .   Ref. p. 10

FILL IN THE APPROPRIATE ANSWERS: (Questions 32-34)

A. Hypertension
B. Death
C. Salt loss hypotension

Changes in the C11 molecule of cortisol result in 32) _____, at C20 result in 33) _____, and at C21 result in 34) _____:
                                         Ref. p. 12

SELECT THE MOST APPROPRIATE ANSWERS:

35. WHICH CAUSES THE GREATEST OPERATIVE RISK?:
     A. Unrecognized preoperative steroid withdrawal
     B. Bilateral adrenal hemorrhage at surgery unrecognized
     C. Bilateral adrenalectomy without steroid replacement
     D. Uncompensated Addison's disease   Ref. p. 12

36. WHICH OF THE FOLLOWING ROUTES OF CORTISOL ACETATE REPLACE-
     MENT IS LEAST EFFECTIVE?:
     A. Intramuscular
     B. Intravenous
     C. Oral
     D. Rectal suppository   Ref. p. 12

ANSWER THE FOLLOWING QUESTIONS BY USING THE KEY
OUTLINED BELOW:
A. If both statement and reason are correct and related cause and effect
B. If both statement and reason are correct but not related cause and effect
C. If statement is true but reason is false
D. If statement is false but reason is true
E. If both statement and reason are false

37. Patients with severe prolonged trauma (i.e. burns, sepsis, infection) die
     with low levels of corticosteroids BECAUSE the chronic stimulus is respon-
     sible for depletion.   Ref. p. 12

38. High levels of corticosteroids in burn patients are ominous findings
     BECAUSE they are indicative of continued stress and ultimate decompensa-
     tion.   Ref. p. 12

39. Aldosterone secretion in the presence of trauma increases even though ACTH
     release remains low BECAUSE Aldosterone secretion is never dependent on
     ACTH stimulation.   Ref. p. 12

SELECT THE MOST APPROPRIATE ANSWER:

40. DURING OPERATIVE TRAUMA WITH THE COMMONLY EMPLOYED
ANESTHETIC AGENTS, WHICH OF THE FOLLOWING APPEARS IN
GREATER CONCENTRATIONS?:
  A. Norepinephrine
  B. Epinephrine
  C. Both are equal   Ref. p. 13

41. FOLLOWING TRAUMA, WHICH CAUSES THE GREATEST STATE OF
WATER RETENTION?:
  A. Renin-Aldosterone   C. ADH
  B. Epinephrine-Norepinephrine   D. ACTH-Cortisol
                                    Ref. p. 14

ANSWER THE FOLLOWING QUESTION BY USING THE KEY
OUTLINED BELOW:
  A. If statement and reason are correct and are related cause and effect
  B. If both statement and reason are correct but not related cause and effect
  C. If statement is true but reason is false
  D. If statement is false but reason is true
  E. If both statement and reason are false

42. The term "Inappropriate ADH Secretion" refers to a low urine output with a
high osmolarity and dilutional hyponatremia BECAUSE this is a frequent
occurrence following head trauma.   Ref. p. 14

SELECT THE MOST APPROPRIATE ANSWER:

43. WHICH OF THE FOLLOWING IS DIABETOGENIC?:
  A. ACTH   D. Glucagon
  B. Growth hormone   E. All of the above
  C. Epinephrine + Norepinephrine   Ref. pp. 14-16

44. WHICH OF THE FOLLOWING HORMONES IS LEAST STIMULATED BY THE
ONSET OF TRAUMA?:
  A. ADH   D. TSH
  B. Growth hormone   E. ACTH
  C. Glucagon   Ref. p. 16

ANSWER THE FOLLOWING QUESTION BY USING THE KEY
OUTLINED BELOW:
  A. If statement and reason are correct and are related cause and effect
  B. If both statement and reason are correct but not related cause and effect
  C. If statement is true but reason is false
  D. If statement is false but reason is true
  E. If both statement and reason are false

45. The Glucose Tolerance Curve in the early post-traumatic period is of
diabetic character BECAUSE of epinephrine secretion.
                                    Ref. p. 17

SELECT THE MOST APPROPRIATE ANSWER:

46. IN THE PYRUVATE-ACETYL COENZYME, A BLOCK AS SEEN IN SEVERE
ANOXIA CAN BE REVERSED BY INCREASING TISSUE PERFUSION BY:
  A. Epinephrine administration   D. Thyroxin administration
  B. Corticosteroid administration E. Angiotensin II
  C. Levarterenol administration   Ref. p. 25 (1st Ed.)

47. THE POST-TRAUMATIC DIABETIC STATE IS AFFECTED BY SUBSTANCES
     WHICH ANTAGONIZE INSULIN. THE MOST POTENT HORMONE WITH
     THIS EFFECT IS?:
     A. Epinephrine, Norepinephrine
     B. Glucagon
     C. Growth homone
     D. ACTH - Cortisol
     E. Aldosterone   Ref. p. 26

48. LIPID MOBILIZATION FOLLOWING SHOCK IS DUE TO_____, WHICH
     ACCELERATES LIPOLYSIS OF TRIGLYCERIDES:
     A. ACTH
     B. TSH
     C. GH
     D. Epinephinre + Norepinephrine
     E. All of the above   Ref. p. 26 (1st Ed.)

49. FOLLOWING TRAUMA, HYPERGLYCEMIA DEVELOPS DUE TO:
     A. Epinephrine inhibition of Insulin secretion and interference with its
         peripheral action
     B. Cortisol secretion
     C. Growth hormone
     D. Glucagon
     E. All of the above   Ref. p. 26

     ANSWER THE FOLLOWING QUESTIONS BY USING THE KEY
     OUTLINED BELOW:
     A. If both statement and reason are correct and related cause and effect
     B. If both statement and reason are correct but not related cause and effect
     C. If statement is true but reason is false
     D. If statement is false but reason is true
     E. If both statement and reason are false

50. A positive nitrogen balance may be ultimately obtained with plasma as the
     only source of protein BECAUSE it provides the highest caloric parenteral
     intake.   Ref. p. 27 (1st Ed.)

51. In hemorrhagic shock and severe anoxia, there is a block in the carbohy-
     drate energy pathway at the pyruvate-acetyl coenzyme A step BECAUSE this
     leads to lactate and pyruvate production.
                                            Ref. p. 27

52. The post-operative Negative Nitrogen balance usually is reversible BECAUSE
     it is possible to administer the essential nutrients intravenously which de-
     crease the period from 3 days to 1 day.   Ref. p. 27

     FILL IN THE APPROPRIATE ANSWERS: (Questions 53-54)
     A.   2 to 3
     B.   11 to 17
     C.   30 to 50
     D.   70 to 100
     E.   120 to 140

     Urinary nitrogen excretion normally is 53) _____ grams daily and follow-
     ing trauma may increase to 54) _____ grams.
                                            Ref. p. 27

55. PROTEIN LOSS AFTER SEVERE TRAUMA OCCURS BECAUSE OF ALL THE
     FOLLOWING, EXCEPT:
     A. Starvation   D. Fever
     B. Increased catabolism   E. None of the above
     C. Bed rest   Ref. pp. 27-28

ANSWER THE FOLLOWING QUESTION BY USING THE KEY BELOW:
A. If both statement and reason are correct and related cause and effect
B. If both statement and reason are correct but not related cause and effect
C. If statement is true but reason is false
D. If statement is false but reason is true
E. If both statement and reason are false

56. Plasma protein decline after injury is primarily in the albumin fraction
BECAUSE of the depressed liver function.

Ref. p. 28

SELECT THE MOST APPROPRIATE ANSWER(S):

57. PROTEIN BREAKDOWN TO ACCOUNT FOR UREA NITROGEN LOSS AFTER
TRAUMA IS PRIMARILY FROM THE:
A. Liver
B. Adipose tissue
C. Skeletal system
D. Dietary intake   Ref. p. 28

58. HYPERCOAGULATION DURING PREGNANCY IS DUE IN PART TO IN-
CREASES IN WHICH OF THE FOLLOWING FACTORS?:
A. Fibrinogen   D. Factor V
B. Prothrombin   E. All of the above
C. Factor VII   Ref. p. 29

59. THE INCIDENCE OF PULMONARY EMBOLISM IN FEMALES ON BIRTH
CONTROL PILLS IS____TIMES GREATER THAN IN WOMEN OF THE
SAME AGE GROUP NOT TAKING PILLS:
A. 3   D. 15
B. 7   E. 19
C. 11   Ref. p. 29

60. DIPHASIC COAGULATION STATES OCCUR IN:
A. Epinephrine administration   D. Pregnancy
B. ACTH + Cortisol administration   E. All of the above
C. Hemorrhage   Ref. p. 29

61. THE PEAK OF HYPERCOAGULABILITY IN HEMORRHAGIC SHOCK IS
REACHED BY_____HOURS AFTER THE ONSET OF BLEEDING:
A. 7   D. 63
B. 24   E. 72
C. 36   Ref. p. 29

62. MOST ALL ACQUIRED BLEEDING DISORDERS CAN BE GROUPED INTO
WHICH OF THE FOLLOWING CATEGORIES?:
A. Thrombocytopenia   E. Hepatic damage
B. Afibrinogenemia   F. All of the above
C. Fibrinolysis
D. Anti-coagulation   Ref. p. 30

63. THE REVERSAL OF COUMADIN EFFECT ON BLOOD CAN BEST BE
ACCOMPLISHED BY:
A. Vitamin C   C. Vitamin K2
B. Vitamin K1   D. Vitamin D
                                     Ref. p. 30

64. TO RETURN THE CLOTTING MECHANISM TO NORMAL BY EXCHANGE
TRANSFUSION_____UNITS OF FRESH WHOLE BLOOD ARE NECES-
SARY:
A. 2-5   D. 15-20
B. 5-10   E. 20-25
C. 10-15   Ref. p. 30

SECTION I - PHYSICAL AND METABOLIC RESPONSE TO TISSUE
              DESTRUCTION AND TRANSPLANTATION

ANSWER THE FOLLOWING QUESTION BY USING THE KEY
OUTLINED BELOW:
A. If both statement and reason are correct and related cause and effect
B. If both statement and reason are correct but not related cause and effect
C. If statement is true but reason is false
D. If statement is false but reason is true
E. If both statement and reason are false

65. Hemorrhage secondary to calcium deficit following multiple blood transfu-
     sions will occur before the onset of tetany BECAUSE tetanic contractions
     appear at calcium levels about 2.5 mg before the development of a coagula-
     tion deficit.   Ref. p. 30

     SELECT THE MOST APPROPRIATE ANSWER:

66. THE DUDRICK FORMULA FOR HYPERALIMENTATION CONTAINS ALL OF
     THE FOLLOWING, EXCEPT:
     A. L-Essential Amino-acids   D. Minerals
     B. Glucose   E. Phosphate
     C. Vitamins   Ref. p. 32

67. TREATMENT OF SEPTIC SHOCK OFTEN REQUIRES WHICH OF THE
     FOLLOWING?:
     A. Phenoxybenzamine   D. Chlorpromazine
     B. Volume replacement   E. All of the above
     C. Antibiotics   Ref. p. 35 (1st Ed.)

68. WHICH OF THE FOLLOWING IS MORE COMMON AFTER MILD
     NON-COMPLICATED TRAUMA?:
     A. Alkalosis
     B. Acidosis
     C. Both equal   Ref. p. 36

69. THE PHYSIOLOGIC MECHANISM WHICH PREVENTS POSTOPERATIVE
     ALKALOSIS IS THE TENDENCY TO CREATE TISSUE HYPOXIA BY:
     A. The effect on the oxy-hemoglobin dissociation curve
     B. Increase in A-V shunting
     C. The effect on vasomotor tone
     D. Increase in cellular catabolism   Ref. p. 36 (p.34)

70. THE BLOOD LACTATE LEVEL IS ELEVATED IN:
     A. Severe metabolic acidosis   D. Respiratory alkalosis
     B. Respiratory acidosis   E. Renal failure
     C. Hepatic failure   Ref. p. 36

71. OF PRIME IMPORTANCE IN DISTINGUISHING COMPENSATED META-
     BOLIC ACIDOSIS FROM UNCOMPENSATED ACID-BASE STATE IS THE:
     A. pH
     B. pCO_2
     C. CO_2 combining power
     D. Buffer base   Ref. p. 36

72. A CO_2 COMBINING POWER BELOW 20 mM/L IS USUALLY FOUND IN
     PATIENTS WITH_____AS THE PRIMARY COMPONENT OF THE
     ACID-BASE IMBALANCE:
     A. Respiratory acidosis
     B. Metabolic acidosis
     C. Mixed respiratory and metabolic acidosis
     D. Respiratory alkalosis
     E. Metabolic alkalosis   Ref. p. 36

73. THE FOLLOWING VALUES DESCRIBE A PATIENT WITH WHICH
CONDITION?:
pH 7.50
pCO_2 25.0
HCO_3 18.4 mM/L
CO_2 Content mM/L 15.7
CO_2 Combining power mM/L 17.5

A. Mixed respiratory acidosis and metabolic alkalosis
B. Metabolic alkalosis with respiratory compensation
C. Mixed respiratory and metabolic acidosis
D. Mixed respiratory alkalosis and metabolic acidosis
Ref. p. 36

ANSWER THE FOLLOWING QUESTIONS BY USING THE KEY
OUTLINED BELOW:
A. If both statement and reason are correct and related cause and effect
B. If both statement and reason are correct but not related cause and effect
C. If statement is true but reason is false
D. If statement is false but reason is true
E. If both statement and reason are false

74. Alkalosis is the more frequent postoperative acid-base imbalance BECAUSE
the primary problem is the respiratory system and its control.
Ref. p. 36

75. Respiratory alkalosis develops as a result of increased pulmonary A-V
shunting with unoxygenated blood BECAUSE hypoxia stimulates increased
ventilation and CO_2 is blown off.   Ref. p. 37

MATCH THE FOLLOWING. EACH LETTERED ITEM MAY BE USED
MORE THAN ONCE:

76. ___ Shock   A. Metabolic acidosis
77. ___ Transfusion (multiple)   B. Respiratory alkalosis
78. ___ Adrenal   C. Respiratory acidosis
79. ___ Atelectasis   D. Metabolic alkalosis
80. ___ Cirrhosis
81. ___ Diabetes mellitus
82. ___ Pyloric obstruction   Ref. pp. 36, 37

SELECT THE MOST APPROPRIATE ANSWER(S):

83. ALL OF THE FOLLOWING STATES ARE INITIATED BY SHOCK, EXCEPT:
A. Hypercoagulation   D. Vasospasm
B. Metabolic acidosis   E. None of the above
C. Lactic acid accumulation   Ref. p. 37

84. THE PRINCIPAL REASON FOR THE USE OF VASODILATORS IN SHOCK
IS TO:
A. Increase peripheral resistance
B. Increase tissue perfusion by lowering peripheral resistance
C. Potentiation of the ionotropic cardiotonic agents
Ref. p. 37

85. WHICH OF THE ELECTROLYTE PROBLEMS ARE OFTEN ASSOCIATED
WITH ALKALOSIS?:
A. Hypocalcemia   D. All of the above
B. Hypokalemia   E. None of the above
C. Hypomagnesemia   Ref. p. 37

86. A COMMON MECHANISM FOR THE INITIATION OF LACTIC ACID
ACIDOSIS IS:
A. The sudden cessation of prolonged hyperventilation
B. Massive infusion of Ringer's Lactate
C. Prolonged Levine tube aspiration
D. Hyperalimentation through feeding jejunostomy
Ref. p. 37

ANSWER THE FOLLOWING QUESTION BY USING THE KEY
OUTLINED BELOW:
A. If both statement and reason are correct and related cause and effect
B. If both statement and reason are correct but not related cause and effect
C. If statement is true but reason is false
D. If statement is false but reason is true
E. If both statement and reason are false

87. Paradoxic aciduria is a postoperative finding due to excessive renal
potassium loss BECAUSE carbonic anhydrase is defective.
Ref. p. 37

SELECT THE MOST APPROPRIATE ANSWER:

88. IDEAL REPLACEMENT THERAPY FOR HYPOKALEMIC METABOLIC
ALKALOSIS DUE TO PYLORIC OBSTRUCTION WOULD INCLUDE:
A. KCL
B. NH_4Cl_2
C. NaCl   Ref. p. 37

89. WHICH OF THE FOLLOWING REPRESENT MECHANISMS FOR THE DE-
VELOPMENT OF ALKALOSIS?:
A. Pulmonary A-V shunting   D. All of the above
B. Cirrhosis   E. None of the above
C. Atelectasis   Ref. p. 37

90. ALL OF THE FOLLOWING MAY BE RESPONSIBLE FOR RESPIRATORY
ALKALOSIS, EXCEPT:
A. Pulmonary A-V shunting
B. Hypoxia
C. Lactic acid
D. Hypotension with carotid and aortic body stimulation
E. Hypoxemia with carotid and aortic body stimulation
Ref. p. 37

91. THE MOST EFFECTIVE METHOD OF PREVENTING LACTIC ACID AC-
CUMULATION IN RESPIRATORY PROBLEMS DUE TO ANESTHESIA IS:
A. Increase the oxygen tension
B. Add carbon dioxide to the gas mixture
C. Add nitrogen to the gas mixture
D. Increase the N_2O concentration   Ref. p. 37

92. LACTIC ACID PRODUCTION APPEARS TO BE DEPENDENT ON WHICH
OF THE FOLLOWING?:
A. Reduction of pH
B. H_2CO_3
C. pCO_2
D. Buffer base   Ref. p. 37

93. A NOTABLE ALKALOSIS DUE TO BLOOD TRANSFUSIONS WITH SODIUM
CITRATE WILL USUALLY REQUIRE_____UNITS, IF RENAL
BICARBONATE EXCRETION IS DEPRESSED:
A. 2   D. 16
B. 4   E. 32
C. 8   Ref. p. 37

94. WHICH OF THE FOLLOWING DISEASED ORGANS MOST AFFECTS THE
DEVELOPMENT OF TRANSFUSION ACIDOSIS?:
A. Renal
B. Hepatic
C. Gastric
D. Small bowel   Ref. p. 37

95. THE CONCENTRATION OF SERUM LACTIC ACID MAY BE CORRELATED
WITH SURVIVAL FROM SHOCK. A PATIENT WITH A LEVEL OF 2 TO 4
mM/L HAS A SURVIVAL RATE OF:
A. 85%
B. 60%
C. 26%
D. 0%   Ref. p. 38

96. IN SEPTIC SHOCK, ALKALOSIS IS AN EXPECTED FINDING. IT IS A(N)
_____PROGNOSTIC FINDING AS COMPARED TO THE ACIDOTIC
STATE:
A. Ominous
B. Good
C. Of no value   Ref. p. 38

97. AN INCREASE IN pCO_2 AND pH WILL:
A. Increase coronary blood flow
B. Decrease coronary blood flow
C. Increase cardiac output
D. Decrease cardiac output   Ref. p. 39

98. WHICH OF THE FOLLOWING HAS A GREATER EFFECT ON CORONARY
BLOOD FLOW AND CARDIAC OUTPUT?:
A. Respiratory alkalosis
B. Respiratory acidosis
C. Metabolic acidosis
D. Metabolic alkalosis   Ref. p. 39

99. THE PRODUCTION OF ADH POSTOPERATIVELY CONTINUES FOR_____
DAYS DEPENDING ON THE SEVERITY OF TRAUMA:
A. 1-2
B. 3-5
C. 6-8
D. 8-10   Ref. p. 39

100. WHICH OF THE FOLLOWING STIMULATES ADH SECRETION?:
A. Nasogastric suction   D. Visceral traction
B. Anesthetic agents   E. All of the above
C. Pre-operative fluid withdrawal Ref. p. 40

101. WHICH OF THE FOLLOWING POSTOPERATIVE FINDINGS ARE ADH
DEPENDENT?:
A. Hyponatremia   D. All of the above
B. Hypernatremia   E. None of the above
C. Water retention + oliguria   Ref. p. 41

102. THE MAJOR MECHANISM OF POTASSIUM LOSS IN HYPOKALEMIC
     ALKALOSIS SECONDARY TO PYLORIC OBSTRUCTION IS:
     A. Starvation
     B. Dilutional
     C. Prolonged suctioning of gastric contents
     D. Renal loss   Ref. p. 42

103. _____IS EFFECTIVE IN SEPTIC SHOCK BECAUSE OF ITS IONOTRO-
     PIC ACTION, PERIPHERAL VASODILATATION AND DECREASE OF POST-
     CAPILLARY PULMONARY RESISTANCE:
     A. Levarterenol   D. Aramine
     B. Epinephrine   E. All of the above
     C. Phenoxybenzamine   Ref. p. 44

104. AMONG THE ANESTHETIC AGENTS CURRENTLY IN USE, CARDIAC AND
     ASSOCIATED COMPENSATORY FUNCTIONS ARE BEST MAINTAINED BY:
     A. Cyclopropane
     B. Ether
     C. Methoxyflurane
     D. Halothane   Ref. p. 45

105. SURGICAL PROCEDURES IN SHOCKY PATIENTS ARE BEST CON-
     DUCTED UNDER:
     A. Cyclopropane
     B. Ether
     C. Halothane
     D. Methoxyflurane   Ref. p. 45

106. WITH ASSISTED RESPIRATION:
     A. O_2 consumption and cardiac output decrease
     B. O_2 consumption and cardiac output increase
     C. O_2 consumption increases and cardiac output decreases
     D. O_2 consumption increases and cardiac output remains the same
     E. O_2 consumption decreases and cardiac output increases
                                           Ref. p. 46

FILL IN THE APPROPRIATE ANSWERS: (Questions 107-108)

     A. Increase(s)(d)
     B. Decrease(s)(d)
     C. No alteration

Metabolic acidosis superimposed on respiratory acidosis 107)_____
the 108)_____cardiac output normally associated with respiratory
acidosis.   Ref. p. 46

SELECT THE MOST APPROPRIATE ANSWERS:

109. "HIGH-OUTPUT RESPIRATORY FAILURE" WHICH PRESENTS WITH POOR
     TISSUE OXYGENATION AND POOR CO_2 EXCRETION IS FOUND IN:
     A. Cirrhosis
     B. Ileus
     C. Pneumonitis
     D. Peritonitis   Ref. p. 46

ANSWER THE FOLLOWING STATEMENT T(RUE) OR F(ALSE):

110. Ventilation with high concentrations of oxygen in both adults and neonates is
     dangerous.   Ref. p. 47

SELECT THE MOST APPROPRIATE ANSWER:

111. HALOTHANE TOXICITY HAS MOSTLY BEEN EXHIBITED IN PATIENTS
     WHO HAVE HAD TWO OR MORE EXPOSURES WITHIN:
     A. 0 to 6 months
     B. 6 to 12 months
     C. 12 to 24 months
     D. 24 to 36 months   Ref. p. 48

112. THE ORGAN MOST FREQUENTLY IMPLICATED IN SHOCK AS CONTRI-
     BUTING TO ITS IRREVERSIBLE STATE IS THE:
     A. Brain   D. Intestine
     B. Heart   E. Kidneys
     C. Liver   Ref. p. 48

113. THE BODY IS ABLE TO METABOLIZE AND ELIMINATE UP TO_____
     GRAMS OF GLUCOSE/Kg/HOUR GIVEN BY PARENTERAL ADMINISTRA-
     TION:
     A. 0.5 gm/Kg/hr
     B. 0.75 gm/Kg/hr
     C. 1.00 gm/Kg/hr
     D. 1.25 gm/Kg/hr   Ref. p. 50 (1st Ed.)

114. A 37 POUND CHILD ADMITTED TO A PEDIATRIC DIVISION REQUIRING
     SHORT TERM MAINTENANCE INTRAVENOUS FLUID AND ELECTRO-
     LYTES WILL REQUIRE_____/24 HOURS:
     A. 1550 cc 5% Dextrose in 1/6 NS + 46 mEq. KCl
     B. 1350 cc 5% Dextrose in NS + 40 mEq. KCl
     C. 1350 cc 5% Dextrose in 1/2 NS + 30 mEq. KCl
     D. 1350 cc 5% Dextrose in 1/4 NS + 27 MEq. KCl
     E. 750 cc 5% Dextrose in 1/2 NS + 22 mEq. KCl
                                      Ref. pp. 52-53 (1st Ed.)

115. WHICH OF THE FOLLOWING GASTROINTESTINAL FLUIDS CONTAINS
     THE HIGHEST CONCENTRATION OF PROTEIN?:
     A. Gastric secretions   D. Small bowel secretions
     B. Pancreatic secretions   E. All of the above
     C. Bilious secretions   Ref. p. 56 (1st Ed.)

116. WHICH OF THE FOLLOWING CONDITIONS RESULTS IN THE GREATEST
     PROTEIN DEPLETION?:
     A. Pyloric obstruction with vomiting
     B. Diarrhea
     C. T-tube drainage with ampullary obstruction
     D. All are equal   Ref. p. 56 (1st Ed.)

117. THE MAJOR LIMITATION TO ACCURATE BLOOD VOLUME DETERMINA-
     TIONS IS:
     A. The type of Isotope utilized
     B. Accurate measurement of patient surface area
     C. The differential hematocrit between lung and capillary
     D. Interstitial fluid volume
     E. Third space sequestration   Ref. p. 60 (1st Ed.)

118. ACUTE DEHYDRATION RESULTING IN A 20% LOSS OF EXTRACELLULAR
     FLUID WILL BE ACCOMPANIED BY WHICH OF THE FOLLOWING FIND-
     INGS?:
     A. Oliguria   D. Postural hypotension
     B. Tachycardia   E. All of the above
     C. Elevated hematocrit   Ref. p. 61 (1st Ed.)

119. DESICCATING DEHYDRATION CAN DEVELOP FROM WHICH OF THE
      FOLLOWING CONDITIONS?:
      A. Hyperemesis gravidarum   D. Tracheostomy
      B. Pyloric stenosis   E. All of the above
      C. Diarrhea   Ref. p. 61 (1st Ed.)

      ANSWER THE FOLLOWING STATEMENT T(RUE) OR F(ALSE):

120. Maximal postoperative fluid sequestration develops by 8-12 hours.
                                         Ref. p. 64 (1st Ed.)

      SELECT THE MOST APPROPRIATE ANSWER:

121. A GENERALIZED DIFFUSE PERITONITIS HAS BEEN COMPARED TO
      SECOND AND THIRD DEGREE BURNS OF_____PER CENT:
      A. 5   D. 45
      B. 15   E. 60
      C. 30   Ref. p. 64 (1st Ed.)

122. TOTAL BODY WATER IN THE AVERAGE MALE PATIENT IS ABOUT_____
      PER CENT OF THE WEIGHT IN Kg:
      A. 10   D. 60
      B. 20   E. 90
      C. 40   Ref. p. 65

123. INTRACELLULAR WATER IS ABOUT_____PER CENT OF THE TOTAL
      BODY WATER:
      A. 10   D. 60
      B. 20   E. 80
      C. 40   Ref. p. 66

      MATCH THE FOLLOWING:

124. ___ Interstitial fluid   A. 3-5%
125. ___ Total body water   B. 18-30%
126. ___ Plasma volume   C. 60%
127. ___ Plasma water content   D. 93%
                                         Ref. p. 66

      SELECT THE MOST APPROPRIATE ANSWER:

128. THE TERM "ANION GAP" FITS WHICH OF THE FOLLOWING DISEASES?:
      A. Renal disease with sulfate and phosphate retention
      B. Diabetic acidosis with keto acids
      C. Shock and adrenal insufficiency with lactic and pyruvic acid accumula-
          tion
      D. Cirrhosis with ammonia accumulation
      E. All of the above   Ref. p. 67

129. TO COMPUTE THE ANION-CATION EQUILIBRIUM, WHICH OF THE
      FOLLOWING FORMULAS SHOULD BE UTILIZED TO ESTABLISH AN
      ACCURACY (+), OR (-) 3 mEq ?:
      A. $(HCO_3)^- + Cl^- = Na+$
      B. $(HCO_3)^- + Cl^- + 10 = Na+$
      C. $Na+ + (HCO_3)^- = Cl^- + 10$ Ref. p. 67

130. THE OSMOLALITY OF PLASMA IS ABOUT_____, (+) OR (-) 10:
      A. 165   D. 315
      B. 175   E. 325
      C. 285   Ref. p. 67

ANSWER THE FOLLOWING QUESTION BY USING THE KEY
OUTLINED BELOW:
A. If both statement and reason are correct and related cause and effect
B. If both statement and reason are correct but not related cause and effect
C. If statement is true but reason is false
D. If statement is false but reason is true
E. If both statement and reason are false

131. Plasma osmolality can be mathematically approximated BECAUSE by
taking twice the serum sodium concentration plus 6 mo, one will attain
that value.   Ref. p. 67

SELECT THE MOST APPROPRIATE ANSWER:

132. WHICH OF THE FOLLOWING MAY BE RESPONSIBLE FOR AN AB-
NORMALLY ELEVATED URINE SODIUM OUTPUT?:
A. Osmotic diuretics   D. Large solute loads
B. Renal tubular diseases   E. All of the above
C. Adrenal insufficiency   Ref. p. 67 (1st Ed.)

133. POSTOPERATIVE FLUID SEQUESTRATION SHOULD BE COMPLETED BY:
A. 8 hours   D. 48 hours
B. 12 hours   E. 72 hours
C. 36 hours   Ref. p. 68 (1st Ed.)

ANSWER THE FOLLOWING QUESTION BY USING THE KEY
OUTLINED BELOW:
A. If both statement and reason are correct and related cause and effect
B. If both statement and reason are correct but not related cause and effect
C. If statement is true but reason is false
D. If statement is false but reason is true
E. If both statement and reason are false

134. Acute respiratory acidosis on alkalosis can exist without any significant
change in CO_2 content of plasma BECAUSE it is primarily affected by the
pCO_2.   Ref. p. 71

ANSWER THE FOLLOWING STATEMENTS T(RUE) OR F(ALSE):

135. Compensation for respiratory acidosis is renal.
                                               Ref. p. 71

136. Respiratory alkalosis is primarily a decrease in pCO_2 below 34 mmHg.
                                               Ref. p. 72

SELECT THE MOST APPROPRIATE ANSWER:

137. COMPENSATION FOR METABOLIC ACIDOSIS RESULTS PRIMARILY
FROM:
A. Respiratory rate and depth increase, with lowering pCO_2
B. Decrease in respiratory rate and depth with elevated pCO_2
C. Renal conservation of ammonia and titratable acidity with increased
    H+ on excretion   Ref. p. 72

138. THE pCO_2 WILL BE_____IN COMPENSATED METABOLIC ALKALO-
SIS (ESPECIALLY WHEN THE CO_2 CONTENT EXCEEDS 35 mEq/l):
A. Increased
B. Decreased
C. Unchanged   Ref. p. 72

MATCH THE FOLLOWING. EACH LETTERED ITEM MAY BE USED
MORE THAN ONCE:

139. ___ Atelectasis
140. ___ Pneumothorax
141. ___ Adrenal insufficiency
142. ___ Postoperative
143. ___ Diabetes mellitus
144. ___ Cushing's disease
145. ___ Chronic lung disease
146. ___ Overuse of diuretics
147. ___ Ureteroenterostomy
148. ___ Respirator hyperventilation

A. Respiratory acidosis
B. Respiratory alkalosis
C. Metabolic acidosis
D. Metabolic alkalosis

Ref. pp. 72-74

149. HOW MANY mEq OF $NaHCO_3$ WILL IT TAKE TO ELEVATE A CO_2 CON-
TENT OF 8 mEq TO 15 mEq IN AN 80 Kg CO_2 PATIENT ?:
A. 44 mEq
B. 88 mEq
C. 124 mEq
D. 224 mEq
E. 324 mEq
Ref. p. 73

150. THE FORMULA FOR CLINICAL BICARBONATE REPLACEMENT IS
BASED ON WHICH OF THE FOLLOWING?:
A. Bicarbonate deficit as reflected by CO_2 content in intravascular com-
partment x 2
B. Bicarbonate deficit in total body water x 2
C. Bicarbonate deficit as reflected by CO_2 content in extracellular com-
partment x 2
D. Bicarbonate deficit in intracellular compartment x 2
Ref. p. 73

151. THE PRIMARY MEANS OF COMPENSATION FOR METABOLIC
ALKALOSIS IS VIA WHICH OF THE FOLLOWING?:
A. Respiratory
B. Renal
C. Both equally
Ref. p. 74 (71)

152. SIGNS OF SIGNIFICANT HYPERKALEMIA ARE FOUND IN WHICH OF THE
FOLLOWING ORGAN SYSTEMS?:
A. Cardiovascular
B. Respiratory
C. Renal
D. Gastrointestinal
E. All of these
Ref. p. 75

153. HYPOKALEMIA IS FREQUENTLY RESPONSIBLE FOR WHICH OF THE
FOLLOWING?:
A. Shortened PR interval, decrease in P-wave amplitude
B. Alkaline urine
C. Paralytic ileus
D. Hyper-reflexia
E. Oliguria
Ref. p. 75

154. HYPOCALCEMIA (BELOW 8.5 mg/100cc) IS FREQUENTLY FOUND IN
WHICH OF THE FOLLOWING STATES?:
A. Hypoproteinemia
B. Hypoxic acidosis
C. Acute pancreatitis
D. Magnesium depletion
E. All of the above
Ref. p. 76

155. OF THE GASTROINTESTINAL SECRETIONS, WHICH ARE MOST NEARLY
      ISOTONIC IN ELECTROLYTE CONTENT TO BLOOD?:
      A. Saliva   D. Distal small bowel
      B. Gastric   E. All are equal
      C. Bile   Ref. p. 76

      ARRANGE THE FOLLOWING IN ORDER OF DESCENDING mEq/L VALUES
      OF POTASSIUM IN THE GASTROINTESTINAL TRACT:

156. A. ___ Saliva   D. ___ Ileum
      B. ___ Bile   E. ___ Pancreatic
      C. ___ Gastric   Ref. p. 76

157. WHICH OF THE FOLLOWING CATIONS AND/OR ANIONS ARE SIGNIFI-
      CANTLY BOUND TO PROTEINS?:
      A. Magnesium   D. Potassium
      B. Sodium   E. Chlorides
      C. Calcium   Ref. p. 76

158. ALL OF THE FOLLOWING ELECTROLYTES ARE SIGNIFICANTLY
      ALTERED BY CHANGES IN pH, EXCEPT:
      A. Magnesium
      B. Sodium
      C. Calcium
      D. Potassium
      E. None of the above   Ref. p. 76

159. OF THE 8,000 TO 10,000 CC OF GASTROINTESTINAL SECRETIONS,
      HOW MUCH IS THE NORMAL BILIOUS OUTPUT?:
      A. 100-250 cc   D. 750-1000 cc
      B. 250-500 cc   E. 1000-1500 cc
      C. 500-750 cc   Ref. p. 76

160. THE TROUSSEAU AND CHVOSTEK SIGNS AS WELL AS HYPER-
      REFLEXIA ARE CHARACTERISTIC OF WHICH OF THE FOLLOWING
      ELECTROLYTE DISTURBANCES?:
      A. Hyponatremia   D. Hypomagnesemia
      B. Hypocalcemia   E. Hypercalcemia
      C. Hypochloremia   Ref. pp. 76,77

      ANSWER THE FOLLOWING STATEMENT T(RUE) OR F(ALSE):

161. Patients on intravenous therapy exceeding 7-10 days are likely to develop
      hypomagnesemia.   Ref. p. 77

      SELECT THE MOST APPROPRIATE ANSWER:

162. COMPLICATIONS OF INTRAVENOUS MAGNESIUM DEPLETION ARE:
      A. Paralytic ileus   D. Hypotension
      B. Sudden potassium fall in serum E. All of the above
      C. Convulsions   Ref. p. 77

163. IN PARATHYROID CRISIS WITH SUDDEN ELEVATIONS OF CALCIUM
      OVER 16 mg/100cc; THE TREATMENT CONSISTS OF:
      A. Intravenous Vitamin D
      B. Parathyroidectomy for removal of adenoma
      C. Thyrocalcitonin
      D. Intravenous bicarbonate
      E. All of the above   Ref. p. 77

164. IN PATIENTS ON CHRONIC INTRAVENOUS FEEDING, THE DAILY
      MAGNESIUM ADMINISTRATION SHOULD BE:
      A. 2.5 to 5 mEq   D. 15 to 20 mEq
      B. 5 to 10 mEq   E. 20 to 30 mEq
      C. 10 to 15 mEq   Ref. p. 77

      FILL IN THE APPROPRIATE ANSWERS: (Questions 165-168)

      A. 1.5 mEq
      B. 2.0 mEq
      C. 2.5 mEq
      D. 5.3 mEq (+) or (-) 0.53 mEq/L

      Serum magnesium levels normally are from 165)_____to 166)_____mEq/L.
      These values are not always reliable in depleted patients. To establish
      such a deficiency, the most accurate tests should include RBC. Magnesium
      levels which are normally 167)_____and urine mEq levels which are below
      168)_____ mEq/L/24 hrs due to efficient renal conservation.
                                          Ref. p. 77

      SELECT THE MOST APPROPRIATE ANSWER:

169. THE "BASE LINE" WATER NEED FOR AN 80 Kg, 6 FOOT 4 INCH MALE
      IS APPROXIMATELY:
      A. 1550 cc   D. 3500 cc
      B. 2000 cc   E. 4000 cc
      C. 2750 cc   Ref. p. 78

      FILL IN THE APPROPRIATE ANSWER: (Questions 170-171)

      A. 20
      B. 42
      C. 102   A. Isotonic
      D. 202   B. Hypertonic
      E. 302   C. Hypotonic
      A solution of 0.3% normal saline contains 170)_____milliosmoles and is
      a(n) 171) _____solution to blood.   Ref. p. 79

      MATCH THE FOLLOWING: EACH LETTERED ITEM MAY BE USED
      MORE THAN ONCE:

172.___ Intraoperatively in otherwise normal patient
173.___ Patient with metabolic alkalosis
174.___ 32 lb. child maintenance
175.___ Diabetic ketoacidosis

                        A. Ringer's lactate
                        B. Normal saline
                        C. 5% glucose/water
                        D. 5% dextrose 1/6 normal saline
                        E. 5% glucose 1.3 normal saline
                            Ref. pp. 79-80

      SELECT THE MOST APPROPRIATE ANSWER(S):

176. EARLIEST CHANGES IN SIMPLE TESTS PERFORMED ON AN HOURLY
      BASIS INDICATING THIRD SPACE SEQUESTRATION ARE IN:
      A. Urine + specific gravity   D. Glucose
      B. BUN   E. All of the above
      C. CBC   Ref. p. 80

177. PREOPERATIVE INTRAVENOUS FLUID THERAPY IS PROBABLY A GOOD
     IDEA BECAUSE_____AND IT PREVENTS DEHYDRATION:
     A. Most patients are placed on N. P. O. the night before
     B. Apprehension decreases the oral intake
     C. Preoperative morphine and meperidine decreases the G. F. R.
     D. The bowel preparation increased fluid loss
     E. All of the above   Ref. p. 80

178. REHYDRATION OF PATIENTS CHRONICALLY DEPLETED CAN BEST BE
     PERFORMED WITH THE HELP OF FLUID ADMINISTRATION:
     A. To increase the urine output to 25-50 cc/hr
     B. To reduce the hematocrit to normal values
     C. To increase the C. V. P. to normal value
     D. All of the above   Ref. p. 80, 83

179. THE ADMINISTRATION OF INTRAVENOUS FAT CAN BE COMPLICATED
     BY WHICH OF THE FOLLOWING:
     A. Changes in liver function
     B. Hypergemitivity
     C. Hemorrhagic tendencies
     D. All of the above   Ref. p. 81 (1st Ed.)

180. IN A 30-YEAR-OLD MALE WITH SYMPTOMATIC HYPONATREMIA,
     WEIGHT = 60 Kg, AND SERUM SODIUM = 120mEq/L, HOW MUCH SODIUM
     WOULD BE NEEDED FOR REPLACEMENT? _____ HOW MUCH SHOULD
     BE ADMINISTERED INITIALLY? _____
     A. 220mEq   D. 720mEq
     B. 360mEq   E. 1000mEq
     C. 580mEq   Ref. p. 81

ANSWER THE FOLLOWING QUESTION BY USING THE KEY
OUTLINED BELOW:
A. If both statement and reason are correct and related cause and effect
B. If both statement and reason are correct but not related cause and effect
C. If statement is true but reason is false
D. If statement is false but reason is true
E. If both statement and reason are false

181. Persistent hyponatremia and postoperative oliguria exceeding 48 hours is
     common BECAUSE it is indicative of third space sequestration.
                                            Ref. pp. 82-84

SELECT THE MOST APPROPRIATE ANSWER:

182. IN THE POSTOPERATIVE OR POST-TRAUMATIC PERIOD ALL OF
     FOLLOWING PROVIDE THE GREATEST INSIGHT INTO BOTH STATIC
     AND DYNAMIC FLUID LOSS, EXCEPT:
     A. Hourly urine volume
     B. Serial hematocrits
     C. Central venous pressure measurements
     D. Blood pressure measurements
     E. None of the above   Ref. p. 84

183. THE MOST FREQUENT WATER AND ELECTROLYTE DISTURBANCE
     SEEN IN SURGICAL PATIENTS IS:
     A. Expanded intracellular volume + hemoconcentration
     B. Dessicating dehydration + hemoconcentration
     C. Desalting water loss + hypernatremia
     D. Expanded extracellular fluid volume + dilutional hyponatremia
                                            Ref. p. 84

184. IN THE POST-OPERATIVE PERIOD, ONE SHOULD BE CATABOLIC AND
THEREFORE LOSING BETWEEN 1/4 TO 1/2 LB./DAY. A WEIGHT GAIN
IN THIS PERIOD USUALLY MEANS:
   A. Volume excess   D. Renal failure
   B. Hypernatremia   E. Respiratory depression
   C. Anabolic state   Ref. p. 84

185. SOLUTE LOADING WITH RESULTING HYPERTONICITY CAN BEST BE
DISTINGUISHED FROM DESSICATING DEHYDRATION BY:
   A. The increase of plasma electrolytes out of proportion to the change
       in hematocrit
   B. The increase in plasma electrolytes + oliguria
   C. Increase in plasma electrolytes in the presence of increased diuresis
   D. The increase in plasma electrolytes + hemoconcentration
                                   Ref. p. 85

186. THE AVERAGE DEPLETED OR COMPLICATED MAJOR SURGICAL PA-
TIENT REQUIRES BETWEEN _____ K CAL/DAY WITH APPROXIMATELY
_____ GRAMS OF NITROGEN:
   A. 0.2 Gm of N + 50 K cal/kg/day
   B. 1000 to 2000 K cal/day + 6 to 12 Gm of N
   C. 2500 to 4000 K cal/day + 12 to 24 Gm of N
   D. 6000 to 10,000 K cal/day + 24 to 36 Gm of N   Ref. p. 88

187. THE COMPLICATIONS OF NAUSEA, VOMITING, AND DIARRHEA ASSOCI-
ATED WITH THE INTAKE OF ELEMENTAL DIETS ARE USUALLY DUE TO:
   A. High osmolarity of the diet
   B. Lack of adequate protein/K cal ratio
   C. Lack of adequate bulk
   D. Electrolyte imbalance   Ref. p. 91

ANSWER THE FOLLOWING STATEMENTS T(RUE) OR F(ALSE):

188. Whole blood is a good source of protein for nutrition.
                                   Ref. pp. 91, 92

189. The assimilation of amino acids and protein hydrolysates is more effi-
ciently utilized if carbohydrates are simultaneously introduced.
                                   Ref. p. 92

190. Negative nitrogen balance will show greater improvement following the
introduction of amino acids and protein hydrolysates simultaneously with
carbohydrates.   Ref. p. 92

SELECT THE MOST APPROPRIATE ANSWER:

191. THE CALORIC VALUE OF 1 LITER OF 7% ALCOHOL IN 5% GLUCOSE
AND WATER IS:
   A. 700 cal   D. 900 cal
   B. 400 cal   E. 1000 cal
   C. 800 cal   Ref. p. 92

192. WHICH ARE INDICATIONS FOR PARENTERAL HYPERALIMENTATION?:
   A. Newborn infants with catastrophic gastrointestinal anomalies, e.g.
       omphalocele, gastroschisis
   B. Adult patients with short bowel syndrome
   C. Patient with prolonged paralytic ileus following major operations
   D. Severe burn patients
   E. Colocutaneous fistulae
   F. All of the above   Ref. p. 92

193. HYPERALIMENTATION PREPARATIONS NORMALLY INCLUDE ALL OF
THE FOLLOWING EXCEPT:
A. 5% protein hydrolysate or amino acids
B. Dextrose to bring 1100 ml. to provide approximately 1000 K cal
C. Electrolytes
D. Fat
E. Multivitamins   Ref. p. 93

ANSWER THE FOLLOWING QUESTION BY USING THE KEY
OUTLINED BELOW:
A. If both statement and reason are correct and related cause and effect
B. If both statement and reason are correct but not related cause and effect
C. If statement is true but reason is false
D. If statement is false but reason is true
E. If both statement and reason are false

194. During hyperalimentation, the urine sugar level should be checked every
6 hours BECAUSE of the possible development of hyperosmolar nonketotic
hyperglycemia.   Ref. pp. 94-95

SELECT THE MOST APPROPRIATE ANSWER:

195. THE USUAL DELAY BEFORE WEIGHT GAIN AND POSITIVE NITROGEN
BALANCE IN PATIENTS ON HYPERALIMENTATION IS ABOUT:
A. 2 days   D. 21 days
B. 7 days   E. 30 days
C. 14 days   Ref. p. 95

ANSWER THE FOLLOWING STATEMENTS T(RUE) OR F(ALSE):

196. In vascular trauma, early platelet adherence is to the vessel endothelium.
Ref. p. 98

197. Platelet aggregation is thought to result from platelet ADP interaction.
Ref. p. 98

198. The mechanism by which prothrombin is activated can be either intrinsic
or extrinsic, the extrinsic being the slower process.
Ref. p. 100

199. Factor XIII, the fibrin stabilizing factor, appears also to have a strong
influence in wound healing.   Ref. p. 101

SELECT THE MOST APPROPRIATE ANSWER(S):

200. THE FIBRINOLYTIC SYSTEM CAN BE ACTIVATED BY WHICH OF THE
FOLLOWING?:
A. Factor XII   D. Prostatic carcinoma
B. Prolonged shock   E. All of the above
C. Ischemia   Ref. pp. 101-102

201. THE MOST COMMON COAGULOPATHY NOTED IN THE SURGICAL
PATIENT IS:
A. Afibrinogenemia   D. Thrombocytopenia
B. Fibrinolysis   E. Factor II deficiency
C. Factor VIII deficiency (Hemophilia A) Ref. p. 102

202. THE MOST COMMON PROBLEM RESULTING IN DEFECTIVE HEMO-
STASIS IS:
A. Increased fibrinolysis   D. Thrombocytopenia
B. Anticoagulants   E. Factor II deficiency
C. Factor VIII deficiency   Ref. p. 102

203.   WHAT IS THE MINIMAL NUMBER OF PLATELETS TO PERMIT ADE-
QUATE SURGICAL HEMOSTASIS?:
A.   20,000 to 30,000 platelets/mm
B.   30,000 to 40,000 platelets/mm
C.   40,000 to 50,000 platelets/mm
D.   50,000 to 60,000 platelets/mm
E.   60,000 to 70,000 platelets/mm   Ref. p. 103

204.   THE MOST EFFECTIVE TEST TO INDICATE A PLATELET DEFICIENCY
IS:
A.   Bleeding time   D.   Lee White clotting time
B.   Rumpel-Leede   E.   All are effective
C.   Clot retraction   Ref. p. 103

205.   CLOT DESTRUCTION IN STATES OF INCREASED FIBRINOLYSIS IS
CONSIDERED POSITIVE IF IT OCCURS WITHIN_____HOURS:
A.   2
B.   4
C.   16
D.   36
E.   48   Ref. p. 104

206.   THE MOST EFFECTIVE SIMPLE SCREENING TESTS FOR "BLEEDERS"
ARE:
A.   Peripheral blood smear   D.   Clot retraction
B.   Whole blood clotting time E.   All of the above
C.   P.T.T. + quick test   Ref. p. 105

207.   LOCALIZED BLEEDING FOLLOWING PROSTATE SURGERY IS A
RESULT OF:
A.   Difficulty in typing of blood vessels of prostatic plexus
B.   Sepsis
C.   Urin-urokinase activation of local tissue plasminogen activation
Ref. p. 107

ANSWER THE FOLLOWING STATEMENT T(RUE) OR F(ALSE):

208.   Defective hemostasis due to thrombocytopenia becomes a prominent factor
after bank blood transfusion of 5 to 9 units.
Ref. p. 107

ANSWER THE FOLLOWING QUESTION BY USING THE KEY
OUTLINED BELOW:
A.   If both statement and reason are correct and related cause and effect
B.   If both statement and reason are correct but not related cause and effect
C.   If statement is true but reason is false
D.   If statement is false but reason is true
E.   If both statement and reason are false

209.   A hemolytic transfusion reaction is easily detected in anesthetized patients
BECAUSE of the sudden onset of oozing in a previously dry operative field.
Ref. p. 107

SELECT THE MOST APPROPRIATE ANSWER(S):

210.   IN A HEMOPHILIAC PATIENT WITH (FACTOR VIII) 10% ACTIVITY, HOW
MUCH FRESH FROZEN PLASMA WILL THEORETICALLY BE NEEDED
TO REACH A LEVEL OF 60% AND MAINTAIN IT FOR 24 HOURS?:
A.   10% of patient's plasma volume
B.   50% of patient's plasma volume
C.   100% of patient's plasma volume
D.   150% of patient's plasma volume
E.   200% of patient's plasma volume   Ref. p. 110

211. BEFORE THE UNDERTAKING OF A TRACHEOSTOMY OR EVEN DENTAL
      CARE IN A HEMOPHILIAC PATIENT, THE FACTOR VIII LEVEL SHOULD
      BE RAISED TO AT LEAST:
      A. 25-30%   D. 75-80%
      B. 35-40%   E. 85-90%
      C. 55-60%   Ref. p. 111

212. FACTORS V, VII, IX AND X DEFICIENCIES:
      A. Are synthesized by the liver
      B. Result in increased PTT and one stage prothrombin
      C. Respond to cryoprecipitate therapy
      D. Occur in patients with prolonged T-tube drainage due to ampullary ob-
          struction
      E. Are only found in male patients   Ref. p. 112

213. FRESH FROZEN PLASMA MAY BE UTILIZED IN WHICH OF THE
      FOLLOWING DEFICIENCIES?:
      A. Classic hemophilia   D. Factor VII deficiency
      B. Von Willebrand's disease   E. Factor X deficiency
      C. Factor V deficiency   Ref. p. 113

214. CONSUMPTION COAGULOPATHY WHICH RESULTS FROM DISSEMINATED
      INTRAVASCULAR COAGULATION CAN ACCOMPANY WHICH OF THE
      FOLLOWING DISEASE STATES?:
      A. Fibrinogenemia   E. Sepsis
      B. Lung surgery   F. All of the above
      C. Shock
      D. Pancreatic surgery   Ref. p. 114

215. THE TREATMENT FOR A CONSUMPTION COAGULOPATHY IS:
      A. Fresh frozen plasma   D. Heparin
      B. Coumadin   E. All of the above
      C. Fibrinogen   Ref. p. 114

216. TO DISTINGUISH A CONSUMPTION COAGULOPATHY FROM FIBRINOLY-
      SIS IN SHOCK, IMPORTANT ASSOCIATED FINDINGS ARE:
      A. Poor clot retraction in the former
      B. Factor V deficiency in the former
      C. Thrombocytopenia in the former
      D. Factor VIII deficiency in the latter
      E. All of the above   Ref. p. 114

217. THE ETIOLOGY FOR INCREASED FIBRINOLYSIS IN CIRRHOSIS AND
      PORTAL HYPERTENSION IS:
      A. Failure to clear sufficient plasmogen activator
      B. Production of deficient fibrinogen
      C. Production of excessive plasminogen
                                            Ref. p. 115

      ANSWER THE FOLLOWING QUESTION BY USING THE KEY
      OUTLINED BELOW:
      A. If both statement and reason are correct and related cause and effect
      B. If both statement and reason are correct but not related cause and effect
      C. If statement is true but reason is false
      D. If statement is false but reason is true
      E. If both statement and reason are false

218. The use of Alpha Amino Epsilon Caproic Acid is essential in fibrinolysis
      but dangerous if used in defibrination due to consumption coagulopathy
      BECAUSE in the latter, the clots formed are mostly insoluble.
                                            Ref. p. 115

SELECT THE MOST APPROPRIATE ANSWER(S):

219.   INDICATIONS FOR SPLENECTOMY IN ITP INCLUDE WHICH OF THE
        FOLLOWING?:
        A. CNS bleeding
        B. The development of leukemia
        C. Contraindications to steroid therapy
        D. Development of polycythemia vera   Ref. p. 116

220.   IN POLYCYTHEMIA VERA, THE MOST COMMON POSTOPERATIVE
        COMPLICATION FOLLOWING MAJOR SURGERY IS:
        A. Thrombosis   D. Hemorrhage
        B. Diabetes insipidus   E. Renal failure
        C. Gastric ulcer   Ref. p. 116

221.   COUMARIN REVERSAL CAN BEST BE PERFORMED WITH:
        A. Protamine sulfate   D. Vitamin K_1
        B. Vitamin K_2 E. Fibrinogen infusion
        C. Bank blood tranfusion   Ref. p. 118

222.   IF EMERGENCY SURGICAL TREATMENT IS REQUIRED IN AN ANTI-
        COAGULATED PATIENT, WHICH OF THE FOLLOWING IS USED? _____
        HOW LONG WILL IT TAKE FOR REVERSAL? _____
                                      A.   2 hours
        A. Vitamin K   B.   4 hours
                                      C.   6 hours
        B. Vitamin K_1 D. 12 hours
                                      E. 24 hours
                                          Ref. p. 119

223.   IN BANKED WHOLE BLOOD, WHICH OF THE FOLLOWING OCCUR
        AFTER 21 DAYS?:
        A. Lactic acid accumulation from 20 mg% to 150 mg%
        B. Ammonia increase from 50 to 680 mg%
        C. Potassium increase from 3 to 30 mEq
        D. Hemolysis resulting in a 20% decrease in RBC
        E. Sodium elevation from 140 to 160 mEq/l
                                          Ref. p. 121

        ANSWER THE FOLLOWING QUESTION BY USING THE KEY
        OUTLINED BELOW:
        A. If both statement and reason are correct and related cause and effect
        B. If both statement and reason are correct but not related cause and effect
        C. If statement is true but reason is false
        D. If statement is false but reason is true
        E. If both statement and reason are false

224.   Rh positive blood should not be transfused to Rh negative females of child-
        bearing age BECAUSE future erythroblastosis may develop in the fetus.
                                          Ref. p. 122

SELECT THE MOST APPROPRIATE ANSWER(S):

225.   INTRAOPERATIVE TRANSFUSION REACTION IS SUGGESTED BY:
        A. Sudden increase in indirect bilirubin
        B. Abnormal bleeding
        C. Drop in haptoglobin level
        D. Hypotension despite adequate replacement
        E. All of the above   Ref. p. 127

226. THE TREATMENT OF ENDOTOXIC SHOCK WHETHER OF LOW OUTPUT
OR HIGH OUTPUT IS:
A. In the former, one uses vasoconstrictors and in the latter, vaso-
dilators
B. In the former one uses vasodilators, and the latter, vasoconstrictors
C. Virtually the same in that both are treated with vasodilators and
volume expanders and antibiotics   Ref. p. 128 (1st Ed.)

227. THE MORTALITY IN ENDOTOXIC SHOCK IS HIGHER IN THE_____
OUTPUT STATE, WHICH IS THE LESS COMMON VARIETY:
A. High
B. Low   Ref. p. 128 (1st Ed.)

228. AIR EMBOLISM IS TREATED BY:
A. Placing the patient on the left side, head down
B. Placing the patient on the right side, head down
C. Immediate right ventricular needle aspiration
D. Immediate patient intubation and administration of 100% oxygen
E. Arterial phlebotomy   Ref. p. 128

229. WHICH OF THE FOLLOWING BACTERIA APPEARS MOST FREQUENTLY
IN ENDOTOXIC SHOCK?:
A. Pseudomonas
B. Aerobacter-Klebsiella
C. E. Coli
D. Strep. viridens
E. Staphylococcus aureus coagulase positive
Ref. p. 130 (1st Ed.)

230. THE ANTIBIOTIC(S) OF CHOICE IN GRAM-NEGATIVE SEPSIS AND
ENDOTOXIC SHOCK IS (ARE):
A. Tetracycline
B. Staphcillin and penicillin
C. Penicillin and Chloromycetin
D. Kanamycin or Coly-mycin
E. Staphcillin, Kanamycin, or Coly-mycin
Ref. p. 130 (1st Ed.)

ANSWER THE FOLLOWING STATEMENT T(RUE) OR F(ALSE):

231. In cardiogenic shock, tissue perfusion and cardiac output can be increased
with vasodilators and the blood pressure can remain reduced.
Ref. p. 130

SELECT THE MOST APPROPRIATE ANSWER:

232. THE ALPHA RECEPTOR STIMULATION TO INITIATE VASOCONSTRIC-
TION IN HYPOTENSIVE STATES IS MEDIATED THROUGH HYPO-
THALAMUS AND RESULTS IN:
A. Adrenal medulla epinephrine secretion
B. Direct effect on the precapillary arteries
C. Sympathetic postganglionic or epinephrine secretions
D. All of the above   Ref. p. 134

233. BETA RECEPTORS ARE RESPONSIBLE FOR:
A. Coronary vasodilatation
B. Myocardial inotropic and chronotropic effect
C. Vasoconstriction of cerebral vessels
D. Vasodilatation
E. All of the above   Ref. p. 134

234.   IN HEMORRHAGIC SHOCK WHICH OF THE FOLLOWING FINDINGS ARE
       USUALLY PRESENT ?:
       A. Decreased cardiac output
       B. Decreased venous pressure (venous return)
       C. Increased peripheral resistance
       D. Peripheral pooling
       E. All of the above   Ref. p. 134

235.   IN HEMORRHAGIC SHOCK THERE IS_____IN THE SYSTOLIC-
       DIASTOLIC DIFFERENTIAL:
       A. Increase
       B. Decrease
       C. No change   Ref. p. 135

236.   IN THE "IRREVERSIBLE SHOCK STATE, " THE_____LEADING TO
       STAGNANT ANOXIA:
       A. Precapillary arteriolar tone is increased and postcapillary venular
           tone is increased
       B. Precapillary arteriolar tone is decreased and postcapillary venular
           tone is increased
       C. Precapillary arteriolar tone is increased and postcapillary venular
           tone is decreased
       D. Precapillary venular tone is decreased and postcapillary venular
           tone is decreased   Ref. p. 136

237.   SURVIVAL OF PATIENTS IN HEMORRHAGIC SHOCK CAN BE INCREASED
       BY:
       A. Rapid retransfusion
       B. Vasodilators such as phenoxybentamine and chlorpromazine
       C. Spinal anesthesia
       D. Total sympathectomies
       E. All of the above   Ref. p. 137

238.   WHICH APPARENTLY HAS A GREATER EFFECT ON THE VENULE
       TONE ?:
       A. Sympathetic stimulation (epinephrine)
       B. Tissue acidosis
       C. More epinephrine   Ref. p. 137

239.   WHICH OF THE FOLLOWING INFECTIVE PROCESSES WILL TEND TO
       SPREAD MORE RAPIDLY ?:
       A. An infection of the toe
       B. An infection of the face   Ref. p. 138 (1st Ed.)

240.   OF THE FOLLOWING STATEMENTS, WHICH WILL LEAST AFFECT THE
       PATHOGENICITY OF AN ORGANISM ?:
       A. The amount of devitalized tissue present
       B. The availability of a good blood supply
       C. The development of an infection in a closed space
       D. All of the above   Ref. p. 138 (1st Ed.)

241.   WHICH OF THE FOLLOWING ARE LEAST PAINFUL ?:
       A. Felon
       B. Retropharyngeal abscess
       C. Abscess of intralobar fissure of lung
       D. Tenosynovitis
       E. All are equal   Ref. p. 138 (1st Ed.)

242. THE "GOLDEN PERIOD" FOR TREATMENT OF OPEN WOUNDS IS_____
      HOURS:
      A. 4   D. 8
      B. 12   E. 20
      C. 16   Ref. p. 139 (1st Ed.)

243. THE "GOLDEN PERIOD" MAY BE EXTENDED BEYOND THE ESTABLISHED
      TIME WITH THE APPLICATION OF LOCAL ANTIBIOTICS, AND ADDI-
      TIONAL EXCEPTIONS TO THE RULE ARE NOTED:
      A. In wounds with an exceptionally good blood supply
      B. In the lower extremity
      C. In minimally contaminated wounds
      D. In upper extremities
      E. None of the above   Ref. p. 139 (1st Ed.)

244. A PATIENT WITH AN OPEN WOUND PRESENTING 10 HOURS AFTER THE
      INJURY SHOULD BE:
      A. Debrided and closed per primum
      B. Closed per primum
      C. Debrided and closed per secundum
      D. Closed per primum, debrided and antibiotics administered
                                        Ref. p. 139 (1st Ed.)

245. WHICH ORGANISMS ARE PREDOMINANTLY FOUND IN PATIENTS WITH
      PERFORATED APPENDICITIS_____, ASCENDING CHOLANGITIS?:
      A. Escherichia
      B. Streptococcus faecales
      C. Both A and B   Ref. p. 140 (1st Ed.)

246. THE LIPOPOLYSACCHARIDE RESPONSIBLE FOR SHOCK IN GRAM-
      NEGATIVE SEPSIS IS FOUND IN:
      A. Necrotic endothelium of the capillaries
      B. Wall of the destroyed white blood cells
      C. Wall of the destroyed red blood cells
      D. Cell wall of the bacteria
      E. All of the above   Ref. p. 140

247. THE MOST RELIABLE SIGN OF A POSITIVE ANTIBIOTIC RESPONSE
      BY THE PATIENT IS:
      A. A slow progressive depression of the leukocyte count
      B. A prompt temperature decrease to normal or near normal limits with-
          in 8-12 hours
      C. A temperature decrease to normal limits within 72 hours
      D. The progressive decrease in the number of colonies at a daily colony
          count for one week
      E. The failure to continue to obtain positive blood cultures
                                        Ref. p. 141 (1st Ed.)

248. THE PRIME CAUSE OF BLOOD PRESSURE DECREASE IN GRAM-
      NEGATIVE SHOCK IS:
      A. Decrease in cardiac output due to intrinsic myocardial disease
      B. Decrease in cardiac output due to peripheral pooling and a decrease in
          venous return
      C. Decrease in cardiac output due to a sudden interstitial fluid accumula-
          tion and decrease in venous return   Ref. p. 141

249. WHICH DISEASE STATE CAN UNDERGO THE MORE RAPID PROGRES-
      SION TO STAGNANT ANOXIA?:
      A. Hemorrhagic shock
      B. Endotoxic shock   Ref. p. 141

ANSWER THE FOLLOWING STATEMENT T(RUE) OR F(ALSE):

250. The end stages of hemorrhagic shock and endotoxic shock are relatively
      the same, resulting in prolonged tissue anoxia.
                                              Ref. p. 141

SELECT THE MOST APPROPRIATE ANSWER:

251. AN INCISION AND DRAINAGE OF AN ABSCESS IS CONSIDERED IN-
      EFFECTIVE IF THE WOUND:
      A. Continues to drain for a period of over 14 days
      B. Continues to drain over a period of 7 days
      C. Remains open for a period of over 21 days
      D. Contains enough bacteria to give persistent positive cultures for over
          14 days   Ref. p. 143 (1st Ed.)

ANSWER THE FOLLOWING STATEMENT T(RUE) OR F(ALSE):

252. In man, endotoxic shock presents with both high and low cardiac outputs
      of which the former is more common.   Ref. p. 144

SELECT THE MOST APPROPRIATE ANSWER:

253. THE DIFFERENCE BETWEEN HIGH OUTPUT AND LOW OUTPUT ENDO-
      TOXIC SHOCK IS:
      A. The former develops AV shunting as a response to endotoxin, and the
          latter presents with peripheral pooling
      B. The former develops peripheral pooling as a response to endotoxin,
          and the latter presents with AV shunting
      C. The former and latter present with peripheral pooling, and the etiology
          of the high output state is not clear   Ref. p. 144

ANSWER THE FOLLOWING STATEMENT T(RUE) OR F(ALSE):

254. In cardiogenic shock, the myocardium is working against an increased
      peripheral resistance.   Ref. p. 145

SELECT THE MOST APPROPRIATE ANSWER:

255. THE "UNITARIAN CONCEPT" OF SHOCK REFERS TO THE RESULTING:
      A. Decreased peripheral vasoconstriction and decreased tissue perfusion
      B. Decreased tissue perfusion and increased peripheral vasoconstriction
      C. Decreased peripheral vasoconstriction and increased tissue perfusion
                                              Ref. p. 147

256. RESTORATION OF WHICH OF THE FOLLOWING HEMODYNAMIC STATES
      APPEAR TO BE MOST IMPORTANT IN SHOCK?:
      A. Blood pressure   D. CVP to 8 cm H_2O
      B. Cardiac output   E. Deficiency in effective circulating
      C. Tissue perfusion   blood volume
                                              Ref. p. 147

MATCH THE FOLLOWING. EACH LETTERED ITEM MAY BE USED
MORE THAN ONCE:

257. ___ Steroids   A. Beta adrenergic stimulation
258. ___ Metaraminol   B. Alpha adrenergic stimulation
259. ___ Chlorpromazine   C. Beta adrenergic blocks
260. ___ Levarterenol   D. Alpha adrenergic blocks
261. ___ Isoproterenol

                               Ref. pp. 150-153

SELECT THE MOST APPROPRIATE ANSWER:

262. ALPHA ADRENERGIC BLOCKING AGENTS_____SURVIVAL IN
ENDOTOXIC SHOCK:
A. Increase
B. Decrease
C. Do not alter   Ref. p. 151

263. WHICH OF THE FOLLOWING IMPROVES THE STATE OF ENDOTOXIC
SHOCK?:
A. Phenoxybenzamine   D. Glucocorticoids
B. Phentolamine   E. All of the above
C. Chlorpromazine   Ref. pp. 151,153

ANSWER THE FOLLOWING QUESTION BY USING THE KEY
OUTLINED BELOW:
A. If both statement and reason are correct and related cause and effect
B. If both statement and reason are correct but not related cause and effect
C. If statement is true but reason is false
D. If statement is false but reason is true
E. If both statement and reason are false

264. It is possible to raise blood pressure by increasing peripheral resistance
but the effects are of short duration BECAUSE of the increase in work
which the heart must perform.   Ref. p. 155

ANSWER THE FOLLOWING STATEMENTS T(RUE) OR F(ALSE):

265. The most important facet in the treatment of cardiogenic shock (i.e.,
failure) is to elevate the blood pressure by increasing myocardial contractility (inotropic drugs only).   Ref. p. 156

266. The recommended therapy in cardiogenic shock is a combination of positive
inotropic myocardial stimulation and peripheral vasodilatation.
Ref. p. 157

SELECT THE MOST APPROPRIATE ANSWER(S):

267. WHICH OF THE FOLLOWING DOES NOT DISTINGUISH EXOTOXINS FROM
ENDOTOXINS?:
A. Exotoxins are primarily a derivative of living bacteria
B. Endotoxins are usually from gram-positive bacteria
C. Endotoxins are primarily a product of dead bacteria
D. All of the above are correct
E. None of the above are correct   Ref. p. 167

268. OF THE FOLLOWING TERMS, THE ONE WHICH BEST DESCRIBES THE
ABILITY OF AN ORGANISM TO DESTROY THE HOST IS:
A. Pathogenicity
B. Saprophytic
C. Virulence   Ref. p. 167

269. WHICH IS CONSIDERED A MORE SERIOUS WOUND:
A. Dog bite
B. Human bite
C. Both are about equal   Ref. p. 168

270. POSITIVE BLOOD CULTURES ARE OBTAINED DURING WHICH TIME
PERIOD DESCRIBED?:
A. Prior to the onset of shaking chills
B. Immediately after the development of shaking chills
C. At the temperature peak whether or not shaking chills accompany the
state
D. During the shaking chills period whether or not a temperature peak is
present
E. None of the above   Ref. p. 168

271.   ALL OF THE FOLLOWING DISEASES MAY BE EASILY DIAGNOSED BY
        BIOPSY MATERIAL, EXCEPT:
        A. Tuberculosis   D. Escherichia coli infection
        B. Mycoses   E. Lymphopathia venereum
        C. Syphilis   Ref. p. 168

272.   WHICH OF THE FOLLOWING IS RESPONSIBLE FOR THE DISTANT
        SPREAD OF A PATHOLOGIC ORGANISM THROUGH THE SYSTEM?:
        A. Cellulitis
        B. Lymphangitis
        C. Suppuration
        D. Septic vascular thrombosis   Ref. p. 169

273.   THE DIFFERENCE BETWEEN A FURUNCLE AND A CARBUNCLE IS:
        A. The presence of staphylococci in the former
        B. The presence of staphylococci in the latter
        C. The presence of a coagulase positive organism in the former
        D. The presence of multiple drainage sites in the latter
                                      Ref. p. 169

        MATCH THE FOLLOWING. EACH LETTERED ITEM MAY BE
        USED MORE THAN ONCE:

274. ___ Cellulitis   A. Staphylococcus aureus coagulase
275. ___ Carbuncle   positive
276. ___ Septic shock   B. Alpha-hemolytic streptococci
277. ___ Meleney's ulcer   C. Beta-hemolytic streptococci
278. ___ Endocarditis   D. Escherichia coli
279. ___ Tonsillitis   E. Microaerophilic nonhemolytic
280. ___ Erysipelas   streptococci
                                   Ref. pp. 169-182

        SELECT THE MOST APPROPRIATE ANSWER(S):

281.   THE MAJOR COMPLICATIONS RESULTING FROM THE ROUTINE PRE-
        OPERATIVE BOWEL PREPARATION ARE:
        A. Colonic perforation
        B. Monilial or staphylococcal overgrowth
        C. Aplastic anemia
        D. Deafness
        E. Anaphylactic shock
        F. All of the above   Ref. p. 171

282.   SUPERINFECTION IS MORE OFTEN ASSOCIATED WITH WHICH OF THE
        FOLLOWING ANTIBIOTIC GROUPS?:
        A. Aminoglycosides   D. Broad spectrum
        B. Griseofulvin   E. Bacitracin
        C. Nystatin   Ref. p. 171

        ANSWER THE FOLLOWING QUESTION BY USING THE KEY
        OUTLINED BELOW:
        A. If both statement and reason are correct and related cause and effect
        B. If both statement and reason are correct but not related cause and effect
        C. If statement is true but reason is false
        D. If statement is false but reason is true
        E. If both statement and reason are false

283.   Chemoprophylaxis is best used intramuscularly 1 to 2 hours prior to sur-
        gery, intravenously during the operation, and postoperatively x1 day,
        BECAUSE there is a reduced incidence of postoperative infection compared
        to the administration of a placebo.   Ref. p. 172

SELECT THE MOST APPROPRIATE ANSWER:

284. INTRAPERITONEAL IRRIGATION WITH WHICH ANTIBIOTIC(S) CAUSES
A POTENTIATION OF THE CURARE EFFECT AND RESULTS IN
RESPIRATORY DISTRESS?:
    A. Neomycin   D. Chloramphenicol
    B. Cephalothin   E. Lincomycin
    C. Kanamycin   Ref. p. 172

MATCH THE FOLLOWING. EACH LETTERED ITEM MAY BE USED
MORE THAN ONCE:

285. ___ Intestinal obstruction   A. Neomycin intraperitoneal
286. ___ Shock   B. Oral penicillin PCNASE resistant
287. ___ Aplastic anemia   C. Intramuscular penicillin PCNASE
288. ___ Acute respiratory   resistant
         depression   D. Intravenous penicillin PCNASE re-
289. ___ Anaphylactic shock   sistant
                                      E. Intravenous chloramphenicol
                                         Ref. pp. 175-177

SELECT THE MOST APPROPRIATE ANSWER:

290. WHICH OF THE FOLLOWING IS AN ANAEROBIC INFECTIVE DISEASE
STATE?:
    A. Clostridial cellulitis
    B. Clostridial myonecrosis (gas gangrene)
    C. Streptococcal myositis
    D. Tetanus
    E. All of the above   Ref. pp. 179-182

FILL IN THE MOST APPROPRIATE ANSWERS: (Questions 291-292)

    A. Anaerobic cellulitis   C. Streptococcal myositis
    B. Clostridial myonecrosis   D. All of the above

In which of the following infections is subcutaneous gas often present
291) _____ and which of the states would have the greatest accumulation 292) _____?:   Ref. pp. 179-182

SELECT THE MOST APPROPRIATE ANSWER:

293. THE MOST LETHAL EXOTOXIN OF THE CLOSTRIDIUM WELCHII
ORGANISM RESPONSIBLE FOR MOST VASCULAR COLLAPSE,
TOXEMIA IS:
    A. Hyaluronidase
    B. Collagenase
    C. Lecithinase
    D. Fibrolysin   Ref. p. 181

294. A SEVERE TOXEMIA IS OFTEN PRESENT IN WHICH OF THE FOLLOW-
ING?:
    A. Anaerobic cellulitis
    B. Clostridial myonecrosis
    C. Streptococcal myositis
    D. All of the above   Ref. p. 182

295. THE INFECTIOUS STATE WHICH IS MOST OFTEN MISTREATED BY
RADICAL SURGERY IS:
    A. Anaerobic clostridial cellulitis
    B. Clostridial myonecrosis
    C. Streptococcal myositis   Ref. p. 182

FILL IN THE MOST APPROPRIATE ANSWERS: (Questions 296-297)

A. Anaerobic cellulitis   C. Streptococcal myositis
B. Clostridial myonecrosis   D. All of the above

The infective state with a high temperature elevation and a disproportion-
ately high pulse rate is 296)_____, that with a proportionately high
pulse is 297)_____.   Ref. p. 182

SELECT THE MOST APPROPRIATE ANSWER(S):

298.   HOW IS IT POSSIBLE TO DISTINGUISH BETWEEN AN ANAEROBIC
       CELLULITIS AND A CLOSTRIDIAL MYONECROSIS?:
       A. The presence of clostridium welchii in the former
       B. The presence of clostridium welchii in the latter
       C. Profuse gas formation without toxemia in the former
       D. Pale and clammy skin in the former
       E. The presence of jaundice in the latter
                                          Ref. p. 182

299.   THE INCUBATION PERIOD FOR TETANUS MAY RANGE FROM____DAYS:
       A. 0 to 7   D. 7 to 21
       B. 0 to 14   E. 3 to 30
       C. 7 to 14   Ref. p. 183

300.   TETANUS IS A DISEASE WHICH IS OFTEN ASSOCIATED WITH WHICH
       OF THE FOLLOWING?:
       A. Wounds due to gun powder injuries
       B. Narcotic addiction
       C. Wounds obtained and fecally contaminated
       D. Compound fractures
       E. Burns
       F. All of the above   Ref. p. 183

301.   THE BASIC SYMPTOMATOLOGY OF TETANUS IS RELATED TO WHICH
       OF THE FOLLOWING?:
       A. Gastrointestinal system
       B. Neurologic system
       C. Skeletal system
       D. Circulatory system   Ref. p. 183

302.   WHICH OF THE FOLLOWING SYMPTOMS ARE CONSIDERED TO BE
       PRODROMAL IN TETANUS?:
       A. Urinary retention
       B. Stiffness and tingling of the jaw muscles
       C. High temperature elevations
       D. Restlessness
       E. Muscular twitching   Ref. pp. 183-184

303.   BOOSTER DOSES OF TETANUS TOXOID AS PROPHYLAXIS SHOULD BE
       GIVEN:
       A. Yearly
       B. Semiannually
       C. Every four to six years
       D. Only necessary within the first three years of life
                                           Ref. p. 184

304.   WHICH OF THE FOLLOWING MEDICATIONS HAS THE LEAST EFFECT
       ON THE DEVELOPMENT OF A TETANUS INFECTION?:
       A. Tetanus toxoid immunization   D. Antibiotics
       B. Human tetanus immune globulin   E. Tetanus antitoxin
       C. Equine antitoxin   Ref. p. 184

IN EACH OF THE FOLLOWING SITUATIONS THE TREATMENT
DESCRIBED MAY BE APPLIED IN ACCORDANCE WITH THE KEY
BELOW. THE SAME ANSWER MAY BE USED MORE THAN ONCE AND
EACH STATE MAY NEED MORE THAN ONE TREATMENT:

A. 0.5 cc tetanus toxoid
B. 250 units human tetanus immune globulin
C. 500 units human tetanus immune globulin
D. Oxytetracycline or penicillin
E. Equine antitoxin (300 units)

305. ___ Tetanus-prone wound in patient previously immunized over six years
         prior and fecal contamination of the area
306. ___ Tetanus-prone wound in a patient previously immunized less than six
         years prior, with minimal contamination
307. ___ A tetanus-prone wound, contaminated, in a patient, when human tetanus
         immune globulin is not available   Ref. p. 185

308. WHICH OF THE MYCOSES IS CHARACTERIZED BY CERVICOFACIAL
     LESIONS, ABDOMINAL CUTANEOUS FISTULAES, PERIAPPENDICEAL
     ABSCESSES?:
     A. Blastomycosis   D. Histoplasmosis
     B. Actinomycosis   E. Moniliasis
     C. Coccidioidomycosis   Ref. pp. 187-188

309. SUBCUTANEOUS NODULES WHICH ARE OFTEN FOUND ABOUT TRAU-
     MATIZED AREAS AND WHICH BREAK DOWN TO FORM ULCERATIONS
     WITH RAGGED MARGINS ARE FOUND IN:
     A. Blastomycosis   D. Histoplasmosis
     B. Actinomycosis   E. Moniliasis
     C. Coccidioidomycosis   Ref. p. 188

310. THE TREATMENT OF CHOICE FOR SYSTEMIC MONILIASIS IS:
     A. Oxytetracycline   D. Amphotericin D
     B. Chloramphenicol   E. All of the above
     C. Amphotericin B   Ref. p. 188

311. THE PRIORITY SYSTEM IN EMERGENCY CARE OF A PATIENT DIC-
     TATES THAT WHICH OF THE FOLLOWING SHOULD BE PERFORMED
     FIRST?:
     A. Control of massive hemorrhage
     B. Initiate treatment of shock with vasopressor
     C. Diagnostic testing plus evaluation
     D. Insertion of an adequate airway   Ref. p. 196

312. THE PREFERRED AIRWAY IN ACUTELY UNCONSCIOUS ADULT
     PATIENTS IS:
     A. Tracheostomy
     B. Cuffed endotracheal tube
     C. Uncuffed endotracheal tube
     D. Ambu bag over oral + nasal passages
                                       Ref. p. 196

313. IN AN ACUTE SITUATION WHERE BLEEDING IS MASSIVE AND THERE
     IS NO TIME TO TYPE AND CROSS MATCH BLOOD, WHICH OF THE
     FOLLOWING SHOULD BE UTILIZED?:
     A. Ringer's Lactate   D. O Rh negative
     B. Type blood AB Rh positive   E. A Rh negative
     C. O Rh positive   Ref. p. 197

314.   WITH ACUTE ARTERIAL HEMORRHAGE FROM A LARGE VESSEL IN AN
       EXTREMITY WHICH OF THE FOLLOWING IS LEAST DESIRABLE ?:
       A. Elevation of extremity
       B. Tourniquet control of bleeding site
       C. Direct digital compression
       D. Ligation, if vessel is superficial   Ref. p. 197

315.   FOLLOWING THE INSERTION OF AN ENDOTRACHEAL TUBE IN A
       PATIENT WITH SEVERE CHEST TRAUMA, IN WHICH IMPROVEMENT
       IS NOT NOTED, WHICH OF THE FOLLOWING COULD NOT BE THE
       CAUSE ?:
       A. Pneumothorax
       B. Hemothorax
       C. Cardiac tamponade
       D. Flail chest
       E. None of the above   Ref. p. 197

316.   IN AN EMERGENCY ROOM, ONE SUSPECTS THE DEVELOPMENT OF A
       PNEUMOTHORAX. WHICH IS THE MOST EFFICIENT WAY TO MAKE
       THE DIAGNOSIS ?:
       A. Chest X-ray (PA)
       B. 18 gauge needle aspiration in anterior axillary line
       C. 18 gauge needle aspiration in posterior axillary line
       D. Chest tube insertion
       E. Measurements of tidal volume   Ref. p. 197

317.   CARDIAC TAMPONADE CAN BE EVACUATED BY ASPIRATION WITH AN
       18 GAUGE NEEDLE IN THE XYPHOID COSTAL ANGLE. WHAT IS THE
       INDICATION FOR SURGICAL INTERVENTION WITH A POSITIVE RESULT ?:
       A. The diagnosis of the condition and a single evacuation
       B. Repeated aspiration x 2
       C. Both   Ref. p. 197

318.   THE TREATMENT OF A FLAIL CHEST IS BEST ACCOMPLISHED BY:
       A. Sand bags
       B. Towel clips to chest + IPPB
       C. Tracheostomy + positive pressure ventilation
                                              Ref. p. 197

319.   A COMATOSE PATIENT WHO HAD SUSTAINED GENERALIZED TRAUMA
       WAS ADMITTED WITH HYPOTENSION. WHICH OF THE FOLLOWING
       WOULD MOST LIKELY EXPLAIN THE HYPOTENSION ?:
       A. Subdural hematoma   D. Hemorrhage
       B. Epidural hematoma   E. All of the above
       C. Neurogenic shock   Ref. p. 198

320.   ANTIBIOTICS ARE MOST EFFECTIVE IN PREVENTING WOUND IN-
       FECTION IF ADMINISTERED:
       A. Postoperatively
       B. Preoperatively or intra-operatively
       C. Equally   Ref. p. 199

321.   THE NORMAL PATIENT TAKING 70 GRAMS OF PROTEIN DAILY WILL
       HAVE A UREA NITROGEN CONTENT OF_____GRAMS. VARIATIONS
       ABOUT THIS FIGURE CAN BE UTILIZED AS AN INDICATION OF POSI-
       TIVE OR NEGATIVE NITROGEN BALANCE IN THE BODY:
       A. 5   D. 20
       B. 10   E. 25
       C. 15   Ref. p. 200

322. WHICH OF THE FOLLOWING VITAMINS APPEAR TO BE ESSENTIAL IN
POSTOPERATIVE PARENTERAL THERAPY?:
A. Vitamin C   D. Thiamine
B. Vitamin A   E. All of the above
C. Vitamin D   Ref. p. 201

323. WHICH OF THE FOLLOWING FACTS IS NOT TRUE WITH REFERENCE
TO AN UNEMPTIED STOMACH AND ANESTHESIA ADMINISTRATION?:
A. Intubation while awake is indicated
B. The use of "crash" induction methods is accompanied by pressure on
the cricoid cartilage to press the esophagus
C. The Mendelson's syndrome is a frequent result of this situation
D. The treatment of chemical pneumonitis due to aspiration requires only
massive irrigation
E. Bronchoscopy is indicated if cyanosis develops following aspirated
foreign material   Ref. p. 202

ANSWER THE FOLLOWING STATEMENTS T(RUE) OR F(ALSE):

324. The incidence of wound infection is inversely proportional to the amount of
irrigation and debridement at the time of injury.
Ref. p. 204

325. All gunshot wounds should undergo delayed primary closure and antibiotics are unnecessary.   Ref. p. 204

SELECT THE MOST APPROPRIATE ANSWER:

326. THE MOST FREQUENT CAUSE OF WOUND INFECTIONS IN TRAUMA
CASES IS:
A. E. Coli   D. Streptococcus
B. Staphylococcus aureus   E. None of the above
C. Pseudomonas aerobacter   Ref. p. 206

327. THE BITE OF A RABID ANIMAL FOUR HOURS OLD IS:
A. Washed with 20% soap solution + 1% Zephiran
B. Debrided
C. Further controlled with rabies antiserum
D. Should receive hyperimmune serum 40 I.U. Kg
E. All of the above   Ref. p. 207

328. WHICH OF THE FOLLOWING IS RESPONSIBLE FOR MORE DEATHS IN
THE UNITED STATES?:
A. Pit vipers' bites
B. Coral snake bites
C. Equal   Ref. p. 212

329. THE PRINCIPLES BEHIND TREATMENT OF POISONOUS SNAKEBITES
INCLUDE ALL, EXCEPT:
A. Tourniquet compressing arterial and venous circulation
B. Cruciate incisions
C. Suction
D. Ice water immersion
E. Crotalidae antivenin polyvalent serum (when indicated)
Ref. p. 212

330. THE MOST SIGNIFICANT FINDING INDICATIVE OF A VENOMOUS
SNAKEBITE IS:
A. Excruciating pain   D. Uncontrolled bleeding
B. Severe local edema   E. Hypotension
C. Paralysis of extremity   Ref. p. 212

ANSWER THE FOLLOWING QUESTION BY USING THE KEY
OUTLINED BELOW:
A. If both statement and reason are correct and related cause and effect
B. If both statement and reason are correct but not related cause and effect
C. If statement is true but reason is false
D. If statement is false but reason is true
E. If both statement and reason are false

331. In the United States, more patients succumb each year to insect bites than
      to snake bites BECAUSE the venom of the former is more potent.
                                              Ref. p. 214

FILL IN THE MOST APPROPRIATE ANSWERS: (Questions 332-333)

A. 12 hours
B. 1 to 2 days
C. 2 to 4 days
D. 4 to 8 days
E. 8 to 12 days

All soft tissue injuries of the neck should be drained for 332)_____
and those involving the esophagus or pharynx should be continued to
333)_____.   Ref. pp. 219-220

SELECT THE MOST APPROPRIATE ANSWER:

334. WHICH IS GREATER IN THE UNITED STATES? MORTALITY FROM:
      A. Blunt abdominal traumas
      B. Sharp penetrating wounds
      C. Both are equal   Ref. p. 220

335. WHICH OF THE FOLLOWING ARE LEAST INDICATIVE OF INTRA-
      ABDOMINAL HEMORRHAGE IN A COMATOSE PATIENT?:
      A. Peritoneal tap with non-clotted blood
      B. Initially hypotensive patient who responds to "push" intravenous fluids
      C. Leukocyte count over 15,000
      D. X-ray of abdomen demonstrating "hazy" abdomen
      E. Negative abdominal tap with rigid abdomen
                                              Ref. p. 221

ANSWER THE FOLLOWING STATEMENT T(RUE) OR F(ALSE):

336. Bullet wounds of the abdomen require surgical exploration in less than
      75% of the cases.   Ref. p. 225

FILL IN THE MOST APPROPRIATE ANSWERS: (Questions 337-338)

A. 70-75
B. 55-60
C. 35-50
D. 25-30
E. 5-10

The retroperitoneal duodenal laceration is difficult to diagnose and carries
a mortality rate of 337)_____. Once explored, the lesion is missed
338)_____ per cent of the time.
                                              Ref. pp. 225-226

SELECT THE MOST APPROPRIATE ANSWER:

339. WHICH OF THE FOLLOWING IS THE LEAST ACCEPTABLE THERAPY
      FOR DUODENAL LACERATION?:
      A. Jejunal patch
      B. Roux-Y-Loop
      C. Pancreatectomy and duodenectomy
      D. Suction controlled fistulae with Foley catheter in duodenum
      E. None of the above   Ref. p. 226

340. COLONIC LACERATIONS DUE TO HIGH-VELOCITY MISSILES REQUIRE:
      A. Resection of damaged bowel and primary closure
      B. Colostomy and exteriorization of damaged area if possible
      C. Neither   Ref. p. 232

341. EXTRAPERITONEAL RECTAL PERFORATIONS BY HIGH-VELOCITY
      MISSILES SHOULD BE TREATED WITH:
      A. Proximal colostomy and debridement and mucous fistulae
      B. Presacral drainage
      C. Both   Ref. p. 232

342. THE OVERALL MORTALITY OF LIVER INJURIES SECONDARY TO
      BLUNT TRAUMA IS ABOUT_____PER CENT:
      A. 10   D. 30
      B. 15   E. 40
      C. 25   Ref. p. 233

343. WHICH OF THE FOLLOWING DOES CONTRIBUTE TO A RELA-
      TIVELY LOWER MORTALITY RATE WITH LIVER TRAUMA THAN IN
      THE PAST?:
      A. Adequate drainage   D. T-tube drainage
      B. Antibiotics   E. All of the above
      C. Liver resection   Ref. p. 233

344. WHICH OF THE ASSOCIATED COMPLICATIONS WITH LIVER RUPTURE
      CARRIES THE WORST PROGNOSIS?:
      A. Thoracic injuries   D. Adrenal injuries
      B. Colonic injuries   E. Gastric injuries
      C. Renal injuries   Ref. p. 235

345. HEMATOBILIA PRESENTS 1 TO 3 WEEKS FOLLOWING HEPATIC
      TRAUMA. IF DISCOVERED, THE TREATMENT MOST LIKELY WOULD
      BE:
      A. Observation plus transfusion
      B. T-tube drainage of the common duct
      C. Intravenous fibrinogen (30 grams)
      D. Immediate exploration plus hepatic resection
      E. Immediate exploration plus suture ligation of bleeding point
                                     Ref. p. 235

346. WHAT IS CONSIDERED A SAFE PERIOD OF TIME TO OCCLUDE THE
      VASCULAR SUPPLY TO THE LIVER, DURING REPAIR IF THE PATIENT
      IS NOT HYPOTHERMIC?:
      A. 75-80 minutes   D. 35-40 minutes
      B. 55-60 minutes   E. 15-20 minutes
      C. 45-50 minutes   Ref. p. 236

347. IN A PANCREATIC LACERATION, THE SERUM AMYLASE:
      A. Does not elevate
      B. Is elevated within two hours
      C. Neither   Ref. p. 238

348.   THE ABDOMINAL ORGAN MOST FREQUENTLY INJURED BY BLUNT
        TRAUMA IS THE:
        A. Liver
        B. Pancreas
        C. Spleen
        D. Bladder
        E. Colon   Ref. p. 242

        ANSWER THE FOLLOWING QUESTION BY USING THE KEY
        OUTLINED BELOW:
        A. If both statement and reason are correct and related cause and effect
        B. If both statement and reason are correct but not related cause and effect
        C. If statement is true but reason is false
        D. If statement is false but reason is true
        E. If both statement and reason are false

349.   Hematuria may represent the best clue to the development of retroperi-
        toneal hematoma BECAUSE bladder damage usually corresponds closely
        to associated retroperitoneal trauma.   Ref. p. 242

        SELECT THE MOST APPROPRIATE ANSWER:

350.   WHICH OF THE FOLLOWING IS NOT TRUE CONCERNING RETROPERI-
        TONEAL HEMATOMAS?:
        A. 80 per cent have gross hematuria
        B. Intraperitoneal abdominal tap may be positive (false positive)
        C. Retroperitoneal bleeding is self-limiting and exploration is not
            warranted
        D. Shock is present in about 40 per cent of the patients
        E. The Grey-Turner sign develops within a few hours
                                                    Ref. p. 243

351.   HEAT TRANSFER WHICH RESULTS IN A BURN IS DEPENDENT UPON
        ALL, EXCEPT:
        A. Local circulation   D. Intensity
        B. Rapidity of heat transfer   E. Local conductivity
        C. Total heat transfer   Ref. p. 253

        FILL IN THE MOST APPROPRIATE ANSWERS: (Questions 352-353)

        A. 30° C
        B. 40° C
        C. 50° C
        D. 65° C
        E. 75° C

        Maintaining a constant duration of exposure, which is the minimal tempera-
        ture that will cause protein denaturation 352)_____? Which will pro-
        duce protein coagulation 353)_____?
                                                    Ref. p. 254
        SELECT THE MOST APPROPRIATE ANSWER:

354.   WHICH OF THE FOLLOWING WILL MOST LIKELY PRODUCE THE
        DEEPEST BURNS?:
        A. Flame burn   D. Immersion scald
        B. Spill scald   E. All are equal
        C. Flash burn   Ref. p. 254

ANSWER THE FOLLOWING QUESTIONS BY USING THE KEY
OUTLINED BELOW:
A. If both statement and reason are correct and related cause and effect
B. If both statement and reason are correct but not related cause and effect
C. If statement is true but reason is false
D. If statement is false but reason is true
E. If both statement and reason are false

355. Immersion scalds are often not as severe as flame burns BECAUSE the
latter often produces deep burns due to prolonged exposure.
Ref. p. 254

356. Immersion scalds will produce the most uniform burn depth BECAUSE a
mixture of full thickness and partial thickness damage is rare.
Ref. p. 254

357. Second degree burns are frequently described as superficial and deep
BECAUSE they vary in their ability to recover by epithelialization.
Ref. p. 254

SELECT THE MOST APPROPRIATE ANSWER:

358. GIVEN A CONSTANT TEMPERATURE AND TIME OF EXPOSURE, THE
LEAST SEVERE BURN WILL PRESENT ON THE:
A. Palm of the hand   D. Face
B. Dorsal skin of the hand   E. All are equal
C. Abdomen   Ref. p. 254

359. THE SKIN OF THE PALM WILL BE LEAST RESISTANT TO A BURN IN
A(N):
A. Adult male foundry worker   D. 2 year-old child
B. 12 year-old school boy   E. All will burn equally
C. Adult female dishwasher   Ref. p. 254

360. WHICH OF THE FOLLOWING WILL BE LEAST HELPFUL IN DISTINGUISH-
ING A THIRD DEGREE FROM A SECOND DEGREE BURN?:
A. Waxy appearance in the former
B. Blistering of skin in the latter
C. Loss of sensitivity in the former
D. Thrombosed veins visible
E. Lack of early cellular inflammatory reaction in the former
Ref. p. 254

361. THE NORMAL UNBURNED PATIENT WILL LOSE 15 TO 21 ml/hour/m^2
OF INSENSIBLE WATER PRIMARILY DUE TO RESPIRATION. HOW
MUCH WILL A PATIENT WITH 40 PER CENT BURNS LOSE?:
A. 20 ml/hour/m^2
B. 40 ml/hour/m^2
C. 60 ml/hour/m^2
D. 80 ml/hour/m^2
E. 100 ml/hour/m^2 Ref. p. 255

362. THE WATER LOSS FROM A BURN BY EVAPORATION IS PRIMARILY:
A. Isotonic
B. Hypotonic
C. Hypertonic
D. Depends on the burn   Ref. p. 255

ANSWER THE FOLLOWING QUESTIONS BY USING THE KEY
OUTLINED BELOW:
A. If both statement and reason are correct and related cause and effect
B. If both statement and reason are correct but not related cause and effect
C. If statement is true but reason is false
D. If statement is false but reason is true
E. If both statement and reason are false

363. The so called "vapor barrier" is totally destroyed in a third degree burn
BECAUSE it results in water evaporation from the skin as if it were merely
an open water basin.   Ref. p. 255

364. Vascular recanalization beneath a second degree burn begins 48 hours after
the burn BECAUSE this is dependent upon the presence or absence of an
underlying infection.   Ref. p. 255

SELECT THE MOST APPROPRIATE ANSWER:

365. WHICH OF THE FOLLOWING ARE NOT TRUE ABOUT BURN WOUND
HEALING?:
A. In third degree burns, new capillary development begins at the end of
the second week
B. The development of vascular tissues is dependent on the presence or
absence of an infection
C. In first degree burns, recanalization of the vascular system begins in
48 hours
D. The major site of burn microorganism is in the hair follicles and
sweat glands
E. All are true   Ref. p. 255

366. THE INITIAL COLONIZATION OF A BURN BY MICROORGANISMS
CONSISTS OF:
A. Pseudomonas   D. Proteus
B. Staphylococcus   E. Mixed flora
C. Escherichia coli   Ref. p. 255

367. THE DEFINITION OF BURN WOUND SEPSIS:
A. Depends on the presence of pathologic organisms
B. Depends on pathogenic organisms and a colony count of over 100,000
organisms per gram of tissue
C. Depends on evidence of bacteria in the blood
D. Depends on bacterial invasion and metastatic spread
E. All constitute "burn sepsis"   Ref. p. 256

ANSWER THE FOLLOWING QUESTIONS BY USING THE KEY
OUTLINED BELOW:
A. If both statement and reason are correct and related cause and effect
B. If both statement and reason are correct but not related cause and effect
C. If statement is true but reason is false
D. If statement is false but reason is true
E. If both statement and reason are false

368. Positive blood culture in a burn patient is uncommon BECAUSE it most
often develops as a result of septic phlebitis from intravenous catheters.
Ref. p. 256

369. Whole blood transfusion is often essential in early burn treatment BECAUSE
as much as 60% of the red cell mass may be destroyed by early hemolysis.
Ref. p. 256

370.   A progressive drop in the hematocrit over 2 to 3 weeks is expected in burn
       patients BECAUSE RBC fragility has been increased and earlier destruc-
       tion of these cells occurs.   Ref. p. 256

371.   Local capillary permeability is affected in burns involving less than 30%
       of the body BECAUSE burns involving a greater surface area cause gen-
       eralized capillary permeability.   Ref. p. 257

       SELECT THE MOST APPROPRIATE ANSWER:

372.   SALT WATER LOSS FROM THE VASCULAR TREE IS CONSISTENT WITH
       WHICH OF THE FOLLOWING?:
       A.   Is lost at a precise rate which can be determined mathematically
       B.   May be delayed by rapid administration of protein fractions early in
            therapy
       C.   In the first 5 hours an 80% loss of plasma volume may occur
       D.   Capillary permeability is not affected
       E.   All of the above are correct   Ref. p. 257

373.   WHICH OF THE FOLLOWING CARDIOVASCULAR EFFECTS ARE NOT
       NOTED TO RESULT FROM A SEVERE BURN?:
       A.   Decrease in cardiac output
       B.   Increase in peripheral vascular resistance
       C.   Increase in the pulse rate
       D.   Decrease in stroke volume
       E.   All are present   Ref. p. 258

374.   THE MOST FREQUENT GASTROINTESTINAL COMPLAINT IN PATIENTS
       WITH BURNS EXCEEDING 30% OF THE BODY IS:
       A.   Acute gastritis   D.   Diarrhea
       B.   Curling's ulcer   E.   None of the above
       C.   Ileus   Ref. p. 258

       ANSWER THE FOLLOWING QUESTIONS BY USING THE KEY
       OUTLINED BELOW:
       A.   If both statement and reason are correct and related cause and effect
       B.   If both statement and reason are correct but not related cause and effect
       C.   If statement is true but reason is false
       D.   If statement is false but reason is true
       E.   If both statement and reason are false

375.   The major post-burn complication involving the kidneys is acute tubular
       necrosis BECAUSE there is a sudden fall in the glomerular filtration rate.
                                   Ref. p. 258

376.   Burns of the pulmonary parenchyma are frequent BECAUSE the inhalation
       of superheated air usually passes the larynx.
                                   Ref. p. 258

377.   Curling's gastric ulcer is a frequent complication of severe burns appear-
       ing in over 25% of cases BECAUSE of the increase in gastric stasis and
       associated hyperacidity.   Ref. p. 259

       ANSWER THE FOLLOWING QUESTION T(RUE) OR F(ALSE):

378.   The requirement of sedation is inversely proportional to the depth of the
       burn.   Ref. p. 259

SELECT THE MOST APPROPRIATE ANSWER:

379.   TRACHEOSTOMY COMPLICATIONS MOST OFTEN ARE RELATED TO:
        A. Tracheal stenosis   D. Erosion of anterior tracheal wall
        B. Sepsis   E. Copious secretions
        C. Sudden obstruction of airway   Ref. p. 259

ANSWER THE FOLLOWING STATEMENT T(RUE) OR F(ALSE):

380.   An organ transplanted into the human is more vulnerable to body defenses
        than the one removed.   Ref. 260 (1st Ed.)

ANSWER THE FOLLOWING QUESTIONS BY USING THE KEY
OUTLINED BELOW:
A. If both statement and reason are correct and related cause and effect
B. If both statement and reason are correct but not related cause and effect
C. If statement is true but reason is false
D. If statement is false but reason is true
E. If both statement and reason are false

381.   The complication of pneumothorax with tracheostomy procedure is not
        infrequent BECAUSE children are most vulnerable.
                                               Ref. p. 260

382.   The "rule of nines" is an accurate method of calculating the involved sur-
        face area in first, second and third degree burns BECAUSE adults are the
        best subjects for application of this formula.
                                               Ref. p. 261

SELECT THE MOST APPROPRIATE ANSWER:

383.   THE PARKLAND FORMULA AVOIDS WHICH OF THE FOLLOWING IN
        THE INITIAL 24-HOUR REPLACEMENT OF FLUID?:
        A. Colloid 0.5ml/Kg body weight x % burn
        B. Ringer's lactate 4ml/Kg body weight x % burn
        C. Dextrose/water
        D. All of the above
        E. None of the above   Ref. p. 261

ANSWER THE FOLLOWING STATEMENT T(RUE) OR F(ALSE):

384.   With significant thermal injury, the obligatory loss of plasma volume con-
        tinues until the rate of infusion exceeds 4.4ml/Kg/hr, at which time plasma
        volume expansion begins.   Ref. p. 261

SELECT THE MOST APPROPRIATE ANSWER:

385.   WHICH OF THE FOLLOWING IS LEAST CORRECT?:
        A. The Brooke Burn Formula is not applicable in first degree burns
        B. The Brooke Burn Formula is not reliable if the burn exceeds 50% of
            the surface area in adults
        C. The Brooke Burn Formula is not reliable in burns exceeding 30% in
            children
        D. The colloid fraction of the burn formula may constitute up to 3000 cc
            of dextrose
        E. The major electrolyte replacement in burns is Ringer's lactate
                                               Ref. p. 261

386.   USING THE BROOKE BURN FORMULA, A 30 YEAR-OLD 70 Kg MALE
        PATIENT WITH 45% SURFACE OF SECOND AND THIRD DEGREE BURNS
        WOULD REQUIRE_____IN THE FIRST 24 HOURS:
        A. 3425 cc Ringer's lactate; 1575 cc colloid; 2000 cc dextrose/water
        B. 4525 cc Ringer's lactate; 1575 cc colloid; 2000 cc dextrose/water
        C. 4725 cc colloid; 1575 cc Ringer's lactate; 2000 cc dextrose/water
        D. 6300 cc Ringer's lactate; 2000 cc colloid
                                               Ref. p. 261

ANSWER THE FOLLOWING QUESTION BY USING THE KEY
OUTLINED BELOW:
A. If both statement and reason are correct and related cause and effect
B. If both statement and reason are correct but not related cause and effect
C. If statement is true but reason is false
D. If statement is false but reason is true
E. If both statement and reason are false

387. A patient with gross hematuria following a 60% burn should be transfused
with whole blood immediately BECAUSE the reduction of hemoglobin results
in defective oxygen transport.   Ref. p. 262

SELECT THE MOST APPROPRIATE ANSWER:

388. TO PREVENT RENAL SHUT-DOWN IN POST-BURN PATIENTS, ALL OF
THE FOLLOWING CAN BE UTILIZED TO AID THE SITUATION, EXCEPT:
A. Maintain urine output between 30 and 50 cc/hour
B. Mannitol administration
C. Alkalinization of the urine
D. Whole blood transfusion   Ref. p. 262

389. CHILDREN UNDER THE AGE OF ONE YEAR SHOULD UNDERGO FLUID
RESUSCITATION FOR BURN THERAPY WITH WHICH OF THE FOLLOW-
ING FLUIDS?:
A. Ringer's lactate
B. Saline
C. Dextrose/water
D. Solution with 40-70 mEq of sodium
E. Solution with 30-40 mEq of sodium   Ref. p. 262

390. WHICH OF THE FOLLOWING ARE NOT ASSOCIATED WITH SILVER
NITRATE (AgNO3) /0.5%/ TREATMENT OF BURNS?:
A. The compresses applied to the burn should always remain moist
B. Debridement of necrotic tissue is essential
C. There is no reduction in overall survival of burn patients when
utilizing the substance
D. The development of hypochloremic hyponatremic alkalosis becomes
most prominent after termination of intravenous therapy in post-burn
patients
E. All of the above are true   Ref. p. 263

ANSWER THE FOLLOWING QUESTIONS BY USING THE KEY
OUTLINED BELOW:
A. If both statement and reason are correct and related cause and effect
B. If both statement and reason are correct but not related cause and effect
C. If statement is true but reason is false
D. If statement is false but reason is true
E. If both statement and reason are false

391. 0.5% silver nitrate solution results in specific loss of sodium BECAUSE of
the precipitation of sodium nitrate on the surface area.
                              Ref. p. 263

392. Sulfamylon (para-aminomethylbenzene sulfonamide) is bacteriostatic
BECAUSE it inhibits bacterial growth and permits continued phagocytosis.
                              Ref. p. 264

SELECT THE MOST APPROPRIATE ANSWER:

393.   WHICH OF THE FOLLOWING ARE DRAWBACKS TO THE USE OF
SULFAMYLON?:
A. Sensitivity in 5% of the cases
B. Strong carbonic anhydrase inhibitor
C. Creates a metabolic acidosis compensated by hyperventilation and a
low CO_2
D. Often results in an elevated urinary specific gravity
E. All of the above   Ref. p. 264

ANSWER THE FOLLOWING QUESTIONS BY USING THE KEY
OUTLINED BELOW:
A. If both statement and reason are correct and related cause and effect
B. If both statement and reason are correct but not related cause and effect
C. If statement is true but reason is false
D. If statement is false but reason is true
E. If both statement and reason are false

394.   Sulfamylon should be utilized cautiously in burn patients with chronic lung
disease BECAUSE the pulmonary tree is the major buffering system when
this drug is used.   Ref. p. 265

395.   Prophylactic antibiotics are often used immediately after the burn
BECAUSE of the frequent development of an overlying pseudomonas infection.   Ref. p. 265

SELECT THE MOST APPROPRIATE ANSWER:

396.   ONE MUST WAIT_____TO ESTABLISH THE SUCCESS OR FAILURE
OF A RENAL GRAFT ON AN IMMUNOLOGIC BASIS:
A. 4 months   D. 72 months
B. 18 months   E. None of the above
C. 36 months   Ref. p. 266 (1st Ed.)

397.   A CIRCULAR ESCHAR OF AN EXTREMITY IN A BURN PATIENT SHOULD
BE TREATED WITH:
A. Antibiotics (systemic)
B. Complete splitting incisions of eschar
C. Radical debridement
D. Elevation of the extremity
E. Addition of silver nitrate   Ref. p. 266

ANSWER THE FOLLOWING QUESTIONS BY USING THE KEY
OUTLINED BELOW:
A. If both statement and reason are correct and related cause and effect
B. If both statement and reason are correct but not related cause and effect
C. If statement is true but reason is false
D. If statement is false but reason is true
E. If both statement and reason are false

398.   A homograft can be applied to a freshly debrided burn area but should be
removed within 72 hours BECAUSE of eventual graft failure and purulent
collections beneath it.   Ref. p. 267

399.   An autograft "take" is noted to give the best results when following a previous homograft of the area BECAUSE the bed of tissue is sterile.
                              Ref. p. 268

SELECT THE MOST APPROPRIATE ANSWER:

400. CURLING'S ULCERS HAVE ALL OF THE FOLLOWING CHARACTERISTICS,
      EXCEPT:
      A. Most commonly gastric
      B. Bleed often
      C. May be multiple
      D. Should almost never have surgical intervention
      E. Occur in 40% of the cases without prodromal symptoms
                                            Ref. p. 269

401. THE TREATMENT OF CHOICE FOR A CURLING'S ULCER IS:
      A. Prophylaxis
      B. Vagotomy and hemigastrectomy
      C. Vagotomy and phyloroplasty
      D. Total gastrectomy
      E. Suture ligation of ulcer base   Ref. p. 269

402. IN BURNS OF THE HAND, WHICH OF THE FOLLOWING AREAS IS
      LEAST LIKELY TO BE FULL THICKNESS?:
      A. Dorsum of the hand
      B. Flexor surface of the tips of the digits
      C. Palm and proximal flexor surface of digits
      D. All are usually equal   Ref. p. 270

ANSWER THE FOLLOWING QUESTIONS BY USING THE KEY
OUTLINED BELOW:
      A. If both statement and reason are correct and related cause and effect
      B. If both statement and reason are correct but not related cause and effect
      C. If statement is true but reason is false
      D. If statement is false but reason is true
      E. If both statement and reason are false

403. Second and third degree burns of the ears may ultimately result in loss of
      the organ BECAUSE of the development of a destructive chondritis.
                                            Ref. p. 270

404. Early autografting of the dorsum of the hand is indicated BECAUSE of the
      development of unsightly contractures.   Ref. p. 270

      SELECT THE MOST APPROPRIATE ANSWER:

405. THE ONLY HUMAN VISCERAL ORGAN CAPABLE OF REGENERATION
      IS THE:
      A. Spleen   D. Intestine
      B. Kidney   E. None of the above
      C. Liver   Ref. p. 275

ANSWER THE FOLLOWING QUESTION BY USING THE KEY
OUTLINED BELOW:
      A. If both statement and reason are correct and related cause and effect
      B. If both statement and reason are correct but not related cause and effect
      C. If statement is true but reason is false
      D. If statement is false but reason is true
      E. If both statement and reason are false

406. Prolongation of homograft survival by present day techniques is not useful
      in cancer patients BECAUSE the tumor is more rapidly propagated.
                                            Ref. p. 276 (1st Ed.)

      SELECT THE MOST APPROPRIATE ANSWER:

407. THE STRENGTH IN SCAR TISSUE IS SUPPLIED PRIMARILY BY_____
      TISSUE:
      A. Epithelial   D. Muscular
      B. Fibrous   E. None of the above
      C. Vascular   Ref. p. 278

ANSWER THE FOLLOWING STATEMENT T(RUE) OR F(ALSE):

408.   A 5 day-old healing wound may histologically appear as a fibrosarcoma.
Ref. p. 278

SELECT THE MOST APPROPRIATE ANSWER:

409.   WHICH OF THE FOLLOWING MAY BE RESPONSIBLE FOR SKIN
CARCINOMA ?:
A. Thermal injuries   D. All of the above
B. Gamma on X-ray   E. None of the above
C. Solar or cosmic radiation   Ref. p. 279

ANSWER THE FOLLOWING STATEMENT T(RUE) OR F(ALSE):

410.   The development of carcinoma induced in wounds is directly proportional
to the wave length.   Ref. p. 279

SELECT THE MOST APPROPRIATE ANSWER(S):

411.   IN A SUTURED OPERATIVE INCISION, HOW LONG WILL IT TAKE FOR
EPITHELIALIZATION TO PRODUCE A WATER TIGHT SEAL ?:
A. 6 hours   D. 36 hours
B. 12 hours   E. 48 hours
C. 24 hours   Ref. p. 280

412.   WHICH CONTAINS A GREATER CONCENTRATION OF HYDROXYPRO-
LINE ?:
A. Collagen
B. Elastin
C. Equal   Ref. p. 282

413.   WHICH OF THE FOLLOWING ALTERS COLLAGEN METABOLISM, AND
MAY REDUCE BURN SCAR CONTRACTURE ?:
A. Vitamin C   D. Mafenide
B. Beta-ammopropionitrite   E. Inorganic silver nitrate
C. Epsilon amino caproic acid   Ref. p. 284

414.   AT WHICH TIME FOLLOWING WOUND TRAUMA DOES THE LEVEL OF
HYDROXYPROLINE INCREASE RAPIDLY ?:
A. 1st day   D. 7th to 8th day
B. 3rd to 4th day   E. 14th to 15th day
C. 4th to 6th day   Ref. p. 287

415.   THE DEVELOPMENT OF SIGNIFICANT TENSILE STRENGTH IN A
WOUND BEGINS ABOUT WHAT POSTOPERATIVE DAY ?:
A. 3rd   D. 12th
B. 5th   E. 21st
C. 9th   Ref. p. 287

416.   WHEN IS THE MAXIMAL COLLAGEN CONTENT OF WOUND TISSUE
NOTED ?:
A. Between 3rd to 5th day
B. Between 6th to 17th day
C. Between 17th to 21st day
D. None of the above   Ref. p. 287

417.   THE SO CALLED "GOLDEN PERIOD" WHICH IS THE TIME ONE CAN
SUCCESSFULLY CLOSE A WOUND FOLLOWING TRAUMA IS_____HOURS:
A. 2
B. 6
C. 12
D. 24
E. Varies with type of injury   Ref. p. 288

418.   WHICH OF THE FOLLOWING SUTURES CONTRIBUTE THE <u>LEAST</u> TO
       WOUND STRENGTH?:
       A. Fibromuscular opposition   D. None of the above
       B. Subcuticular opposition   E. All are equal
       C. Skin coaptation   Ref. p. 289

419.   SKIN ERYTHEMA IN CHILDREN AND TEENAGERS SHOULD NEVER BE
       AN INDICATION FOR REVISION BECAUSE:
       A. It is always temporary
       B. It may last for several years and then disappear
       C. Both of the above
       D. None of the above   Ref. p. 289

       FILL IN THE MOST APPROPRIATE ANSWERS: (Questions 420-422)

       A. Full thickness (Wolff)
       B. Split thickness (Thiersh)
       C. Neither

       The 420)_____thickness skin graft will take more successfully than
       421)_____thickness. It is also noted that a better cosmetic result
       will be obtained by a 422)_____thickness graft.
                                             Ref. pp. 291-292

       ANSWER THE FOLLOWING QUESTIONS BY USING THE KEY
       OUTLINED BELOW:
       A. If both statement and reason are correct and related cause and effect
       B. If both statement and reason are correct but not related cause and effect
       C. If statement is true but reason is false
       D. If statement is false but reason is true
       E. If both statement and reason are false

423.   In female donors, the kidney of choice is the right BECAUSE it has a
       longer renal vein.   Ref. p. 292 (1st Ed.)

424.   An appendectomy is routinely carried out in the recipient along with a
       nephrectomy BECAUSE appendicitis may be confused with the clinical
       findings of homograft rejection.   Ref. p. 295 (1st Ed.)

       SELECT THE MOST APPROPRIATE ANSWER:

425.   THE SIMPLEST RENAL TRANSPLANT TO PERFORM TECHNICALLY IS:
       A. Right kidney on the left side
       B. Left kidney on the right side
       C. Right kidney on the right side
       D. Left kidney on the left side
       E. None of the above   Ref. p. 295 (1st Ed.)

426.   ARTERIAL ANASTOMOSIS IN RENAL TRANSPLANTATION INCLUDES
       ALL, <u>EXCEPT</u>:
       A. Renal artery to renal artery
       B. Renal artery to hypogastric artery
       C. Renal artery to external iliac artery
       D. Renal artery to common iliac artery
       E. Renal artery to aorta   Ref. p. 296 (1st Ed.)

427.   IMMEDIATE VIGOROUS SWELLING OF THE RENAL TRANSPLANT ON
       ITS OWN OR AFTER COMPRESSION OF THE RENAL VEINS AT SURGERY:
       A. Indicates potential renal failure
       B. Is not prognostic
       C. Indicates potential success   Ref. p. 297 (1st Ed.)

ANSWER THE FOLLOWING QUESTION BY USING THE KEY
OUTLINED BELOW:
A. If both statement and reason are correct and related cause and effect
B. If both statement and reason are correct but not related cause and effect
C. If statement is true but reason is false
D. If statement is false but reason is true
E. If both statement and reason are false

428. Postoperative care includes preventing the patient from lying in the op-
      posite side of the transplant BECAUSE the graft is not attached to adjacent
      tissues at surgery.   Ref. p. 298 (1st Ed.)

SELECT THE MOST APPROPRIATE ANSWER:

429. WHICH OF THE FOLLOWING HAVE HAD THE GREATEST RISE IN MOR-
      TALITY RATES OVER THE PAST 40 YEARS?:
      A. Gastric carcinoma   D. Lung carcinoma
      B. Pancreatic carcinoma   E. Leukemia
      C. Colorectal carcinoma   Ref. p. 298

FILL IN THE MOST APPROPRIATE ANSWERS: (Questions 430-431)

      A. Lung   A. 10%
      B. Colon-rectum   B. 25%
      C. Breast   C. 44%
      D. Skin   D. 80%
      E. Stomach   E. 94%

The most frequent carcinoma presenting in the human is 430)_____.
Its virulence and spread permit it to be controlled 431)_____per cent
of the time.   Ref. p. 299

SELECT THE MOST APPROPRIATE ANSWER:

432. THE CANCER MOST UNCONTROLLABLE AND RESULTING IN THE
      LOWEST SURVIVAL RATE IS:
      A. Leukemia
      B. Hodgkin's disease
      C. Uterine
      D. Lung
      E. Gastric   Ref. p. 299

433. SILVER CLIPS ARE ATTACHED ROUTINELY TO THE HOMOGRAFT
      CAPSULE DURING THE OPERATION TO HELP ESTABLISH THE
      DIAGNOSIS OF:
      A. Acute rejection   D. Venous thrombosis
      B. Arterial occlusion   E. All of the above
      C. Acute tubular necrosis   Ref. p. 300 (1st Ed.)

THE ETIOLOGY OF CANCER IS TO A LARGE PART DEPENDENT UPON
ENVIRONMENTAL AND CONGENITAL INFLUENCES. MATCH THE
FOLLOWING TUMORS AND ETIOLOGIC FACTORS:

434. ___ Bladder   carcinoma   A. Uranium mine workers
435. ___ Burkitt's lymphoma   B. Burn
436. ___ Marjolin's ulcer   C. Virus
437. ___ Lung carcinoma   D. Ultraviolet light
438. ___ Thyroid carcinoma in children   E. Schistosomiasis
439. ___ Colon   cancer-polyps   F. Radiation of thymus
440. ___ Lip carcinoma   G. Congenital
                                             Ref. pp. 300-301

MATCH THE CARCINOGEN WITH THE DISEASE IT INITIATES:

441. ___ Aromatic amines   A. Skin carcinoma
442. ___ Benzene   B. Mesotheliomas
443. ___ Coal tar, pitch   C. Sinus and laryngeal carcinoma
444. ___ Isopropyl oil   D. Leukemia
445. ___ Asbestos   E. Urinary tract
                                   Ref. pp. 300-301

SELECT THE MOST APPROPRIATE ANSWER:

446. DAUGHTERS OF WOMEN WITH BREAST CANCER:
A. Have no greater incidence of carcinoma onset
B. Develop breat carcinoma at a younger age than their mothers
C. Neither   Ref. p. 301

MATCH THE ANTIGEN OR SUBSTANCE WITH THE ASSOCIATED TUMOR:

447. ___ α-Fetoglobulin   A. GI cancers (colon)
448. ___ Carcinoembryonic antigen B. Thyroid medullary carcinoma
449. ___ Calcitonin   C. Hepatoma
                                   Ref. p. 303

SELECT THE MOST APPROPRIATE ANSWER:

450. WHICH OF THE FOLLOWING CONDITIONS IS PRECANCEROUS?:
A. Regional ileitis   D. Diabetes mellitus
B. Neurofibromatosis   E. All of the above
C. Polyarteritis nodosa   Ref. p. 303

451. THE MEASUREMENT OF TUMOR DOUBLING TIME IS BEST FOL-
LOWED BY:
A. Roentgenograms
B. Chemical analysis electrophoretic pattern
C. Both
D. Neither   Ref. p. 303

ANSWER THE FOLLOWING STATEMENT T(RUE) OR F(ALSE):

452. Tumor doubling time, i.e. the time it takes a tumor to double in volume,
appears to be an accurate method for comparing the biologic aggressiveness
of neoplasms.   Ref. p. 303

SELECT THE MOST APPROPRIATE ANSWER:

453. WHICH IS CONSIDERED MORE IMPORTANT IN CONTROLLING TUMOR
REJECTION?:
A. Cellular immune response   C. Both are equal
B. Humoral immune response   D. Neither
                               Ref. p. 306

454. "TRANSPLANT LUNG" IS A SYNDROME CHARACTERIZED BY:
A. Alveolar capillary block with minimal lung findings on physical ex-
amination
B. X-ray pattern of miliary tuberculosis
C. Treatment for above conditions - prednisone
D. Low pO_2 normal CO_2
E. Is autoimmune phenomenon
F. All of the above   Ref. p. 307 (1st Ed.)

455. WHICH OF THE FOLLOWING USUALLY INCREASES THE FREQUENCY
AND GROWTH RATE, AND SHORTENS THE LATENCY PERIOD, FOR
VIRAL AND CARCINOGEN-INDUCED NEOPLASMS IN EXPERIMENTAL
ANIMALS?:
A. Irradiation   D. Steroids
B. Neonatal thymectomy   E. Antilymphocyte globulin
C. Chemotherapy   F. All of these
                               Ref. p. 307

456. THE CONCEPT OF IMMUNE SURVEILLANCE DEPENDS ON:
      A. The immune system to recognize the foreignness of tumor-specific
         antigens on neoplastic cells
      B. The immune system to totally destroy the tumor tissue as it is being
         produced
      C. Cellular mediated response   Ref. p. 307

457. TUMOR-SPECIFIC ANTIGENS HAVE BEEN DEMONSTRATED IN ALL OF
      THE FOLLOWING EXCEPT:
      A. Malignant melanoma   D. Colon carcinoma
      B. Gastric carcinoma   E. Breast carcinoma
      C. Osteosarcoma   Ref. p. 309

458. THE MAXIMAL ADVANTAGE IN FOLLOWING A CEA (CARCINOEMBRYONIC
      ANTIGEN) LEVEL IN COLON CANCER PATIENTS IS THAT IT IS:
      A. Tumor-specific and establishes the presence or absence of the tumor
      B. A highly accurate method of detecting an early tumor of the colon
      C. Useful in postoperative follow-up to indicate the onset of a recurrence of
         the tumor   Ref. p. 310

459. THE RESPONSE TO DNCB (DINITROCHLOROBENZENE) MEASURES THE
      PATIENT'S CELL-MEDIATED IMMUNITY AND IS OF VALUE FOR:
      A. Tumor destruction   C. Prognosis
      B. Tumor recurrence detection   D. None of these
                                        Ref. pp. 310, 311

460. TUMORS WHICH HAVE A TENDENCY TOWARD DIRECT EXTENSION
      THROUGH TISSUE SPACES INCLUDE ALL EXCEPT:
      A. Adenocarcinoma of esophagus   C. Hodgkin's
      B. Adenocarcinoma of stomach   D. Soft tissue sarcomas
                                        Ref. p. 314

ANSWER THE FOLLOWING STATEMENT T(RUE) OR F(ALSE):

461. In the pregnant female, renal transplantation represents a contraindication
      to a normal vaginal delivery.   Ref. p. 315 (1st Ed.)

FILL IN THE MOST APPROPRIATE ANSWERS: (Questions 462-463)

      A. Blood stream   A. Liver
      B. Lymphatics   B. Lung
      C. Local invasion   C. Opposite kidney
      D. Preaortic lymph nodes   D. Bone marrow

Initially renal carcinoma metastasizes via (the) 462)_____and therefore 463)_____is frequently the first organ to be involved.
                                        Ref. p. 315

ANSWER THE FOLLOWING STATEMENT T(RUE) OR F(ALSE):

464. The route of hematogenous spread and therefore the organ to which meta-
      stases develops first is often dictated by the venous blood flow to the
      portal or caval circulation.   Ref. p. 315

ANSWER THE FOLLOWING QUESTION BY USING THE KEY
OUTLINED BELOW:
      A. If both statement and reason are correct and related cause and effect
      B. If both statement and reason are correct but not related cause and effect
      C. If statement is true but reason is false
      D. If statement is false but reason is true
      E. If both statement and reason are false

465. The greater the quantity of protein in the urine, THE GREATER the de-
      gree of histoincompatibility.   Ref. p. 317 (1st Ed.)

SELECT THE MOST APPROPRIATE ANSWER:

466. TISSUE BIOPSY IS THE MOST DEFINITIVE DIAGNOSTIC TOOL OF THE
PHYSICIAN. A 1/2 cm PIGMENTED LESION OF THE SHOULDER IN A
25 YEAR-OLD FEMALE IS PREPARED FOR SURGERY; WHICH OF THE
FOLLOWING IS INDICATED?:
A. Needle biopsy
B. Incisional biopsy
C. Excisional biopsy
D. Erosion technique with papanicolaou studies
E. None of the above   Ref. p. 319

467. STAGING OF HODGKIN'S DISEASE SHOULD INCLUDE WHICH OF THE
FOLLOWING?:
A. Exploratory laparotomy   D. Celiac lymph node biopsy
B. Splenectomy   E. All of these
C. Liver biopsy   Ref. p. 320

468. PRESENT DAY METHODS OF MAINTAINING PATIENTS WITH HEPATIC
FAILURE INCLUDE ALL, EXCEPT:
A. Exchange transfusion   D. Partial hepatectomy
B. Plasmaphoresis   E. Cross circulation
C. Extracorporeal hepatic perfusion   Ref. pp. 321-323 (1st Ed.)

469. THE MOST SUCCESSFUL MEANS OF DEALING WITH CANCER, AS LONG
AS IT REMAINS LOCALIZED TO THE PRIMARY SITE AND REGIONAL
NODES, IS:
A. Surgery   C. Both A and B
B. Radiation   D. Neither A nor B
                                   Ref. p. 321

470. PALLIATION OF A PATIENT WITH CANCER SHOULD INCLUDE WHICH
OF THE FOLLOWING?:
A. Relief of obstruction
B. Relief of pain
C. Restore function
D. Repair disfiguring appearance
E. All of the above   Ref. p. 321

471. THE LOCAL RECURRENCE RATE IN THE SUTURE LINE FOR RESECTED
COLONIC CARCINOMA MAY BE REDUCED BY USING:
A. "No touch" technique
B. Umbilical tape ties proximal and distal to the tumor
C. Local irrigation of cut ends of colon with bichloride of mercury solution
D. Iodized sutures
E. All of the above   Ref. p. 322

472. THE RATE OF LOCAL RECURRENCE IN THE SUTURE LINE FOLLOWING
RESECTION FOR COLONIC CARCINOMA IS ABOUT _____ PERCENT:
A. 1   D. 40
B. 10   E. 60
C. 20   Ref. p. 322

473. THE MOST COMMON SITE OF INFECTION IN A RECIPIENT IN
IMMUNOSUPPRESSIVE THERAPY IS THE:
A. Graft itself
B. Injection site
C. Lungs   Ref. p. 328 (1st Ed.)

474. WHICH OF THE FOLLOWING LESIONS IS MOST AMENABLE TO RADIA-
TION?:
A. Colon carcinoma   D. Wilms' tumor
B. Hodgkin's disease   E. Skin tumors
C. Seminoma   Ref. p. 328

475.   THE FUNCTION OF ANIMAL TRANSPLANTS (RENAL, LIVER, LUNG,
       HEART) WITHOUT IMMUNOSUPPRESSIVE THERAPY HAS A MEAN OF
       _____ DAYS:
       A. 2-4   D. 16-18
       B. 6-8   E. 20-22
       C. 10-12   Ref. pp. 330-333 (1st Ed.)

       FILL IN THE MOST APPROPRIATE ANSWERS: (Questions 476-477)

       A. Hodgkin's disease   A. Nitrogen mustard
       B. Choriocarcinoma   B. Actinomycin D
       C. Prostatic carcinoma   C. Fluorouracil
       D. Endometrial carcinoma   D. Methotrexate
       E. Breast carcinoma   E. Estrogens

       Chemotherapy has to date only been curative in 476)_____. The
       agent utilized is 477)_____.   Ref. p. 335

       SELECT THE MOST APPROPRIATE ANSWER:

478.   THE MOST COMMONLY USED ANTIMETABOLITE FOR BREAST CANCER
       HAS BEEN ____. MOST RECENTLY (1974), THE USE OF ____ IN PRE-
       MENOPAUSAL WOMEN WITH APPARENT SURGICAL CURES OR EVEN
       LOW NODE INVOLVEMENT HAS BEEN STATISTICALLY HELPFUL.
       A. Phenylalanine mustard   C. 5-Fluorouracil
       B. Cyclophosphamide   D. Methotrexate
                                        Ref. p. 337

479.   IN CHILDREN, A 5 YEAR SURVIVAL IS NOT A USEFUL INDICATION OF
       CURE SINCE THE EARLIEST CANCER CELL COULD NOT HAVE
       STARTED PRIOR TO CONCEPTION. IF ONE CELL AND ITS SUBSE-
       QUENT GENERATION GREW AT A CONSTANT RATE IT WOULD REACH
       THE SAME SIZE OF THE TUMOR FOUND AFTER:
       A. 9 months plus double the age of the child at treatment
       B. Double the age of the child minus 9 months
       C. 18 months plus double the child's age
       D. 9 months plus triple the child's age
       E. None of the above   Ref. p. 342

480.   A "SECOND SET REACTION" AS DESCRIBED BY MEDAWAR IS MOST
       LIKELY CHARACTERIZED BY ALL OF THE FOLLOWING, EXCEPT:
       A. More rapid onset than "First Set Reaction"
       B. Increase in circulating antibody
       C. Destruction of vascular endothelium and infarction
       D. Lack of round cells
       E. Can be prolonged as long as donor and recipient remain in cross cir-
           culation   Ref. p. 351

481.   MATCH THE FOLLOWING CELL TYPES WITH THEIR IMMUNOLOGIC
       FUNCTION:

       (1) ___ B cells   A. Responsible for manufacturing circulating im-
       (2) ___ T cells   munoglobulins and thus for humoral immunity
                                B. Responsible for cellular immunity and immuno-
                                    competent cell population
                                        Ref. p. 354

       ANSWER THE FOLLOWING STATEMENT T(RUE) OR F(ALSE):

482.   Graft versus host (GVH) reaction is responsible for "Runt" disease in
       mice.   Ref. p. 355

ANSWER THE FOLLOWING QUESTION BY USING THE KEY
OUTLINED BELOW:
A. If both statement and reason are correct and related cause and effect
B. If both statement and reason are correct but not related cause and effect
C. If statement is true but reason is false
D. If statement is false but reason is true
E. If both statement and reason are false

483. Blood or lymph irradiation through an A-V shunt has caused prolonged
graft survival BECAUSE circulating lymphocytes are more radiosensitive
than the other blood elements.   Ref. p. 372

SELECT THE MOST APPROPRIATE ANSWER(S):

484. ALL OF THE FOLLOWING METHODS OF IMMUNOSUPPRESSION RE-
DUCE CELLULAR IMMUNOCOMPETENCE, EXCEPT:
A. Azathioprine   D. Thymectomy in adults
B. Prednisone   E. Actinomycin C
C. Antilymphocytic globulin   Ref. pp. 372-374

485. "TOLERANCE" IS PROPORTIONATE TO THE VOLUME OF ANTIGENIC
CELLS AND THE POPULATION OF HOST IMMUNOCYTES AND CAN BE
INCREASED IN:
A. Massive irradiation of the recipient
B. Injections of methotrexate
C. The neonate injected with adult spleen cells
                                   Ref. pp. 379-380

486. WHICH TWO METHODS ARE USED TO ESTABLISH HISTOCOMPATIBILITY
BEFORE TRANSPLANTATION IS UNDERTAKEN?:
A. Terasaki typing   D. Mixed cell agglutination
B. Lymphocyte cytotoxicity   E. Jerne Plaque technique
C. Mixed lymphocyte culture typing   Ref. p. 382

487. THE ANTISERA OF THE LEUKOCYTE TYPING TECHNIQUES ARE
COLLECTED FROM:
A. Women who have multiple pregnancies and are immunized against
their fetus
B. Patients immunized following multiple transfusions
C. Patients who have received multiple skin grafts
D. Patients who have received other transplants
E. All of the above   Ref. p. 382

488. THE MOST COMMON HOMOGRAFT IS:
A. Bone   D. Lung
B. Kidney   E. Heart
C. Blood   Ref. p. 383

489. THE MOST COMMON CAUSE OF POSTOPERATIVE JAUNDICE FOLLOW-
ING GASTRECTOMY IS:
A. Hemolytic jaundice
B. Common duct obstruction due to local edema
C. Misplaced tie about common duct
D. None of the above   Ref. p. 385 (1st Ed.)

ANSWER THE FOLLOWING QUESTIONS BY USING THE KEY
OUTLINED BELOW:
A. If both statement and reason are correct and related cause and effect
B. If both statement and reason are correct but not related cause and effect
C. If statement is true but reason is false
D. If statement is false but reason is true
E. If both statement and reason are false

490. Tendon grafts are almost nonantigenic BECAUSE the cellular elements of
the immunologic system are present with the tissues.
                                   Ref. p. 385

491. Reimplantation of the upper extremities is more successful than of the
lower BECAUSE nerve regeneration is greater in the arm.
                                   Ref. p. 387

FILL IN THE MOST APPROPRIATE ANSWERS: (Questions 492-493)

A. Median nerve
B. Ulnar nerve

Motor recovery in the 492)_____nerve is greater than in the
493)_____nerve.   Ref. p. 387

SELECT THE MOST APPROPRIATE ANSWER:

494.   POSTOPERATIVE COMPLICATIONS IN REIMPLANTATION PROCE-
       DURES INCLUDE WHICH OF THE FOLLOWING?:
       A. Slough of graft   D. Sepsis
       B. Osteomyelitis   E. All of the above
       C. Acidosis   Ref. p. 388

495.   AFTER TRANSPLANTATION OF THE PANCREAS IN ALLOXAN-
       PRODUCED DIABETIC RATS, THE DIABETES:
       A. Improves
       B. Remains the same
       C. Gets worse   Ref. p. 390

496.   THE BEST CANDIDATES FOR HEPATIC TRANSPLANTATION SEEM
       TO BE:
       A. Children with biliary atresia
       B. Patients with primary cancer
       C. Adults with Laennec's cirrhosis
       D. Adults with post-hepatic cirrhosis   Ref. p. 394

497.   WHICH OF THE FOLLOWING ANASTOMOSES ARE ESSENTIAL IN
       AUXILIARY LIVER TRANSPLANTATIONS?:
       A. Infrahepatic vena cava (VC) of transplant to vena cava of host
       B. Portal vein of transplant to superior mesenteric vein of host
       C. Celiac artery or aorta of donor to aorta of host
       D. Gall bladder to small bowel of host
       E. All of the above   Ref. p. 396

498.   WHICH OF THE FOLLOWING ARE OPERATIVE COMPLICATIONS ASSOCI-
       ATED WITH LIVER TRANSPLANTATION?:
       A. Bleeding
       B. Ligation of cystic duct along with common duct
       C. Paralysis of right diaphragm
       D. Hypothermia
       E. All of the above   Ref. pp. 396, 397

499.   IMMUNOSUPPRESSION IN LIVER TRANSPLANTATION IS PRESENTLY
       INITIATED WITH:
       A. Azathioprine
       B. Antilymphocyte serum (ALS)
       C. Prednisone   Ref. p. 398

ANSWER THE FOLLOWING QUESTIONS BY USING THE KEY
OUTLINED BELOW:
A. If both statement and reason are correct and related cause and effect
B. If both statement and reason are correct but not related cause and effect
C. If statement is true but reason is false
D. If statement is false but reason is true
E. If both statement and reason are false

500.   Reinnervation of the cardiac transplant occurs within six months after sur-
       gery BECAUSE there is improved cardiac function.
                                        Ref. p. 399

501.   Cardiac rejection is best illustrated by EKG voltage decrease BECAUSE it
       serves as a guide for immunosuppressive therapy.
                                        Ref. p. 401

502.   Ligation of the bronchial artery does alter function of the lung BECAUSE it
       contributes to bronchostenosis.   Ref. p. 402

SELECT THE MOST APPROPRIATE ANSWER:

503. DIVISION OF THE PULMONARY ARTERY ALONE RESULTS IN_____
OF THE LUNG:
A. Fibrosis
B. Necrosis
C. Infection
D. Bronchiostenosis   Ref. p. 402

504. THE ONLY ABSOLUTE CONTRAINDICATIONS TO RENAL TRANSPLANTA-
TION ARE:
A. Pancytopenia   D. Malignant disease not under control
B. Active infection   E. Low socioeconomic group
C. Severe malnutrition   Ref. p. 404

ANSWER THE FOLLOWING QUESTION BY USING THE KEY
OUTLINED BELOW:
A. If both statement and reason are correct and related cause and effect
B. If both statement and reason are correct but not related cause and effect
C. If statement is true but reason is false
D. If statement is false but reason is true
E. If both statement and reason are false

505. Patients with glomerulonephritis and antibodies to the glomerulus basement
membrane should not be transplanted until a nephrectomy has been performed and antibodies have reached low levels BECAUSE there is a higher
incidence of graft rejection.   Ref. p. 405

SELECT THE MOST APPROPRIATE ANSWER(S):

506. RENAL HOMOGRAFTS ARE NOT GREATLY AFFECTED BY WHICH PRE-
EXISTING DISEASE IN THE RECIPIENT?:
A. Proliferative glomerulonephritis
B. Tuberculosis
C. Polyarteritis nodosa
D. Hypertensive nephrosclerosis
E. Childhood nephritis with nephrotic syndrome
Ref. pp. 405; 429

507. WHICH OF THE FOLLOWING PATIENTS WOULD BE LEAST AMENABLE
TO TRANSPLANTATION?:
A. Chronic glomerulonephritis   D. Gout
B. Polyarteritis   E. Diabetes mellitus
C. Nephrocalcinosis   Ref. p. 405

508. IN CHOOSING A DONOR FOR RENAL TRANSPLANTATION IN A FEMALE,
THE WORST DONOR WOULD BE:
A. Her son   D. An unrelated donor
B. Her father   E. Her twin sister
C. Her husband   Ref. pp. 408-409

509. EVALUATION OF LIVING RENAL TRANSPLANT DONORS SHOULD IN-
CLUDE WHICH OF THE FOLLOWING?:
A. Preoperative renal angiogram
B. Donor should be over 21 years of age and under 55 years of age
C. ABO blood type compatibility
D. Should not have cancer
E. All of the above   Ref. pp. 409; 411

510. COMPLIMENTARY OPERATIONS OF RENAL TRANSPLANT RECIPIENTS
TO PREVENT ASSOCIATED COMPLICATIONS INCLUDE:
A. Splenectomy   D. Appendectomy
B. Parathyroidectomy   E. Adrenalectomy
C. Thymectomy   Ref. p. 413

ANSWER THE FOLLOWING QUESTION BY USING THE KEY
OUTLINED BELOW:
A. If both statement and reason are correct and related cause and effect
B. If both statement and reason are correct but not related cause and effect
C. If statement is true but reason is false
D. If statement is false but reason is true
E. If both statement and reason are false

511. Post-transplant massive diuresis is common BECAUSE it is prognostically
always a good sign.   Ref. p. 414

SELECT THE MOST APPROPRIATE ANSWER:

512. ACUTE TUBULAR NECROSIS IS MORE COMMON IN_____TRANS-
PLANTS:
A. Cadaver
B. Nonrelated living donor
C. Related living donor   Ref. p. 417

513. IF HYPERACUTE REJECTION APPEARS AT THE OPERATING TABLE
ONE SHOULD:
A. Immediately remove the homograft
B. Irradiate the homograft
C. Initiate steroids
D. Selectively perfuse the homograft with a high concentration of
azathioprine   Ref. p. 417

514. IN THE FACE OF DEVELOPING ACUTE TUBULAR NECROSIS IN THE
HOMOGRAFT_____SHOULD BE REDUCED:
A. Prednisone
B. Radiation
C. Azathioprine
D. All of the above   Ref. p. 418

515. TRANSPLANT REJECTION IS MOST LIKELY TO OCCUR_____IN
LIVING DONOR GRAFTS THAN IN CADAVER GRAFTS:
A. Earlier
B. Later
C. No difference   Ref. p. 418

516. ACUTE HOMOGRAFT REJECTION IS CHARACTERIZED BY:
A. Swelling of the kidney
B. Abrupt reduction in urine volume
C. Progressive decrease in urine volume over 4-5 days
D. High sodium concentration in urine
E. All of the above   Ref. p. 418

517. THE MOST DEPENDABLE DAILY SIGN OF IMPENDING REJECTION IS:
A. Depression of renal blood flow
B. Elevation of urinary immunoglobulins
C. Increase in heterophil
D. Oliguria and elevation of BUN
E. All of the above   Ref. p. 418

518. REJECTION PHENOMENA INCLUDE:
A. Lymphocytes in the urine
B. Urine and blood LDH changes
C. Change in size of the kidney
D. Depression of CO_2 fraction of complement
E. All of the above   Ref. p. 418

519. THE MOST IMPORTANT PARAMETER TO FOLLOW IN ORDER TO DIF-
FERENTIATE RENAL ALLOGRAFT REJECTION IS:
A. Serum creatinine   D. Urine specific gravity
B. BUN   E. Renal arteriogram
C. Uric acid   Ref. p. 419

520. THE MOST RELIABLE CONFIRMATORY TEST OF RENAL FUNCTIONAL
DETERIORATION IS:
A. Serum creatinine   D. Renal radiogram
B. IVP   E. Renal arteriogram
C. Renal biopsy   Ref. p. 419

521. IN RENAL TRANSPLANT PATIENTS, THE MOST IMPORTANT PARA-
METER TO FOLLOW IS:
A. BUN   D. Creatinine level in serum
B. Creatinine clearance   E. Protein in urine
C. WBC   Ref. p. 419

522. THE GROUP WITH THE WORST PROGNOSIS FOR RENAL TRANSPLANT
SURVIVAL IS:
A. Patients with no rejection and no proteinuria
B. Patients with rejection episodes over 30 days or within the first week
of transplant
C. Patients with two or more acute rejection episodes
D. Patients with a solitary acute rejection episode   Ref. p. 421

FILL IN THE MOST APPROPRIATE ANSWERS: (Questions 523-524)

A. 100
B. 87
C. 50
D. 27
E. 15

On the basis of clinical criteria for graft acceptance, a patient having
more than one acute rejection during the first four months post-transplant,
has a long term prognosis of 523)____per cent and if the rejection episodes develop after the four month period or during the first week postoperative, the prognosis is 524)____per cent.
Ref. p. 421

ANSWER THE FOLLOWING QUESTIONS BY USING THE KEY
OUTLINED BELOW:
A. If both statement and reason are correct and related cause and effect
B. If both statement and reason are correct but not related cause and effect
C. If statement is true but reason is false
D. If statement is false but reason is true
E. If both statement and reason are false

525. A major problem in renal transplants in identical twins is the high incidence of glomerulonephritis in the proliferative recipient when this has
been the primary disease state BECAUSE the disease continues to develop.
Ref. pp. 421-422

526. The use of antibiotics in renal transplant patients should be avoided
BECAUSE the associated medications predispose to fungal infections.
Ref. p. 423

SELECT THE MOST APPROPRIATE ANSWER:

527. SEPSIS IS RESPONSIBLE FOR_____PER CENT OF THE RENAL
      TRANSPLANT PATIENTS WHO EXPIRE:
      A. 20   D. 70
      B. 30   E. 80
      C. 50   Ref. p. 423

528. THE MOST COMMON COMPLICATION OF IMMUNOSUPPRESSION IS:
      A. GI bleeding   D. Allograft rejection
      B. Glomerulonephritis   E. Onset of malignant neoplasm
      C. Infection   Ref. p. 423

      ANSWER THE FOLLOWING QUESTIONS BY USING THE KEY
      OUTLINED BELOW:
      A. If both statement and reason are correct and related cause and effect
      B. If both statement and reason are correct but not related cause and effect
      C. If statement is true but reason is false
      D. If statement is false but reason is true
      E. If both statement and reason are false

529. Patients with cancer are included as donors BECAUSE the cancer
      can be transmitted to the recipient.   Ref. p. 423

530. Post-transplantation hemoglobin levels return to normal BECAUSE of a
      return of the erythropoietin level.   Ref. p. 426

      SELECT THE MOST APPROPRIATE ANSWER:

531. LONG TERM FUNCTION OF LIVING DONOR TRANSPLANTS IS_____
      THAN IN THE CADAVER TRANSPLANT RECIPIENT:
      A. Longer
      B. Less
      C. Same as   Ref. p. 426

532. INCIDENCE OF REJECTION PHENOMENON IN RELATED-LIVING
      DONOR TRANSPLANTS IS:
      A. 55%   D. 85%
      B. 65%   E. 95%
      C. 75%   Ref. p. 427

533. ANNUAL MORTALITY RATE IN TRANSPLANTED PATIENTS IS ABOUT:
      A. 5%
      B. 10%
      C. 15%
      D. 20%   Ref. pp. 428-429

      FILL IN THE MOST APPROPRIATE ANSWERS: (Questions 534-535)

      A. 50
      B. 60
      C. 70
      D. 80
      E. 90

      The number of patients surviving related liver donor transplantation either
      because of a functioning graft or assist with hemodialysis is about 534)____
      per cent, and in cadaver donors about 535)____per cent.
                                      Ref. pp. 428-429

SELECT THE MOST APPROPRIATE ANSWER:

536. INCIDENCE OF REJECTION PHENOMENON IN CADAVER DONOR
      TRANSPLANTS IS:
      A. 55%   D. 85%
      B. 65%   E. 95%
      C. 75%   Ref. p. 429

      ANSWER THE FOLLOWING QUESTION BY USING THE KEY
      OUTLINED BELOW:
      A. If both statement and reason are correct and related cause and effect
      B. If both statement and reason are correct but not related cause and effect
      C. If statement is true but reason is false
      D. If statement is false but reason is true
      E. If both statement and reason are false

537. The presence of a previous transplant rejection speaks greatly against
      success of a retransplantation BECAUSE of a higher antigen titer.
                                       Ref. pp. 430-431

SELECT THE MOST APPROPRIATE ANSWER:

538. EXPLOSIVE ANESTHETIC AGENTS FOLLOW ALL OF THE FOLLOWING
      RULES, EXCEPT:
      A. Should not be used with surgical electrocautery
      B. Are generally less of a cardiovascular depressant than the non-
          explosive anesthetics
      C. Produce a greater physiological alteration than do non-explosive
          anesthetics
      D. Are more useful for deep levels of anesthesia
      E. Are better for intraabdominal surgery
                                       Ref. p. 444

539. WHICH OF THE FOLLOWING PLAY A ROLE IN THE SELECTION OF AN
      ANESTHETIC FOR A PATIENT ?:
      A. Patient's condition
      B. Physiologic effect of the agent
      C. Experience of anesthesiologist
      D. Skill of surgeon
      E. Site and type of surgical procedure
      F. All of the above   Ref. p. 444

540. THE MOST FREQUENT CAUSE OF CARDIAC ARREST DUE TO OPERA-
      TIVE ANESTHESIA IS:
      A. Inadequate ventilation
      B. Vascular collapse
      C. Renal failure
      D. Central nervous system depression
      E. Direct myocardial irritability   Ref. p. 444

541. WHICH OF THE FOLLOWING CONDITIONS CONTRAINDICATES THE
      USE OF GENERAL ANESTHESIA ?:
      A. Hemorrhagic shock
      B. Septic shock
      C. Inadequate airway
      D. Chest trauma with left pulmonary collapse
      E. Cardiac tamponade   Ref. p. 444

542. THE MOST RELIABLE CLINICAL ESTIMATE OF HYPOXIA AND CO_2
RETENTION DURING ANESTHESIA IS:
A. Respiratory rate
B. Pulse rate
C. Color of skin
D. Tidal volume
E. Blood pressure
F. None of the above
G. All of the above
Ref. p. 445

ANSWER THE FOLLOWING QUESTIONS BY USING THE KEY
OUTLINED BELOW:
A. If both statement and reason are correct and related cause and effect
B. If both statement and reason are correct but not related cause and effect
C. If statement is true but reason is false
D. If statement is false but reason is true
E. If both statement and reason are false

543. Clinical estimates of anesthetic hypoxia are not accurate BECAUSE the
most reliable method is arterial blood gas tensions.
Ref. p. 445

544. The only method to guarantee patency of the airway is by endotracheal
intubation BECAUSE direct observation of the vocal cords is essential.
Ref. p. 445

MATCH THE FOLLOWING. EACH LETTERED ITEM MAY BE USED
MORE THAN ONCE:

545. ___ Ether
546. ___ Halothane
547. ___ Cyclopropane
548. ___ Nitrous oxide
A. Non-explosive
B. Ventricular irritability
C. More effective with anoxia
D. Greatest safety range
E. ADH secretion stimulated
Ref. pp. 445-450

SELECT THE MOST APPROPRIATE ANSWER(S):

549. NITROUS OXIDE DELETERIOUSLY AFFECTS THE_____SYSTEM:
A. Respiratory
B. Cardiovascular
C. Renal
D. Hepatic
E. None of the above
Ref. p. 445

550. THE USE OF NITROUS OXIDE DURING SURGERY REQUIRES WHICH OF
THE FOLLOWING?:
A. Premedication
B. Electrocautery not be utilized
C. Frequent monitoring of gas tensions
D. Relative anoxia
E. All of the above
Ref. p. 445

551. NITROUS OXIDE IS OF GREATEST USE:
A. By itself
B. With oxygen
C. As a supplement
D. None of the above
Ref. p. 446

552. WHICH OF THE FOLLOWING ARE SIGNIFICANT DIFFERENCES BE-
TWEEN NITROUS OXIDE AND MORPHINE ANALGESIA?:
A. The former does not depress the cardiovascular system
B. The former does not depress the respiratory system
C. The former is rapidly reversible
D. All of the above
E. None of the above
Ref. p. 446

553.   CYCLOPROPANE (C3H6) ANESTHESIA IS OFTEN ASSOCIATED WITH:
        A. Metabolic alkalosis   D. Respiratory acidosis
        B. Metabolic acidosis   E. None of the above
        C. Respiratory alkalosis   Ref. p. 446

        ANSWER THE FOLLOWING QUESTIONS BY USING THE KEY
        OUTLINED BELOW:
        A. If both statement and reason are correct and related cause and effect
        B. If both statement and reason are correct but not related cause and effect
        C. If statement is true but reason is false
        D. If statement is false but reason is true
        E. If both statement and reason are false

554.   Nitrous oxide should be used carefully in patients with intestinal obstruc-
        tion and pneumothorax BECAUSE there is a tendency for it to accumulate
        within airfilled cavities which result in volume expansion.
                                           Ref. p. 446

555.   Cyclopropane causes respiratory depression BECAUSE it decreases the
        threshold of the respiratory center to CO_2.
                                           Ref. p. 446

556.   With cyclopropane there is an increased catecholamine stimulation
        BECAUSE of the peripheral sympathetic effect.
                                           Ref. p. 447

557.   Cyclopropane is contraindicated in open-heart surgery BECAUSE the
        myocardial irritability is primarily ventricular.
                                           Ref. p. 447

        SELECT THE MOST APPROPRIATE ANSWER:

558.   ONE OF THE MAJOR ADVANTAGES OF CYCLOPROPANE IN A POOR
        RISK PATIENT IS:
        A. Permits easy respiratory control
        B. Maintenance of blood pressure
        C. Stimulates renal blood flow
        D. Decreases epinephrine release
        E. All of the above   Ref. p. 447

559.   DIETHYL ETHER PRODUCES WHICH OF THE FOLLOWING FIRST?:
        A. Respiratory depression
        B. Cardiovascular collapse
        C. Both simultaneously   Ref. p. 448

560.   WHICH OF THE FOLLOWING AGENTS IS CONSIDERED BEST FOR PA-
        TIENTS IN A PEDIATRIC CATEGORY?:
        A. Cyclopropane
        B. Diethyl ether
        C. Halothane
        D. Nitrous oxide   Ref. p. 448

561.   ETHER IS AN EFFECTIVE ANESTHETIC FOR SURGERY WITH CONCEN-
        TRATIONS OF OXYGEN UP TO_____PER CENT:
        A. 46   D. 96
        B. 66   E. 100
        C. 86   Ref. p. 449

562.   WHICH OF THE FOLLOWING ANESTHETICS IS HEPATOTOXIC?:
        A. Diethyl ether   D. Nitrous oxide
        B. Cyclopropane   E. Penthrane
        C. Halothane   Ref. p. 449

563.   DIETHYL ETHER PRODUCES WHICH OF THE FOLLOWING METABOLIC
STATES ?:
A.   Metabolic alkalosis
B.   Metabolic acidosis
C.   Respiratory alkalosis
D.   Respiratory acidosis   Ref. p. 449

564.   IN WHICH OF THE FOLLOWING PATIENTS WOULD DIETHYL ETHER
BE THE ANESTHETIC OF CHOICE ?:
A.   A diabetic
B.   A patient with lactic acid acidosis
C.   A pediatric patient undergoing abdominal surgery
D.   A patient with pheochromocytoma   Ref. p. 449

565.   WHICH OF THE FOLLOWING METABOLIC CONDITIONS IS ASSOCIATED
WITH DIETHYL ETHER ADMINISTRATION ?:
A.   Hyperglycemia
B.   Metabolic alkalosis
C.   Increase in serum glucagon
D.   Decrease in catecholamines
E.   Decrease in anaerobic pathway function
Ref. p. 449

ANSWER THE FOLLOWING QUESTION BY USING THE KEY
OUTLINED BELOW:
A.   If both statement and reason are correct and related cause and effect
B.   If both statement and reason are correct but not related cause and effect
C.   If statement is true but reason is false
D.   If statement is false but reason is true
E.   If both statement and reason are false

566.   The combination of halothane and nitrous oxide is frequently used
BECAUSE it decreases the incidence of arterial hypotension found fre-
quently with the former anesthetic agent alone.
Ref. p. 449

SELECT THE MOST APPROPRIATE ANSWER(S):

567.   WHICH OF THE FOLLOWING ANESTHETIC AGENTS WITH MYOCARDIAL
DEPRESSANT ACTIONS ALSO STIMULATES A COMPENSATORY SYSTEM ?:
A.   Halothane   D.   Ether
B.   Cyclopropane   E.   All of the above
C.   Nitrous oxide   Ref. p. 449

568.   A PATIENT WHO UNDERWENT GENERAL ANESTHESIA WAS OPERATED
ON AT 9 A.M.   SUDDENLY AT 8 P.M. HE DEVELOPS A FEVER OF
102º F. WHAT IS THE MOST LIKELY DIAGNOSIS ?:
A.   Acute thrombophlebitis   D.   Anastomotic leakage
B.   Wound infection   E.   Wound dehiscence
C.   Atelectasis   Ref. p. 461

569.   WHICH OF THE FOLLOWING FACTORS FAILS TO CORRELATE WELL
WITH THE INCIDENCE OF WOUND DEHISCENCE ?:
A.   Age   D.   Anemia
B.   Hypoproteinemia   E.   Obesity
C.   Atelectasis   Ref. p. 462

FILL IN THE MOST APPROPRIATE ANSWERS: (Questions 570-571)

A. 30
B. 18
C. 10
D. 3.6
E. 0.6

An abdominal operation carried on for 30 minutes has a postoperative infection rate of 570)_____per cent and one which persists for 6 hours runs
a risk of 571)_____per cent.   Ref. p. 463

SELECT THE MOST APPROPRIATE ANSWER(S):

572.   WOUND INFECTIONS GENERALLY APPEAR ON THE:
       A. First day postoperative
       B. Second to fourth day
       C. Fifth to seventh day
       D. Seventh to fourteenth day
       E. None of the above   Ref. p. 463

573.   THE USE OF DRAINS IN AREAS WHERE BLEEDING IS EXPECTED IS:
       A. A wise move
       B. Not indicated
       C. Neither of the above   Ref. p. 464

574.   A POSTOPERATIVE PATIENT PRESENTING WITH DECREASED VENTI-
       LATION, AN ARTERIAL pO_2 OF 80 mmHg AND pCO_2 OF 50 mmHg MOST
       LIKELY HAS:
       A. Atelectasis
       B. Hypoventilation syndrome
       C. Pulmonary embolus
       D. Pulmonary edema   Ref. p. 465

575.   A POSTOPERATIVE PATIENT WITH AN ARTERIAL pO_2, 80 mmHg AND
       pCO_2, 35 mmHg HAVING A TEMPERATURE DEVIATION AND TACHY-
       CARDIA WOULD MOST LIKELY HAVE:
       A. Atelectasis
       B. Hypoventilation syndrome
       C. Pulmonary embolus
       D. Pulmonary edema   Ref. p. 468

576.   OF THE FOLLOWING, EXPERIMENTALLY, WHICH APPEARS TO PLAY
       THE LEAST ROLE IN ATELECTASIS DEVELOPMENT IN POSTOPERA-
       TIVE PATIENTS?:
       A. Bronchial obstruction
       B. Inspiratory insufficiency
       C. Diminished surfactant   Ref. p. 468

577.   WHICH OF THE FOLLOWING ANESTHETIC AGENTS ARE ASSOCIATED
       WITH A HIGHER THAN NORMAL INCIDENCE OF CARDIAC
       ARRHYTHMIAS?:
       A. Halothane   D. Cyclopropane
       B. Ether   E. All of the above
       C. Nitrous oxide   Ref. p. 470

578. OVER-DIGITALIZATION IS A FREQUENT CAUSE OF INTRAOPERATIVE
      ARRHYTHMIAS. THE TREATMENT WOULD INCLUDE WHICH OF THE
      FOLLOWING ?:
      A. Potassium chloride
      B. Procaineamide
      C. Discontinue additional digitalis administration
      D. Quinidine
      E. Intravenous calcium chloride   Ref. p. 471

579. A PATIENT WHO IS A BRITTLE DIABETIC IS BROUGHT TO THE
      OPERATING ROOM; WHICH OF THE FOLLOWING SHOULD BE DONE ?:
      A. Serial blood glucose levels in the operating room
      B. Serial blood acetone levels in the operating room
      C. Serial urine glucose levels in the operating room
      D. The administration of insulin preoperatively and postoperatively
      E. Regular insulin coverage by adding some to the intravenous bottle
                                                Ref. p. 473

580. THE MOST FREQUENT ASSOCIATED INJURY WITH FAT EMBOLIZATION
      IS INJURY TO THE:
      A. Hip
      B. Humerus
      C. Ribs
      D. Vertebrae
      E. Tibia   Ref. p. 475

581. THE MORTALITY RATE ASSOCIATED WITH FAT EMBOLISM IS_____
      PER CENT:
      A. 20-30   D. 80-90
      B. 40-50   E. 100
      C. 60-70   Ref. p. 475

582. THE AFFERENT LOOP SYNDROME IS ACCOMPANIED BY ALL OF THE
      FOLLOWING, EXCEPT:
      A. Postcibal vomiting
      B. Vitamin B$_{12}$ deficiency
      C. Develops more frequently in gastric ulcers than duodenal ulcers
      D. Emesis without bile is characteristic
      E. Rarely total obstruction   Ref. p. 482

583. THE PERIOD IN WHICH THE DUODENAL STUMP BLOWOUT MOST
      LIKELY DEVELOPS FOLLOWING GASTRECTOMY WITH A BILLROTH II
      ANASTOMOSIS IS:
      A. 2nd - 7th day
      B. 8th - 14th day
      C. 14th - 21st day
      D. Over 21 days   Ref. p. 484

584. IN WHICH OF THE FOLLOWING WILL THE GREATEST FLUID AND
      ELECTROLYTE ABNORMALITIES DEVELOP ?:
      A. Distal ileal fistula   D. Duodenal fistula
      B. Sigmoidocutaneous fistula   E. Gastric fistula
      C. Proximal small bowel fistula   Ref. p. 485

ANSWER THE FOLLOWING QUESTION BY USING THE KEY OUTLINED
BELOW:
A. If both statement and reason are correct and related cause and effect
B. If both statement and reason are correct but not related cause and effect
C. If statement is true but reason is false
D. If statement is false but reason is true
E. If both statement and reason are false

585. Respiratory failure is tolerated longer than circulatory arrest BECAUSE
the circulatory system stores more than twice as much oxygen as the lungs.
Ref. p. 492

SELECT THE MOST APPROPRIATE ANSWER(S):

586. IN WHICH OF THE FOLLOWING WOULD ARTERIAL HYPOXEMIA
BE SEEN?:
A. Emphysema   D. Cystic fibrosis
B. Asthma   E. Severe mitral stenosis
C. Pulmonary embolism   Ref. p. 493

587. THE DIFFERENCE IN THE PARTIAL PRESSURE OF OXYGEN FROM THE
ALVEOLI TO THE ARTERIAL BLOOD IS CALLED:
A. Tidal volume   D. Functional residual capacity
B. Alveolar-arterial oxygen gradient   E. Pulmonary transit time
C. Lung compliance   Ref. p. 494

588. A DIAGNOSIS OF ACUTE RESPIRATORY FAILURE IS MADE WHEN THE
ARTERIAL OXYGEN TENSION FALLS BELOW _____, IF THERE IS NO
PRIOR LUNG DISEASE OR INTRACARDIAC DEFECT:
A. 20 mmHg   D. 80 mmHg
B. 40 mmHg   E. 90 mmHg
C. 60 mmHg   Ref. p. 494

589. WHICH OF THE FOLLOWING MAY CAUSE SEVERE HYPOXEMIA?:
A. Shunting of unsaturated blood to arterial system
B. Injury to pulmonary capillary endothelium
C. Increased interstitial lung water
D. Insufficient pulmonary surfactant
E. All of the above   Ref. p. 494

590. THE USE OF A RESPIRATOR WITH CONTINUOUS POSITIVE-PRESSURE
BREATHING DOES WHICH OF THE FOLLOWING?:
A. Reduces the cost of respiratory work
B. Decreases dead space
C. Increases hypoxemia
D. Decreases shunting by ventilating more alveoli
E. Increases pulmonary surfactant   Ref. p. 494

591. THE PULSE PRESSURE, OR DIFFERENCE BETWEEN SYSTOLIC AND
DIASTOLIC BLOOD PRESSURE, OFTEN:
A. Narrows in the face of increased total peripheral resistance
B. Widens in the face of increased total peripheral resistance
C. Is not a useful variable in peripheral resistance evaluation
Ref. p. 494

592. NORMAL MIXED VENOUS BLOOD IS 75% SATURATED WITH A PARTIAL
PRESSURE OF 40 mmHg. LOWER LEVELS INDICATE INCREASED OXY-
GEN DEMANDS CANNOT BE MET BY:
A. Increasing cardiac output
B. Decreasing available arterial oxygen
C. Decreasing cardiac output
D. All of the above   Ref. p. 495

593. WHICH OF THE FOLLOWING TEND TO SHIFT THE OXYHEMOGLOBIN DISSOCIATION CURVE TO THE RIGHT WHERE MORE OXYGEN IS RELEASED AT HIGHER TISSUE OXYGEN TENSION?:
    A. Heat
    B. Hypoxic acidosis
    C. CO_2
    D. All of these
    E. None of these
    Ref. p. 495

594. IN BANK BLOOD, THE RED CELL DIPHOSPHOGLYCERATE (DPG) IS:
    A. Reduced
    B. Increased
    C. Unchanged
    Ref. p. 495

595. BLOOD LACTATE LEVELS INDICATE:
    A. Aerobic metabolism is predominant
    B. Anaerobic metabolism is present
    C. Both
    D. Neither
    Ref. p. 497

596. A BLOOD LACTATE INCREASE FROM 1.5 mEq/L TO LEVELS ABOVE 10 mEq/L INDICATES:
    A. An improving state
    B. A grave prognosis unless reversed
    C. Neither
    Ref. p. 497

ANSWER THE FOLLOWING STATEMENT (T)RUE OR (F)ALSE:

597. The Codman Apnea Alarm is a 10-compartment air mattress with sensors to detect the air displacement associated with respiration, and therefore, if an infant stops breathing, an alarm is set off.   Ref. p. 497

ANSWER THE FOLLOWING QUESTION BY USING THE KEY OUTLINED BELOW:
A. If both statement and reason are correct and related cause and effect
B. If both statement and reason are correct but not related cause and effect
C. If statement is true but reason is false
D. If statement is false but reason is true
E. If both statement and reason are false

598. An increased alveolar-arterial gradient on 100% oxygen is very useful BECAUSE it is an early warning sign for many post-operative problems.
    Ref. p. 498

SELECT THE MOST APPROPRIATE ANSWER(S):

599. THE TOTAL OXYGEN CONSUMPTION NORMALLY USED TO PROVIDE ENERGY FOR BREATHING IS _____%; _____% IN POST-OP PATIENTS:
    A. 2
    B. 20
    C. 50
    D. 60
    E. 80
    Ref. p. 498

600. HIGH CENTRAL VENOUS PRESSURE READINGS (OVER 15 CM H_2O) MOST OFTEN INDICATE:
    A. Unsuspected pneumothorax
    B. The development of pulmonary emboli
    C. Inability of right ventricle to handle venous returns
    D. Increase in venous capacitance   Ref. p. 501

601. THE SWAN-GANZ BALLOON-TIP CATHETER IS DESIGNED TO:
    A. Float into the pulmonary artery and obtain its wedge pressure
    B. Measure left ventricular pressure directly by passage through the subclavian artery
    C. Be a reliable guide of left ventricular end-diastolic pressure
    Ref. p. 502

602. WHICH IS MORE RELIABLE AS AN INDEX OF LEFT VENTRICULAR
FUNCTION?:
A. Central venous pressure catheter
B. Swan-Ganz catheter
C. Both are equal
D. Neither   Ref. p. 502

603. THE RATIONALE BEHIND DIRECT SKELETAL MUSCLE pH ELECTRODE
IMPLANTATION IS:
A. A lag of acid metabolite washout from tissues into peripheral circulation
B. Skeletal muscle tolerates hypoxia, and its blood supply tends to shut off
early in critical states, shifting to anaerobic glycolysis
C. Both
D. Neither   Ref. p. 508

SELECT THE MOST APPROPRIATE ANSWER(S):

604. WHICH OF THE FOLLOWING IS ABSORBED THROUGH THE SKIN AND
      REMAINS THERAPEUTICALLY ACTIVE ?:
      A. Cortisone acetate   D. Hydrocortisone
      B. Heavy metals   E. Sodium and calcium
      C. Insulin   Ref. p. 514

605. WHICH OF THE FOLLOWING DISEASE STATES RESPONDS BEST TO
      SYMPATHECTOMY ?:
      A. Raynaud's disease   D. Diabetes mellitus
      B. Buerger's disease   E. Acrocyanosis
      C. Hydroadenitis   Ref. p. 514

606. THE CURATIVE TREATMENT OF CHRONIC HYPERHIDROSADENITIS
      SUPPURATIVA AXILLARIS IS:
      A. Incision and drainage
      B. Excision of axillary
      C. Radiation
      D. Excision of involved area plus skin graft
      E. Atropinization   Ref. p. 516

607. CHILDREN WITH RAPIDLY EXPANDING HEMANGIOMAS (STRAWBERRY
      MARKS) SHOULD:
      A. Have an immediate incisional biopsy to establish diagnosis
      B. Undergo excision of the lesion because of malignant potential
      C. Be observed, since complete regression is often the rule
      D. Undergo radiation
      E. Be inspected with sclerosing agents
                                         Ref. p. 518

608. GLOMUS TUMORS ARE FOUND TO BE HISTOLOGICALLY IN WHICH
      OF THE FOLLOWING ?:
      A. Mesodermal
      B. Ectodermal
      C. Endodermal
      D. Neuroectodermal   Ref. p. 518

609. WHICH OF THE FOLLOWING DISEASE STATES MAY BE ASSOCIATED
      WITH NEUROFIBROMATOSIS ?:
      A. Pheochromocytoma   D. Gliomas
      B. Sarcoma   E. All of the above
      C. Meningiomas   Ref. p. 519

610. WHICH OF THE FOLLOWING LESIONS HAS A GREATER MALIGNANT
      POTENTIAL ?:
      A. Basal cell carcinoma
      B. Squamous cell carcinoma
      C. Neither   Ref. p. 520

611. WHICH OF THE FOLLOWING IS NOT USUALLY PRESENT IN SQUAMOUS
      CELL CARCINOMA ?:
      A. Satellite nodules
      B. Induration
      C. Pearls expressed from the ulcer
      D. Telangiectasia
      E. Central ulceration with irregular base
                                         Ref. p. 520

612. WITH WHICH OF THE FOLLOWING IS THE CURE RATE FOR SQUAMOUS
CELL CARCINOMA HIGHER?:
A. Radiation
B. Surgical excision
C. Neither   Ref. p. 520

613. THE FIVE YEAR SURVIVAL RATE FOR SQUAMOUS CELL CARCINOMA
OF THE SKIN IS:
A. 20%   D. 80%
B. 40%   E. 95%
C. 60%   Ref. p. 521

614. THE HIGHEST INCIDENCE OF MALIGNANT MELANOMA IS FOUND IN
WHICH OF THE FOLLOWING?:
A. Compound nevus   C. Junctional nevus
B. Intradermal nevus   D. Blue nevus
                          Ref. p. 521

615. THE MOST COMMON NEVUS IN CHILDREN PRIOR TO PUBERTY IS
WHICH OF THE FOLLOWING?:
A. Junctional nevus
B. Compound nevus
C. Equal   Ref. p. 521

616. WHICH OF THE FOLLOWING CHEMOTHERAPEUTIC AGENTS IS
UTILIZED FOR MALIGNANT MELANOMA?:
A. TSPA (Triethylene Thiophosphoramide)
B. Nitrogen mustard
C. Fluorouracil
D. Phenylalanine mustard
E. All of the above   Ref. p. 524

617. FIVE YEAR PROGNOSIS RATE OF A SUPERFICIAL MELANOMA LESS
THAN 2 CM IN DIAMETER IS:
A. 90%   D. 30%
B. 70%   E. 10%
C. 50%   Ref. p. 525

618. WHAT PERCENT OF CANCER IN FEMALES IS OF BREAST ORIGIN?:
A. 5   D. 25
B. 10   E. 40
C. 15   Ref. p. 533

619. THE PEAK INCIDENCE OF BREAST CARCINOMA APPEARS IN PATIENTS
BETWEEN_____YEARS OF AGE:
A. 35-45   D. 65-75
B. 45-55   E. 75-85
C. 55-65   Ref. p. 533

620. THE MOST FREQUENT SITE FOR THE DEVELOPMENT OF SCIRRHOTIC
ADENOCARCINOMA OF THE BREAST IS:
A. Upper outer quadrant
B. Lower outer quadrant
C. Upper inner quadrant
D. Lower inner quadrant   Ref. p. 535

621. STAGING OF BREAST CARCINOMA IN ACCORDANCE WITH THE AMERI-
CAN JOINT COMMITTEE ON CANCER WILL PLACE A 3 CM BREAST
LESION IN THE UPPER OUTER QUADRANT WITH ASSOCIATED SKIN
DIMPLING, NO CHEST WALL ADHERENCE AND A SOLITARY AXILLARY
LYMPH NODE. NO EVIDENCE OF METASTATIC SPREAD. WHICH OF
THE FOLLOWING STAGES BEST APPLIES?:
A. Stage I T1 N1 M0   D. Stage III T2 N1 M0
B. Stage II T1 N1 M0   E. Stage IV T2 N1 M1
C. Stage II T2 N1 M0   Ref. p. 536

622. IN A PATIENT WITH CHRONIC CYSTIC MASTITIS, ASPIRATION IS AN
ACCEPTABLE PROCEDURE TO CONFIRM THE DIAGNOSIS IN ALL,
EXCEPT:
A. Clear brown-green fluid is present
B. No palpable mass is present after aspiration
C. Close follow-up biannually with no development
D. About 50% of the cases will not recur
E. All are correct   Ref. p. 538

623. THE INCIDENCE OF CARCINOMA OF THE BREAST IN PATIENTS WITH
A SANGUINOUS NIPPLE, DISCHARGE IS_____PER CENT:
A. 0-10   D. 30-40
B. 10-20   E. 40-50
C. 20-30   Ref. p. 538

624. THE MOST DIFFICULT BREAST LESION(S) TO GROSSLY DISTINGUISH
FROM CARCINOMA IS (ARE):
A. Fat necrosis   D. Fibroadenoma
B. Granular cell myoblastoma   E. Chronic cystic mastitis
C. Sclerosing adenosis   Ref. p. 538

625. WHICH OF THE FOLLOWING DISEASE STATES IS REPRESENTATIVE
OF "MONDOR'S DISEASE"?:
A. Sclerosing adenosis
B. Thrombophlebitis of breast veins
C. Granular cell myoblastoma
D. Fibrosarcoma of the breast
E. Chronic cystic mastitis   Ref. p. 538

626. PAGET'S DISEASE OF THE BREAST HAS ALL OF THE FOLLOWING,
EXCEPT:
A. Nipple scaling
B. More often post-menopausal
C. Sanguinous nipple discharge
D. Constitutes 1% of all breast carcinomas
E. Arises from the ductal tissue about the nipple
                                        Ref. p. 539

627. THE FIVE YEAR SURVIVAL RATE WITH INTRADUCTAL NON-
INFILTRATING CARCINOMA OF THE BREAST IS:
A. 10-20%   D. 70-80%
B. 30-40%   E. 90-100%
C. 50-60%   Ref. p. 539

628. THE TREATMENT OF CHOICE IN CYSTOSARCOMA PHYLLOIDES IS:
A. Radical mastectomy
B. Simple mastectomy
C. Local excision
D. Radiation
E. Bilateral oophorectomy   Ref. p. 540

629. WHICH OF THE FOLLOWING HAS A GREATER FIVE YEAR SURVIVAL
     RATE ?:
     A. Scirrhous carcinoma of the breast
     B. Medullary carcinoma of the breast
     C. Both are equal   Ref. p. 540

630. THE HAAGENSEN "TRIPLE BIOPSY" INCLUDES ALL OF THE FOLLOW-
     ING, EXCEPT:
     A. Biopsy of primary breast lesion
     B. Biopsy of highest axillary nodes
     C. Biopsy of internal mammary nodes
     D. Biopsy of supraclavicular nodes on the side of the lesion
                                              Ref. p. 541

631. PRESERVATION OF WHICH OF THE FOLLOWING STRUCTURES IS CON-
     SIDERED MOST IMPORTANT IN A RADICAL MASTECTOMY ?:
     A. Pectoralis minor   D. Long thoracic nerve
     B. Thoracodorsal nerve   E. All are essential
     C. Pectoralis major   Ref. pp. 542-543

632. POSTOPERATIVE RADIATION OF THE AXILLA, SUPRACLAVICULAR
     AND INTERNAL MAMMARY LYMPH NODES RESULT IN WHICH OF THE
     FOLLOWING ?:
     A. An increase in five year survival   D. All of the above
     B. A decrease in local recurrence   E. None of the above
     C. A decrease in metastatic spread   Ref. p. 544

633. FIVE YEAR SURVIVAL RATE OF BREAST CARCINOMA IS GREATER
     WITH WHICH OF THE FOLLOWING PROCEDURES ?:
     A. Simple mastectomy plus radiation
     B. Radical mastectomy
     C. The results of both are equal   Ref. p. 544

634. THE FIVE YEAR SURVIVAL RATE IN PATIENTS WITHOUT AXILLARY
     LYMPH NODES FOLLOWING RADICAL MASTECTOMY IS ABOUT:
     A. 50-55%   D. 80-85%
     B. 60-65%   E. 90-95%
     C. 70-75%   Ref. p. 547

635. THE FIVE YEAR SURVIVAL RATE IN PATIENTS WITH AXILLARY
     LYMPH NODES FOLLOWING RADICAL MASTECTOMY IS:
     A. 10-15%   D. 40-45%
     B. 20-25%   E. 50-55%
     C. 30-35%   Ref. p. 547

636. RECURRENT BREAST CARCINOMA WITH PAINFUL BONE AND SUB-
     CUTANEOUS METASTASES IN A PREMENOPAUSAL FEMALE FOLLOW-
     ING A RADICAL MASTECTOMY SHOULD HAVE WHICH OF THE
     FOLLOWING NEXT ?:
     A. Bilateral adrenalectomy   D. Bilateral oophorectomy
     B. Hypophysectomy   E. Estrogen administration
     C. Chemotherapy plus 5 fluorouracil Ref. p. 549

637. IN THE SAME PATIENT THE REMISSION RATE WOULD BE:
     A. 10-30%
     B. 30-50%
     C. 50-70%
     D. 70-80%
     E. 80-90%   Ref. p. 549

638. IN A POST-MENOPAUSAL PATIENT WITH RECURRENT BREAST CAR-
CINOMA INVOLVING THE BONES AND SUBCUTANEOUS TISSUES WHICH
THERAPEUTIC TRIAL WOULD BE INITIATED?:

A. Bilateral adrenalectomy   D. Bilateral oophorectomy
B. Hypophysectomy   E. Estrogen administration
C. 5 fluorouracil   Ref. p. 550

639. IF THE POST-MENOPAUSAL PATIENT DOES NOT RESPOND TO THE
CORRECT FIRST LINE THERAPY, WHAT WOULD BE THE NEXT STEP?:

A. Bilateral adrenalectomy   D. Bilateral oophorectomy
B. Hypophysectomy   E. Estrogen administration
C. Chemotherapy with fluorouracil   Ref. p. 550

640. WHICH OF THE FOLLOWING HAS GREATER SENSITIVITY TO THE
TREATMENT WITH RESPECT TO TIME?:

A. Early treatment of an asymptomatic breast lesion
B. Late treatment of a symptomatic lesion
C. The lesions respond equally   Ref. p. 551

641. WHAT IS THE REMISSION RATE TO CHEMOTHERAPY ON THE PRE-
MENOPAUSAL FEMALE FOLLOWING INITIAL THERAPY?:

A. 10-20%   D. 40-50%
B. 20-30%   E. 50-60%
C. 30-40%   Ref. p. 551

SELECT THE MOST APPROPRIATE ANSWER(S):

642. WHARTON'S DUCTS ARE ASSOCIATED WITH WHICH OF THE FOLLOW-
ING ?:
A. Sublingual gland   D. Pancreas
B. Submaxillary gland   E. Liver
C. Parotid gland   Ref. p. 557

643. WHICH OF THE FOLLOWING CONDITIONS IS AN ETIOLOGIC FACTOR IN
LINGUAL CARCINOMA ?:
A. Syphilis   D. Telangectasia
B. Senile keratosis   E. "Hairy tongue"
C. Hyperkeratosis   Ref. p. 558

644. IN WHICH ANATOMIC POSITION ARE BRONCHIAL CLEFT CYSTS MOST
LIKELY TO PRESENT ?:
A. Along the posterior border of the sternocleidomastoideus muscle
B. Along the anterior border of the sternocleidomastoideus muscle
C. Lateral to the sternocleidomastoid muscle and inferior to the omohyoid
muscle
D. None of the above   Ref. p. 558

645. NEEDLE AND FRAGMENT BIOPSIES OF CERVICAL AND ORAL TUMORS
ARE ACCEPTABLE FOR ALL, EXCEPT:
A. Tonsillar carcinoma   D. Lymphoma
B. Carcinoma of the lip   E. Hyperkeratotic lip changes
C. Peutz Jegher pigmented spots Ref. p. 561

FILL IN THE MOST APPROPRIATE ANSWERS: (Questions 646-647)

A. Transitional cell   A. Cigarette smokers
B. Adenocarcinoma   B. Mailmen
C. Squamous cell carcinoma   C. Textile workers
D. Fibrosarcoma   D. Fishermen

Tumors of the lip are commonly 646)_____and have a predilection
for 647) _____ .   Ref. p. 561

SELECT THE MOST APPROPRIATE ANSWER:

648. WHICH OF THE FOLLOWING IS CONSIDERED TO BE A PREMALIGNANT
LIP LESION ?:
A. Peutz-Jegher pigmentation   D. Hyperkeratosis
B. Telangectasia   E. None of the above
C. Neuroma   Ref. p. 562

649. THE TREATMENT OF CHOICE FOR CARCINOMA OF THE LIP IS (LESS
THAN 1 CM DIAMETER):
A. Radiation
B. Excision
C. Both A and B   Ref. p. 563

650. WHICH OF THE FOLLOWING APPEAR TO INFLUENCE THE DEVELOP-
MENT OF ORAL CARCINOMA ?:
A. Alcoholism   D. Poor oral hygiene
B. Smoking   E. All of the above
C. Syphilis   Ref. p. 564

651.   A LESION IN THE FLOOR OF THE MOUTH ARISING FROM OBSTRUC-
        TION OF A MINOR SALIVARY GLAND IS CALLED:
        A. Dermoid   D. Meleney's ulcer
        B. Mixed cell tumor   E. Ranula
        C. Rodent ulcer   Ref. p. 565

652.   ALL OF THE FOLLOWING ARE CONSISTENT WITH DERMOIDS OF
        THE ORAL CAVITY, EXCEPT:
        A. Are usually located in the midline
        B. Significant malignant degeneration
        C. Have a definite capsule
        D. Should be shelled out if possible
        E. May present in the submental triangle
                                         Ref. p. 565

653.   THE MOST COMMONLY PRESENTING TUMOR OF THE SALIVARY
        GLANDS ARE:
        A. Wharton's tumor
        B. Mucoepidermoid carcinoma
        C. Cylindroma
        D. Mixed cell tumors
        E. Acinar cell adenocarcinoma   Ref. p. 566

        ANSWER THE FOLLOWING QUESTIONS BY USING THE KEY
        OUTLINED BELOW:
        A. If both statement and reason are correct and related cause and effect
        B. If both statement and reason are correct but not related cause and effect
        C. If statement is true but reason is false
        D. If statement is false but reason is true
        E. If both statement and reason are false

654.   Patients with oral dyskeratosis have a malignant potential BECAUSE five
        per cent of the patients will eventually develop a malignancy.
                                         Ref. p. 568

655.   Carcinoma of the tongue most often develops centrally BECAUSE it begins
        in an area of hyperkeratosis.   Ref. p. 568

656.   The metastatic spread of a lingual carcinoma from the tongue always
        follows a similar path BECAUSE the submental lymph nodes drain the
        tumors from the distal portion of the tongue.
                                         Ref. p. 568

        SELECT THE MOST APPROPRIATE ANSWER:

657.   WHAT PERCENTAGE OF LINGUAL TUMORS HAVE LYMPH NODE
        METASTASES AT THE TIME THEY ARE DISCOVERED?:
        A. 10%   D. 70%
        B. 40%   E. 80%
        C. 60%   Ref. p. 568

        MATCH THE ORIGIN OF THE TUMOR WITH THE INITIAL SITE OF
        METASTASES:

658.___ Cervical lymph nodes   A. Tip of tongue
659.___ Submaxillary lymph nodes   B. Borders of the tongue
660.___ Submental lymph nodes   C. Floor of the mouth
661.___ Submandibular lymph nodes   D. Posterior third of the tongue
                                         Ref. pp. 568-572

SELECT THE MOST APPROPRIATE ANSWER:

662. IN WHICH CONDITION(S) WILL A RADICAL NECK DISSECTION BE IN-
     DICATED WHEN REGIONAL LYMPH NODE SPREAD HAS OCCURRED?:
     A. Carcinoma of the tongue without obvious lymph node spread
     B. Carcinoma of the floor of the mouth
     C. Gingival carcinoma without obvious cervical node spread
     D. Carcinoma of the epiglottis
     E. Carcinoma of the tonsil   Ref. pp. 568-572

663. WHICH OF THE FOLLOWING POTENTIATES THE INVASION OF A
     GINGIVAL TUMOR?:
     A. Radiation   D. None of the above
     B. Chemotherapy   E. All of the above
     C. Extraction of a tooth   Ref. p. 569

664. CARCINOMA OF THE OROPHARYNX IS MOST COMMONLY FOUND
     IN THE:
     A. Tonsils
     B. Posterior third of the tongue
     C. Soft palate
     D. Epiglottis   Ref. p. 571

665. TONSILLAR LYMPHOSARCOMAS COMPRISE ONE PER CENT OF THE
     MALIGNANT LESIONS; THE TREATMENT OF CHOICE IS:
     A. Excision
     B. Wide excision, ipsilateral radical neck
     C. Wide excision, bilateral radical neck
     D. Radiation
     E. Chemotherapy   Ref. p. 571

666. THE MOST FREQUENTLY OBSERVED SYMPTOM RELATED TO
     LARYNGEAL CARCINOMA IS:
     A. Pain   D. Hemoptysis
     B. Chronic cough   E. Horner's syndrome
     C. Hoarseness   Ref. p. 573

667. WHICH OF THE FOLLOWING AREAS HAS THE GREATEST INCIDENCE
     OF EPIDERMOID CARCINOMA?:
     A. Glottic region of the larynx
     B. Supraglottic region of the larynx
     C. Subglottic region of the larynx   Ref. p. 573

668. WHICH CHARACTERISTICS BEST DESCRIBE THE GLOTTIC
     CARCINOMAS?:
     A. Preceded by hyperkeratosis
     B. Very well differentiated
     C. Slow-growing
     D. Often may be cured by cobalt therapy
     E. All of the above
     F. All except D   Ref. p. 573

669. THE TREATMENT OF CHOICE FOR CANCER OF THE TRUE CORD
     (LOCALIZED) IS:
     A. Local excision
     B. Excision plus ipsilateral radical neck dissection
     C. Laryngectomy
     D. Laryngectomy plus ipsilateral radical neck dissection
     E. High voltage radiation   Ref. p. 574

670. THE FIVE YEAR SURVIVAL FOR CARCINOMA OF THE VOCAL CORD
     (STAGES I AND II) IS:
     A. 20 per cent   D. 70 per cent
     B. 40 per cent   E. 90 per cent
     C. 50 per cent   Ref. p. 575

671. TUMORS OF THE NASOPHARYNX WHICH ARE RADIOSENSITIVE ARE:
     A. Epidermoid carcinoma
     B. Lymphosarcoma
     C. Both equally   Ref. p. 579

672. THE INTEGRATION OF COBALT IRRADIATION AND SURGICAL EXCI-
     SION OF TUMORS IN THE NASAL SINUSES PERMITS A FIVE YEAR
     SURVIVAL OF_____PER CENT (MAXILLARY SINUSES):
     A. 5-10   D. 45-55
     B. 15-25   E. 65-75
     C. 30-35   Ref. p. 580

673. IN LESIONS OF THE PAROTID GLAND, WHICH CRANIAL NERVE IS
     OFTEN INVADED?:
     A. Trigeminal   D. Facial
     B. Spinal accessory   E. Auditory
     C. Hypoglossal   Ref. p. 580

674. THE MANDIBULAR BRANCH OF THE FACIAL NERVE MAY BECOME
     INVADED BY EITHER A LESION OF THE PAROTID OR SUBMAXILLARY
     GLAND. TO TEST ITS FUNCTION ONE MUST:
     A. Establish an area of loss of sensation
     B. Establish a loss of taste at the tip of the tongue
     C. Determine if the patient is able to pucker his (her) lips
     D. Determine if the patient is able to balloon his (her) cheek
                                             Ref. p. 580

675. WHICH OF THE FOLLOWING NERVES LIES CLOSEST TO WHARTON'S
     DUCT?:
     A. Facial nerve   D. Lingual nerve
     B. Hypoglossal   E. Alveolar nerve
     C. Spinal accessory   Ref. p. 581

676. TO DISTINGUISH PATHOLOGICALLY BETWEEN A PAROTID MIXED
     TUMOR AND WHARTON'S TUMOR, ONE MUST IDENTIFY_____IN
     THE LATTER:
     A. Pseudocartilage structures
     B. Lymphoid tissue with germinal centers
     C. Mixoid type cells
     D. Pseudostratified epithelium
     E. All of the above   Ref. p. 581

677. THE MOST COMMON MALIGNANT LESION OF THE PAROTID GLAND IS:
     A. Squamous cell carcinoma
     B. Adeno cystic carcinoma cylindroma
     C. Acinar cell adenocarcinoma
     D. Mucoepidermoid carcinoma
     E. Anaplastic adenocarcinoma   Ref. p. 582

678. WHICH OF THE BENIGN LESIONS OF THE SALIVARY GLANDS HAVE
     MALIGNANT POTENTIAL?:
     A. Wharton's tumor   D. None of the above
     B. Mikulicz's disease   E. All of the above
     C. Mixed tumors   Ref. p. 582

679. BIOPSIES OF THE SALIVARY GLANDS SHOULD:
    A. Always be excisional   D. None of
    B. Always be incisional   E.
    C. Be primarily needle aspirations   Ref. p. 583

680. MOST MALIGNANT TUMORS OF THE NECK ARE:
    A. Of thyroid origin
    B. Metastatic in nature
    C. Lymphomas
    D. Adenocarcinomas   Ref. p. 584

MATCH THE SOURCE OF THE TUMOR WITH THE LYMPH NODES MOST
FREQUENTLY INVOLVED:

681. ___ Gastric carcinoma   A. Upper cervical chain
682. ___ Right lung and left lower   B. Cervical lymph nodes in the middle
       lobe of the lung   third of the neck
683. ___ Nasopharynx, lateral   C. Left supraclavicular lymph nodes
       pharyngeal walls   (Virchow's)
684. ___ Hypopharynx, thyroid,   D. Right scalene fat pad lymph nodes
       larynx   Ref. p. 584

SELECT THE MOST APPROPRIATE ANSWER:

685. CHEMODECTOMAS ARE CHARACTERIZED BY ALL OF THE FOLLOW-
ING, EXCEPT:
    A. Paraganglionic tissue   D. Hypoglossal nerve paralysis
    B. Malignant degeneration   E. Pain
    C. Dysphagia   Ref. p. 585

686. THE TUMOR MOST OFTEN ENCOUNTERED IN THE NECKS OF
CHILDREN IS:
    A. Thyroid carcinoma   D. Neuroblastoma
    B. Lymphoma   E. Teratoma
    C. Fibrosarcoma   Ref. p. 585

MATCH THE FOLLOWING. EACH LETTERED ITEM MAY BE USED
ONLY ONCE:

687. ___ Flail chest
688. ___ Normal alveolar pCO_2
689. ___ High concentration of alveolar
        O_2 with bronchial obstruction
690. ___ More likely associated with
        hemoptysis
691. ___ Chief lymph drainage from
        lungs
692. ___ Pores of Kohn
693. ___ Paralysis of hemidiaphragm

A. Ruptured pulmonary artery
B. Ruptured bronchial artery
C. 35-45 mmHg
D. Paradoxical motion
E. 95-100 mmHg
F. Helps favor atelectasis
G. Helps prevent atelectasis
H. Right thoracic duct
I. Left thoracic duct
        Ref. pp. 597-598

ANSWER THE FOLLOWING STATEMENTS T(RUE) OR F(ALSE):

694. An abnormally elevated CVP can result in respiratory failure due to lymph
     accumulation.   Ref. p. 599

695. Cyanosis requires greater than 5 grams of reduced Hb.
                                      Ref. p. 601

696. Endogenous lipoid pneumonia is most commonly encountered from intake
     of mineral oil in the elderly.   Ref. p. 509 (1st Ed.)

SELECT THE MOST APPROPRIATE ANSWER:

697. DISPLACEMENT OF THE MEDIASTINUM IN THE ADULT PATIENT
     USUALLY AFFECTS WHICH OF THE FOLLOWING SYSTEMS THE MOST ?:
     A. Respiratory
     B. Arterial
     C. Venous   Ref. pp. 597-598

698. THE PULMONARY FUNCTION TEST WHICH YIELDS THE MOST VALU-
     ABLE INFORMATION TO A CLINICIAN IS:
     A. Vital capacity (VC)   D. Residual air (RA)
     B. Timed vital capacity (TVC)   E. No one test is effective
     C. Maximum breather capacity (MBC) Ref. p. 600

699. WHICH OF THE FOLLOWING DISEASE STATES ARE RESPONSIBLE
     FOR HEMOPTYSIS?:
     A. Klebsiella pneumonia   D. Pneumococcal pneumonia
     B. Bronchiectasis   E. All of the above
     C. Mitral stenosis   Ref. p. 601

700. SURGICAL INDICATIONS FOR PECTUS EXCAVATUM REPAIRS ARE
     USUALLY OF_____ORIGIN:
     A. Cardiac
     B. Respiratory
     C. Psychological   Ref. p. 603

701. THE PRIMARY FACTOR IN RESUSCITATION OF ARRESTED PATIENTS
     IS:
     A. Cardiac compression
     B. Intravenous initiation
     C. Adequate airway
     D. All are equal   Ref. p. 604

702. TREATMENT OF CHOICE IN FLAIL CHEST WITH COMPROMISE OF
      VENTILATION IS:
      A. Tracheostomy
      B. Towel clips to elevate ribs
      C. Assisted ventilation with positive pressure
      D. Intercostal block to decrease pain
      E. All together   Ref. p. 604

703. COSTAL CHONDRITIS RESULTS FROM THE STRIPPING OF PERICHON-
      DRIUM AND THE INTRODUCTION OF PYOGENIC ORGANISMS TO AN
      AVASCULAR CARTILAGE. WHICH ORGANISM PRODUCES THE MOST
      FREQUENT INFECTION?:
      A. Streptococci   D. Actinomyces
      B. Staphylococci   E. Blastomyces
      C. Tuberculosis   Ref. p. 605

704. ALL OF THE FOLLOWING MAY RESULT IN LYTIC COSTAL LESIONS,
      EXCEPT:
      A. Hyperparathyroid adenoma D. Radiation necrosis
      B. Chondrosarcoma   E. Paget's disease
      C. Eosinophilic granuloma   Ref. p. 606

705. TIETZI SYNDROME OF THE COSTAL CARTILAGES USUALLY DEVELOPS
      AT THE:
      A. Second costal cartilage
      B. Fifth costal cartilage
      C. Eighth costal cartilage
      D. All costal cartilages develop equally
                                    Ref. p. 606

706. THE MOST COMMON COSTAL LESION IS:
      A. Eosinophilic granuloma
      B. Fibroma
      C. Chondrosarcoma
      D. Osteochondroma
      E. Fibrous dysplasia (bone cyst)   Ref. p. 608

707. THE BLOOD SUPPLY TO THE VISCERAL PLEURA IS DERIVED FROM
      THE VASCULAR SYSTEM THROUGH THE:
      A. Bronchial artery   D. Aortic offshoots
      B. Pulmonary artery   E. All of the above
      C. Intercostal arteries   Ref. p. 610

708. THE "ELASTIC RECOIL" OF A LUNG GOVERNS THE INTRAPLEURAL
      PRESSURE. IN ATELECTASIS, THE PRESSURE IS:
      A. More negative
      B. Less negative
      C. Unchanged   Ref. p. 611

709. TRANSMEDIASTINAL PLEURAL HERNIATION OCCURS RARELY. ITS
      SITE OF OCCURRENCE IS GENERALLY:
      A. Retrosternal
      B. Anterior to vertebral column
      C. Both   Ref. p. 612

710. A SPONTANEOUS PNEUMOTHORAX EXCEEDING_____PER CENT OF
      THE CHEST CAVITY SHOULD HAVE A CHEST TUBE INSERTED:
      A. 25   D. 55
      B. 35   E. 65
      C. 45   Ref. p. 612

711. PLEURAL EFFUSION OFTEN APPEARS IN WHICH OF THE FOLLOWING
     DISEASE STATES?:
     A. Pancreatitis
     B. Meig's syndrome
     C. Acute mediastinitis
     D. Right heart failure
     E. All of the above   Ref. p. 614

     ANSWER THE FOLLOWING QUESTIONS BY USING THE KEY
     OUTLINED BELOW:
     A. If both statement and reason are correct and related cause and effect
     B. If both statement and reason are correct but not related cause and effect
     C. If statement is true but reason is false
     D. If statement is false but reason is true
     E. If both statement and reason are false

712. The absorption coefficient of CO_2 is about 21 times that of O_2; THERE-
     FORE, a PCO_2 alveolar-arterial gradient usually exceeds 8 mmHg.
                                             Ref. p. 600

713. A bronchopleural fistula usually develops as a result of extrapulmonary
     pathology entering the bronchus acutely BECAUSE hepatic abscesses are
     the most common cause.   Ref. p. 616

714. Closed tube drainage in patients with empyema is often converted to open
     tube drainage BECAUSE 80 to 85 per cent of the out-flow becomes thick and
     solid.   Ref. p. 616

715. Air in an empyemic cavity rules out the presence of a bronchopleural
     fistula BECAUSE it usually is present in enclosed cavities with Escherichia
     coli.   Ref. p. 618

716. Decortication of the lung is a surgical procedure to remove the visceral
     pleura of the lung BECAUSE it maintains the lung in an expanded state.
                                             Ref. p. 619

717. Tuberculous empyema and pyogenic empyema are treated the same
     BECAUSE both respond favorably to closed tube drainage.
                                             Ref. p. 620

718. Tuberculous empyema is occasionally treated by open drainage BECAUSE
     persistent bronchopleural fistula forces one to open it.
                                             Ref. p. 620

719. Agenesis of the right lung has a poorer prognosis than that of the left
     BECAUSE of the loss of functional pulmonary tissue.
                                             Ref. p. 622

720. In infants lobar obstructive emphysema on one side may be accidentally
     diagnosed as atelectasis of the opposite side BECAUSE of contralateral
     bronchus obstruction.   Ref. p. 624

721. Blunt trauma of the lung should often have a pulmonary resection BECAUSE
     the resulting non-viable tissue slowly undergoes necrosis and is difficult
     to detect.   Ref. p. 627

722. Saccular bronchiectasis has a better prognosis than tubular bronchiectasis
     BECAUSE the former type has a loss of elasticity.
                                             Ref. p. 629

FILL IN THE MOST APPROPRIATE ANSWERS: (Questions 723-724)

A. Staphylococcal
B. Pneumococcal
C. Streptococcal
D. Enterococcus
E. Friedlander's bacillus

The most common bacterial empyema seen in the 1930's was 723) _____ ,
because of antibiotic therapy. The etiology of this disease has changed to
724) _____ .   Ref. p. 615

SELECT THE MOST APPROPRIATE ANSWER(S):

725. PLEURAL FLUID WITH THE APPEARANCE OF "ANCHOVY SAUCE" IS
      CHARACTERISTIC OF:
      A. Escherichia coli   D. Ecchinococcus
      B. Endamoeba histolytica   E. None of the above
      C. Staphylococcus aureus   Ref. p. 615

726. THE PRIMARY TREATMENT OF EMPYEMA WHICH RESULTS FROM
      TUBERCULOSIS IS:
      A. Open tube drainage   D. Thoracoplasty
      B. Systemic antibiotic therapy E. Thoracentesis
      C. Closed tube drainage   Ref. p. 616

727. THE DIFFERENTIAL DIAGNOSIS OF AN ENCAPSULATED EMPYEMA
      VERSUS THE INFECTED SOLITARY CYST INCLUDES ALL OF THE
      FOLLOWING, EXCEPT:
      A. In the latter, the patient suffers from frequent previous respiratory
          illness
      B. The contour of the fluid in the former is triangular or fusiform,
          whereas in the latter, it is rounded in both properties
      C. Little pleural thickening is present in the latter
                                       Ref. p. 616

728. THE MOST COMMON ERROR IN PERFORMING A THORACOPLASTY FOR
      DRAINAGE OF EMPYEMA IS:
      A. The drainage site not performed in the most dependent area of the
          empyema
      B. Insufficient removal of rib to accommodate adequate drainage
      C. Failure to perform the procedure in an upright position in a patient
          with bronchopleural fistula
      D. Failure to biopsy empyema wall
      E. Failure to stage the procedure   Ref. p. 617

729. FAILURE TO ESTABLISH ADEQUATE DRAINAGE IN AN EMPYEMA WITH
      A BRONCHOPLEURAL FISTULA PRESENT IS INDICATED BY:
      A. Drainage less than 100 cc/day
      B. Hemorrhagic drainage less than 100 cc/day
      C. The development of hemoptysis
      D. Continued productive cough with purulent material
      E. All of the above   Ref. p. 619

730. CALCIFICATION OF THE PLEURA USUALLY REPRESENTS A STATE OF
      CHRONIC PLEURITIS WITH MASSIVE FIBROUS THICKENING OVER THE
      PLEURAL SURFACES. THE MOST AFFECTED PLEURA IS:
      A. Parietal
      B. Visceral
      C. Both   Ref. p. 620

731. HEMORRHAGIC PLEURAL EFFUSION WITH A MASS ADHERENT TO THE
     CHEST WALL MOST LIKELY IS:
     A. Tuberculosis   D. Mesothelioma
     B. Bronchiogenic carcinoma   E. Histoplasmosis
     C. Pulmonary infarction   Ref. p. 621

732. PLEURAL CALCIFICATION IS OFTEN INDICATIVE OF:
     A. Chronic empyema   D. Non-tuberculous empyema
     B. Tuberculous empyema   E. All of the above
     C. Bronchopleural fistula   Ref. p. 621

733. THE MOST COMMON MALIGNANT PLEURAL TUMOR IS A:
     A. Fibrosarcoma   D. Mesothelioma
     B. Adenocarcinoma   E. Chondrosarcoma
     C. Lymphosarcoma   Ref. p. 621

734. IN THE PATIENT WITH A MESOTHELIOMA, ONE OFTEN FINDS:
     A. Hypoglycemia   D. All of the above
     B. An association with asbestosis E. None of the above
     C. Pleural effusion is hemorrhagic Ref. p. 621

735. PROGRESSIVE HYPOGLYCEMIA ASSOCIATED WITH PLEURAL MESO-
     THELIOMA IS BEST TREATED BY:
     A. Excision of tumor
     B. Glucagon infusion
     C. 17 hydroxycorticosteroids
     D. Temporary intravenous glucose therapy
     E. Radiation of the tumor   Ref. p. 621

736. WHICH OF THE FOLLOWING ARTERIO-VENOUS FISTULA IS NOT
     ASSOCIATED WITH CARDIAC ENLARGEMENT AND HYPERTROPHY?:
     A. A-V fistula of femoral vessels
     B. A-V fistula of renal artery and vein
     C. A-V fistula of pulmonary vessels
     D. A-V fistula of radial vessels
     E. All A-V fistula are associated with cardiac enlargement and hypertrophy
                                        Ref. p. 623

737. WHICH OF THE FOLLOWING DISEASE STATES ARE MOST OFTEN CON-
     FUSED WITH THE CONDITION IN THE ABOVE QUESTION?:
     A. Polycythemia vera   D. Congenital heart disease
     B. Acquired heart disease   E. Leriche's syndrome
     C. Polyarteritis nodosum   Ref. p. 623

738. CAVITY FORMATION IS INFLUENCED BY:
     A. Hyperinflation or pulmonary defect
     B. Local pulmonary destruction
     C. Developmental anomaly
     D. All of the above   Ref. p. 625

739. BRONCHIECTASIS MAY DEVELOP FROM ALL OF THE FOLLOWING,
     EXCEPT:
     A. Chronic pulmonary infection
     B. Congenital malformation
     C. Retained bronchial foreign body
     D. Chronic pleural effusion
     E. Tuberculosis   Ref. p. 628

740. THE "MIDDLE LOBE SYNDROME" REFERS TO:
      A. Bronchial compression of the right middle lobe by lymph nodes result-
          ing in atelectasis
      B. Middle lobe pneumonitis following cardiac surgery
      C. Vascular anomaly of the hemizygous vein with resulting bronchial com-
          pression
      D. Bronchus obstruction due to selective invasion of a bronchus by bron-
          chiogenic carcinoma   Ref. p. 630

741. PULMONARY ABSCESSES SECONDARY TO ASPIRATION ARE MOST
      OFTEN SEEN IN THE:
      A. Anterior upper lobe
      B. Posterior upper lobe
      C. Posterior lower lobe
      D. Apical lower lobe   Ref. p. 631

742. THE MOST COMMON CONGENITAL ANOMALY ASSOCIATED WITH A
      TRACHEO-ESOPHAGEAL FISTULA IS:
      A. Jejunal atresia   D. Esophageal atresia
      B. Imperforate anus   E. None of the above
      C. Hypospadius   Ref. p. 635

743. THE SURGICAL TREATMENT OF PULMONARY TUBERCULOSIS:
      A. Depends on the results obtained from months of chemotherapy
      B. Often terminated the disease if done early with no need of follow-up
          chemotherapy
      C. Should not be performed unless sputum contains resistant tubercle
          bacilli
      D. Can now be avoided if adequate chemotherapy is administered
      E. None of the above   Ref. p. 636

744. THE MOST COMMON FUNGAL DISEASE CONFUSED WITH TUBERCU-
      LOSIS IS:
      A. Coccidioidomycosis   D. Nocardiosis
      B. Histoplasmosis   E. Blastomycosis
      C. Actinomycosis   Ref. p. 638

745. ACTINOMYCOSIS IS MOST FREQUENTLY FOUND IN WHICH OF THE
      FOLLOWING AREAS?:
      A. Abdomen   D. Renal
      B. Thoracic   E. Extremities
      C. Cervico-facial   Ref. p. 639

746. THE PRIME DANGER OF HYDATID CYST RUPTURE DURING ITS
      REMOVAL IS:
      A. Spread of cysts to pleural cavity
      B. Anaphylactic reaction
      C. Spread of cysts to myocardium
      D. Spread of cysts to liver
      E. None of the above   Ref. p. 640

747. WITH PARTIAL BRONCHIAL OBSTRUCTION, FLUOROSCOPY MAY
      DEMONSTRATE MEDIASTINAL SHIFT TOWARD WHICH SIDE?:
      A. Central lateral
      B. Same
      C. Neither   Ref. p. 641

748. THE MOST COMMONLY FOUND BRONCHIAL ADENOMA IS:
      A. Cylindroma (adenocystic carcinoma)
      B. Mucoepidermoid
      C. Carcinoid
      D. None of the above   Ref. p. 642

749. THE MOST COMMON VARIETY OF PULMONARY TUMOR DEVELOPS
      FROM WHICH OF THE FOLLOWING?:
      A. Tracheal wall
      B. Visceral pleura
      C. Pulmonary parenchyma
      D. Bronchial wall
      E. Parietal pleura   Ref. p. 642

      ANSWER THE FOLLOWING QUESTION BY USING THE KEY
      OUTLINED BELOW:
      A. If both statement and reason are correct and related cause and effect
      B. If both statement and reason are correct but not related cause and effect
      C. If statement is true but reason is false
      D. If statement is false but reason is true
      E. If both statement and reason are false

750. Hematoma of the lung frequently degenerates to carcinoma and should
      THEREFORE be removed.   Ref. p. 642

      SELECT THE MOST APPROPRIATE ANSWER(S):

751. BRONCHIAL ADENOMA IS MOST FREQUENTLY 90% OF WHICH OF
      THE FOLLOWING?:
      A. Mainstem bronchi (Lucas)
      B. Bronchiolus
      C. Trachea
      D. Periphery of pulmonary parenchyma
                                                   Ref. p. 644

752. WHICH IS THE MOST COMMON ENDOCRINE SITE OF METASTATIC
      BRONCHIOGENIC CARCINOMA?:
      A. Thyroid   D. Pancreas
      B. Parathyroid   E. Ovaries
      C. Adrenal   Ref. p. 646

753. WHICH OF THE FOLLOWING METABOLIC PROBLEMS FREQUENTLY
      DEVELOP IN ASSOCIATION WITH BRONCHIOGENIC CARCINOMA?:
      A. Hypercalcemia   D. Hypoglycemia
      B. Hyponatremia   E. All of the above
      C. Serotonin production   Ref. p. 647

754. WHICH PULMONARY LESION MOST OFTEN METASTASIZES TO THE
      OPPOSITE LUNG?:
      A. Adenocarcinoma   D. Cylindroma
      B. Alveolar cell carcinoma   E. Carcinoid
      C. Epidermoid cell carcinoma   Ref. p. 648

755. ALVEOLAR CELL LUNG CARCINOMA IS:
      A. Found more frequently in males
      B. Found equally in males and females
      C. Frequently causes hemoptysis early
      D. Multicentric in origin
      E. Easily diagnosed with bronchoscopy
                                                   Ref. p. 648

756. THE FIVE YEAR SURVIVAL RATE IN PATIENTS EXPLORED FOR
      BRONCHIOGENIC CARCINOMA IS:
      A. 5%   D. 25%
      B. 15%   E. 35%
      C. 20%   Ref. p. 649

757. THE SCALENE NODE BIOPSY HAS A GREATER NUMBER OF POSITIVES
      IN PREVIOUSLY UNDIAGNOSED:
      A. Bronchiogenic carcinoma
      B. Boeck's sarcoid
      C. Tuberculosis
      D. Gastric carcinoma   Ref. p. 650

758. IN PATIENTS WHO UNDERGO PNEUMONECTOMY, WHICH OF THE
      FOLLOWING IS TRUE?:
      A. I.V. fluids should be enough to keep the urine output 60 cc/hour
      B. Patient should be kept on the dehydrated side
      C. Accurate replacement   Ref. p. 652

759. IN A PNEUMONECTOMY, THE EARLY LIGATION OF THE PULMONARY
      VEIN IS IMPORTANT TO:
      A. Prevent the spread of carcinoma due to manipulation
      B. Prevent increased stress on the left side of the heart
      C. Prevent excessive bleeding during the remaining procedure
      D. Permit easy access to the mainstem bronchus
                                               Ref. p. 652

760. THE IMPORTANT POSTOPERATIVE FINDINGS INDICATING MEDIA-
      STINAL SHIFT ARE:
      A. Tracheal shift
      B. Palpatory and auscultatory shift of cardiac apex
      C. X-ray evidence
      D. Paradoxical respiration
      E. All of the above   Ref. p. 655

761. THE MOST RELIABLE INDICATION OF MEDIASTINAL SHIFT IS:
      A. Tracheal shift
      B. Palpatory and auscultatory shift of cardiac apex
      C. X-ray evidence
      D. Paradoxical respiration
      E. All of the above   Ref. p. 656

      ANSWER THE FOLLOWING QUESTION BY USING THE KEY
      OUTLINED BELOW:
      A. If both statement and reason are correct and related cause and effect
      B. If both statement and reason are correct but not related cause and effect
      C. If statement is true but reason is false
      D. If statement is false but reason is true
      E. If both statement and reason are false

762. Bronchoscopy in children is more dangerous than in adults BECAUSE
      tracheal trauma and resulting mucosal swelling blocks the comparatively
      small trachea.   Ref. p. 658

      SELECT THE MOST APPROPRIATE ANSWER:

763. HOW DOES A TENSION PNEUMOTHORAX DISPLACE THE MEDIASTINUM?:
      A. Toward the same side
      B. Toward the opposite side
      C. Does not cause a shift   Ref. p. 660

764. THE MOST COMMON CAUSE OF MEDIASTINITIS IS:
      A. Cervical cellulitis
      B. Osteomyelitis of vertebrae
      C. Pleural empyema
      D. Ruptured esophagus (perforation)
      E. Pericarditis   Ref. p. 660

ANSWER THE FOLLOWING STATEMENT T(RUE) OR F(ALSE):

765. Bilateral pleural effusion is a common result of mediastinitis.
                                        Ref. p. 661

SELECT THE MOST APPROPRIATE ANSWER(S):

766. THE PRIMARY REASON FOR SURGICAL REMOVAL OF AN INTRA-
      THORACIC GOITER IS:
      A. Tracheal compression
      B. High degree of malignant degeneration
      C. Increased tendency toward hyperthyroidism
      D. All of the above   Ref. p. 664

767. THE MOST COMMON ANTERIOR MEDIASTINAL TUMOR IS (ARE):
      A. Dermoid   D. Pleuropericardial cysts
      B. Thymic   E. Lymphosarcomas
      C. Hodgkin's disease   Ref. p. 665

768. THE PATENT DUCTUS ARTERIOSUS IS REPRESENTED BY WHICH OF
      THE FOLLOWING VASCULAR RINGS?:
      A. 2nd   D. 5th
      B. 3rd   E. 6th
      C. 4th   Ref. p. 677

769. THE DEVELOPMENT OF THE HEART IN THE FETAL STAGE OCCURS
      BETWEEN THE_____WEEK:
      A. 1st and 3rd   D. 10th and 20th
      B. 3rd and 5th   E. 20th and 30th
      C. 5th and 8th .   Ref. p. 677

770. THE MOST COMMON CONGENITAL HEART DISEASE IN THE NEWBORN
      IS:
      A. Atrial septal defect
      B. Ventricular septal defect
      C. Patent ductus arteriosus
      D. Coarctation of the aorta
      E. Pulmonary valvular stenosis   Ref. p. 678

771. IN WHICH OF THE FOLLOWING STATES IS PULMONARY HYPERTEN-
      SION MOST APT TO DEVELOP?:
      A. Pulmonary valvular stenosis
      B. Coarctation of the aorta
      C. Aortic valvular stenosis
      D. Atrio-septal defect with left to right shunt
      E. All of the above   Ref. p. 679

772. THE TERM "DIASTOLIC OVERLOAD" AS OPPOSED TO "SYSTOLIC
      OVERLOAD" RESULTS IN WHICH OF THE FOLLOWING PATHOLOGIC
      CHANGES INITIALLY?:
      A. Cardiac dilatation   D. All of the above
      B. Cardial hypertrophy   E. None of the above
      C. Bacterial endocarditis   Ref. p. 679

773. PULMONARY HYPERTENSION IS BEST EVALUATED BY:
      A. Measure of pulmonary vascular resistance
      B. Measure of pulmonary vascular pressures
      C. Measure of pulmonary vascular flow
                                     Ref. p. 679

774. WHICH OF THE FOLLOWING STATEMENTS ARE TRUE?:
      A. Cardiac output is increased in a left to right shunt
      B. Cardiac output is not increased in a right to left shunt
      C. Cardiac failure is rare in left to right shunts
      D. Cardiac failure is rare in right to left shunts
      E. All of the above are true   Ref. p. 680

775. IN A PATIENT WITH A HEMOGLOBIN (Hb) OF 10 GRAMS, WHAT DE-
      CREASE IN ARTERIAL OXYGENATION FROM A NORMAL OF 95 PER
      CENT WILL BE NECESSARY TO CREATE A CYANOTIC STATE?:
      A. 42% oxygen   D. 72% oxygen
      B. 52% oxygen   E. 85% oxygen
      C. 62% oxygen   Ref. p. 680

776. WHICH OF THE FOLLOWING ARE INDICATIVE OF CENTRAL CYANOSIS
      AS OPPOSED TO PERIPHERAL CYANOSIS?:
      A. Measuring the left atrial O_2 saturation and finding it below 95%
      B. Measuring the left atrial pressure and finding it above 25 mmHg
      C. Sudden improvement in cyanotic condition following 100% O_2 breathing
      D. All of the above
      E. None of the above   Ref. p. 680

777. WHICH OF THE FOLLOWING CAUSES LEFT ATRIAL ENLARGEMENT?:
      A. (VSD) Ventricular septal defect   D. Tricuspid atresia
      B. Mitral insufficiency   E. Ebstein's malformation
      C. Patent ductus arteriosus   Ref. p. 681

ANSWER THE FOLLOWING STATEMENT T(RUE) OR F(ALSE):

778. The term "gracile" habitus refers to a frail underweight child with either
      an atrio-septal defect or patent ductus arteriosus.
                                        Ref. p. 680

ANSWER THE FOLLOWING QUESTIONS BY USING THE KEY
OUTLINED BELOW:
      A. If both statement and reason are correct and related cause and effect
      B. If both statement and reason are correct but not related cause and effect
      C. If statement is true but reason is false
      D. If statement is false but reason is true
      E. If both statement and reason are false

779. Ventriculo-septal defect carries the highest incidence of pulmonary hyper-
      tension BECAUSE the most important responsible factor is the pressure
      load and not the flow rate.   Ref. p. 680

780. The squatting position commonly found in the tetralogy of Fallot tempor-
      arily improves the patient's condition BECAUSE it increases the peri-
      pheral vascular resistance with a resulting increase in pulmonary flow.
                                        Ref. p. 681

781. Hemoptysis in patients with tetralogy of Fallot is common BECAUSE of the
      increase in pulmonary flow.   Ref. p. 681

MATCH THE FOLLOWING WITH THE APPROPRIATE PRESSURE:

782. ___ Normal right atrial pressure   A. 15-30 mmHg
783. ___ Normal left atrial pressure   B. 5-10 mmHg
784. ___ Normal left ventricular pressure   C. 0-5 mmHg
785. ___ Normal right ventricular pressure   D. 80-130 mmHg
                                              Ref. p. 684

SELECT THE MOST APPROPRIATE ANSWER:

786. THE MOST COMMON CONGENITAL DEFECT ASSOCIATED WITH
      PULMONARY STENOSIS IS:
      A. Right bundle branch block
      B. Ventricular-septal defect
      C. Atrial septal defect
      D. Patent foramen ovale
      E. Patent ductus arteriosus   Ref. p. 686

ANSWER THE FOLLOWING STATEMENT T(RUE) OR F(ALSE):

787. Infundibular pulmonic stenosis which accounts for 5-10 per cent of the
      pulmonic stenosis patients usually presents with a post-stenotic dilatation
      earlier than the true pulmonary stenosis.
                                            Ref. p. 686

SELECT THE MOST APPROPRIATE ANSWER(S):

788. THE DIAGNOSIS OF PULMONARY STENOSIS SHOULD INCLUDE WHICH
      OF THE FOLLOWING?:
      A. Loud systolic murmur   D. Cyanosis
      B. Weak pulmonic second sound   E. Diastolic murmur
      C. Right ventricular enlargement Ref. p. 688

789. THE RIGHT VENTRICULAR PRESSURE NORMALLY_____FOLLOW-
      ING PULMONIC VALVE SURGICAL CORRECTION:
      A. Drops but still remains high
      B. Does not change
      C. Returns to normal baseline level   Ref. p. 689

790. WHICH OF THESE FACTS ARE TRUE ABOUT CONGENITAL AORTIC
      VALVULAR STENOSIS?:
      A. More common in females
      B. Calcification is common below age of 17-18 years of age
      C. Post-stenotic dilatation is common
      D. Rheumatic fever is a frequent cause
      E. All of the above   Ref. p. 690

791. A PEAK SYSTOLIC GRADIENT BETWEEN THE LEFT VENTRICLE AND
      THE AORTA OF 70 mmHg INDICATES WHICH OF THE FOLLOWING?:
      A. Mild disability not requiring surgery
      B. Moderate disability requiring surgery
      C. Severe disability requiring surgery
      D. Severe disability requiring no surgery
                                            Ref. p. 690

792. IN PREDUCTAL (INFANTILE) COARCTATION OF THE AORTA, WHICH
      OF THE FOLLOWING MAY OCCUR?:
      A. Cyanosis of the lower half of the body
      B. Pulmonary congestion
      C. Left to right shunt
      D. Right to left shunt
      E. All of the above   Ref. p. 696

793. POSTOPERATIVE COMPLICATIONS FROM SURGICAL REPAIR OF
      AORTIC COARCTATION INCLUDE:
      A. Hoarseness
      B. Paradoxical hypertension
      C. Paraplegia
      D. Abdominal pain with developing intestinal necrosis
      E. All of the above   Ref. p. 698

794. THE INNOMINATE ARTERY EMBRYOLOGICALLY DEVELOPS FROM
WHICH OF THE FOLLOWING?:

A. 2nd   D. 5th
B. 3rd   E. 6th
C. 4th   Ref. p. 701

795. WHICH DEFECTS ARE COMMONLY ASSOCIATED WITH OSTIUM PRIMUM
DEFECTS AND ATRIOVENTRICULAR CANAL MALFORMATIONS?:

A. Mitral insufficiency   D. Tricuspid insufficiency
B. Aortic stenosis   E. Mitral stenosis
C. Pulmonary stenosis   Ref. p. 704

ANSWER THE FOLLOWING QUESTION BY USING THE KEY
OUTLINED BELOW:

A. If both statement and reason are correct and related cause and effect
B. If both statement and reason are correct but not related cause and effect
C. If statement is true but reason is false
D. If statement is false but reason is true
E. If both statement and reason are false

796. Atrial septal defect is not commonly picked up in many adults BECAUSE
the shunting of blood does not develop until full muscular development of
the left ventricle occurs.   Ref. p. 704

SELECT THE MOST APPROPRIATE ANSWER(S):

797. CONTRAINDICATIONS TO SURGERY IN PATIENTS WITH AN ATRIAL
SEPTAL DEFECT ARE:

A. Patients over 50 years of age
B. Pulmonary hypertension with increased pulmonary vascular resistance
C. Pulmonary blood flow one to two times greater than systemic flow
D. Pulmonary hypertension without increased pulmonary vascular resist-
ance
E. All of the above   Ref. p. 705

798. TOTAL ANOMALOUS DRAINAGE OF PULMONARY VEINS IS:

A. Not compatible with life
B. Occurs almost always with an ASD which permits survival
C. Not differentiated from ASD by X-ray or cardiac catheterization
D. None of the above   Ref. p. 707

799. THE PRINCIPAL PROBLEM IN THE REPAIR OF OSTIUM PRIMUM
DEFECT IS RELATED TO:

A. Inadequate repair of mitral insufficiency
B. Failure to close the septal defect
C. Production of heart block without recognition
D. Inadequate repair of tricuspid insufficiency
E. All of the above   Ref. p. 711

800. THE TERM CYANOTIC TETRALOGY OF FALLOT RESULTS FROM:

A. A pulmonary blood flow greater than the systemic blood flow
B. A systemic blood flow greater than the pulmonary blood flow
C. None of the above   Ref. p. 714

801. THE SIZE OF THE SHUNT IN A VENTRICULAR SEPTAL DEFECT CAN
BE CALCULATED BY:

A. An increase in oxygen saturation by 100% from right atrium to right
ventricle
B. Ratio between the pulmonary and systemic blood flow
C. Cardiac catheterization with measurement of pressures in right and
left ventricles
D. None of the above
E. All of the above   Ref. p. 714

ANSWER THE FOLLOWING QUESTIONS BY USING THE KEY
OUTLINED BELOW:
A. If both statement and reason are correct and related cause and effect
B. If both statement and reason are correct but not related cause and effect
C. If statement is true but reason is false
D. If statement is false but reason is true
E. If both statement and reason are false

802. Ventricular septal defects frequently develop pulmonary hypertension
      BECAUSE they go into cardiac failure early.
                                              Ref. p. 714

803. The life expectancy in patients with a ventricular septal defect is about
      40 years BECAUSE this is the time it takes for the pulmonary flow to be-
      come twice the systemic.   Ref. p. 714

      SELECT THE MOST APPROPRIATE ANSWER(S):

804. WHICH OF THE FOLLOWING STATEMENTS CONCERNING PATIENTS
      WITH VSD IS NOT VALID?:
      A. Endocarditis is not a complication
      B. Pulmonary hypertension frequently develops
      C. Cardiac failure is often present
      D. The life expectancy in an uncorrected VSD is about 40 years
      E. All of the above are correct   Ref. p. 714

805. THE OPERATION OF CHOICE IN A TWO-MONTH OLD INFANT WITH
      CONGESTIVE HEART FAILURE DUE TO A VENTRICULAR SEPTAL
      DEFECT IS:
      A. Patch repair of defect
      B. Banding of pulmonary artery
      C. Create an atrial defect 1/2 the size of the VSD
      D. None of the above   Ref. p. 715

806. WHICH OF THE FOLLOWING FACTORS WOULD ENCOURAGE A
      SURGEON TO OPERATE EARLIER ON A VSD?:
      A. Retardation of growth in a child
      B. The development of cyanosis
      C. The development of bacterial endocarditis
      D. Development of pulmonary hypertension
      E. Pulmonary vascular resistance of greater than 1/2 the systemic
          vascular resistance   Ref. p. 715

807. THE STIMULUS FOR CLOSURE OF A PATENT DUCTUS ARTERIOSUS IS:
      A. Expansion of the lungs
      B. Change in arterial CO_2 tension
      C. Change in arterial pH
      D. Change in arterial oxygen tension
      E. All combined   Ref. p. 716

808. WHICH CONGENITAL HEART DEFECTS SIGNIFICANTLY INCREASE THE
      INCIDENCE OF BACTERIAL ENDOCARDITIS?:
      A. VSD
      B. ASD
      C. Pulmonary valvular stenosis
      D. Patent ductus arteriosus
      E. All of the above   Ref. p. 718

ANSWER THE FOLLOWING QUESTIONS BY USING THE KEY
OUTLINED BELOW:
A. If both statement and reason are correct and related cause and effect
B. If both statement and reason are correct but not related cause and effect
C. If statement is true but reason is false
D. If statement is false but reason is true
E. If both statement and reason are false

809. The development of bacterial endocarditis when relative to congenital heart
lesions is universally uncommon BECAUSE it appears to be related to
blood flow under a high pressure system.
Ref. p. 718

810. Surgery for a patent ductus arteriosus is almost always indicated
BECAUSE the contraindication is the development of cyanosis.
Ref. p. 719

SELECT THE MOST APPROPRIATE ANSWER:

811. THE PRIMARY CAUSE OF EARLY DEATH IN TETRALOGY OF
FALLOT IS:
A. Brain abscess
B. Gastrointestinal hemorrhage
C. Cerebral vascular accident due to thrombus formation
D. Bacterial endocarditis
E. All of the above are equally responsible
Ref. p. 722

MATCH THE FOLLOWING TO DIFFERENTIATE TETRALOGY OF FALLOT
FROM THE FOLLOWING DISEASE STATES:

812. ___ Tricuspid atresia
813. ___ Pulmonary valve stenosis
plus patent foramen ovale
814. ___ Transposition of great
vessels
815. ___ Tetralogy of Fallot

A. Normal heart size
B. Left axis deviation on EKG
C. Right cardiac enlargement (CHF)
D. Increase in pulmonary vascular
markings
Ref. p. 723

SELECT THE MOST APPROPRIATE ANSWER:

816. THE MOST COMMON INDICATION FOR POSTOPERATIVE REEXPLORA-
TION FOLLOWING REPAIR OF A TETRALOGY IS:
A. Cardiac failure
B. Hemorrhage
C. Inadequate repair of VSD
D. Pulmonary insufficiency
E. Aortic obstruction
Ref. p. 727

817. THE MOST FREQUENT CAUSE OF DYSPNEA IS:
A. Left heart failure
B. Myocardial infarction
C. Pulmonary infarction
D. Anxiety
E. Mitral stenosis
Ref. p. 750

818. SYNCOPE AS A COMPLICATION OF HEART DISEASE APPEARS IN ALL
OF THE FOLLOWING, EXCEPT:
A. Aortic stenosis
B. Mitral stenosis
C. Tetralogy of Fallot
D. Heart block
E. Pulmonary valve stenosis
Ref. p. 750

819. THE MOST FREQUENT CAUSE OF HEMOPTYSIS IS:
A. Bronchiogenic carcinoma
B. Pulmonary tuberculosis
C. Pulmonary embolism
D. Mitral stenosis
E. Bronchiectasis
Ref. p. 750

820. A BOUNDING PULSE IS THE RESULT OF A WIDE PULSE PRESSURE.
     THIS CAN BE FOUND IN ALL, <u>EXCEPT</u>:
     A. Aortic insufficiency   D. Pregnancy
     B. Patent ductus arteriosus   E. Hypothyroidism
     C. Peripheral A-V fistula   Ref. p. 751

821. A HARSH HOLOSYSTOLIC MURMUR FOUND ALONG THE LOWER LEFT
     STERNAL BORDER IS INDICATIVE OF:
     A. Patent ductus arteriosus
     B. Atrial septal defect
     C. Ventricular septal defect
     D. Pericarditis
     E. All of the above   Ref. p. 751

822. WHICH OF THE FOLLOWING X-RAY VIEWS WOULD BEST DEMON-
     STRATE LEFT VENTRICULAR ENLARGEMENT ?:
     A. Right anterior oblique position
     B. Left anterior oblique position
     C. Lateral view
     D. Posterior anterior view
     E. None of the above   Ref. p. 751

823. THE PRESENCE OF "KERLEY LINES" IS INDICATIVE OF:
     A. Pulmonary edema
     B. Left atrial pressures over 20 mmHg
     C. Increased pulmonary resistance
     D. Tetralogy of Fallot
     E. Pulmonary hypertension   Ref. p. 752

824. IN AORTIC OR MITRAL INSUFFICIENCY, WHICH OF THE FOLLOWING
     IS MOST VALUABLE ?:
     A. Sones technique
     B. Cardiac catheterization and differential oxygen changes
     C. Cardiac catheterization and differential chamber pressures
     D. Cineangiography
     E. All are equally useful   Ref. p. 752

825. WHAT IS THE MORTALITY RATE DUE TO CEREBRAL EMBOLISM OF
     UNOPERATED PATIENTS WITH MITRAL STENOSIS WHO ARE
     FIBRILLATING ?:
     A. 5%   D. 45%
     B. 15%   E. 65%
     C. 25%   Ref. p. 752

826. THE DEVELOPMENT OF DYSPNEA, SYNCOPE AND CHEST PAIN IN
     ASSOCIATION WITH AORTIC STENOSIS IS AN INDICATION FOR IM-
     MEDIATE SURGERY BECAUSE OF THE DEVELOPMENT OF WHICH OF
     THE FOLLOWING ?:
     A. Sudden death
     B. Cerebral embolism
     C. Atrial fibrillation
     D. Severe decompensation with pulmonary hypertension
     E. All of the above   Ref. p. 752

     ANSWER THE FOLLOWING QUESTION BY USING THE KEY
     OUTLINED BELOW:
     A. If both statement and reason are correct and related cause and effect
     B. If both statement and reason are correct but not related cause and effect
     C. If statement is true but reason is false
     D. If statement is false but reason is true
     E. If both statement and reason are false

827. In patients with aortic stenosis the worst prognostic sign is frequent
     anginal episodes BECAUSE few patients with this survive over one to two
     years.   Ref. p. 752

SELECT THE MOST APPROPRIATE ANSWER:

828. PULMONARY HYPERTENSION IN ACQUIRED MITRAL STENOSIS AS
OPPOSED TO THAT ASSOCIATED WITH CONGENITAL VENTRICULAR
SEPTAL DEFECT APPLIES TO WHICH OF THE FOLLOWING?:
   A. Never improves after surgery
   B. Is a contraindication for surgery
   C. Carries a lower mortality rate
   D. Improves after surgery
   E. Indicates that a heart lung machine is not essential for an adequate
      repair   Ref. p. 753

829. THE PRESENT DAY PUMP OXYGENATORS FOR BYPASS CREATE
_____FLOW:
   A. Nonpulsatile
   B. Pulsatile
   C. Both   Ref. p. 753

830. WHICH OF THE FOLLOWING REQUIRES THE LEAST BLOOD IN
"PRIMING" THE PUMP OXYGENATOR?:
   A. Disc oxygenator
   B. Screen oxygenator
   C. Bubble oxygenator
   D. All are about equal   Ref. pp. 753-754

831. WHICH OF THE FOLLOWING IS MORE IMPORTANT WITH A PATIENT
ON BYPASS?:
   A. Mean arterial pressure
   B. Flow rate
   C. Both are equal   Ref. p. 753

832. THE MOST IMPORTANT GUIDE FOR TAKING A PATIENT OFF BYPASS
IS WHICH OF THE FOLLOWING?:
   A. Central venous pressure of 6 cm H_2O
   B. A left atrial pressure between 15 and 20 mmHg
   C. A hematocrit of at least 32%
   D. A blood pressure of at least 100/80 mmHg
                                            Ref. p. 754

833. IMMEDIATE COMPLICATION OF EXTRACORPOREAL BYPASS INCLUDES:
   A. Renal insufficiency   D. Psychosis
   B. Respiratory insufficiency   E. All of the above
   C. Bleeding tendency   Ref. p. 755

834. WHICH OF THE FOLLOWING IS OF THE GREATEST VALUE IN FOL-
LOWING THE POSTOPERATIVE CARE AFTER CARDIAC SURGERY?:
   A. Intra-arterial pressure   D. Electrocardiogram
   B. Central venous pressure   E. Serial hematocrits
   C. Left atrial pressure   Ref. p. 755

835. THE NORMAL MIXED VENOUS OXYGEN SATURATION SHOULD BE
GREATER THAN_____PER CENT:
   A. 40-45
   B. 50-60
   C. Over 60   Ref. p. 756

836. THE PERICARDIOTOMY SYNDROME OF DRESDALE CLINICALLY
PRESENTS WITH:
A. Fever
B. Friction rub
C. Pericardial effusion or pleural effusion
D. Lymphatic round cell infiltration
E. All of the above   Ref. p. 758

837. THE MOST APPROPRIATE TREATMENT OF THE PERICARDIOTOMY
SYNDROME IS:
A. Heparin   D. Peritoneal dialysis
B. Prednisone   E. Blood transfusions
C. Epsilon aminocaproic acid Ref. p. 758

838. THE FIRST STEP IN CARDIAC RESUSCITATION IS:
A. Cardiac massage   D. Vasopressor instillation
B. Bicarbonate administration E. Hypothermia
C. Ventilation   Ref. p. 760

ANSWER THE FOLLOWING STATEMENT T(RUE) OR F(ALSE):

839. In mitral stenosis, the indication to perform the operative procedure on
bypass is often a result of the fibrosis and shortening of the chordae
tendini.   Ref. p. 762

SELECT THE MOST APPROPRIATE ANSWER:

840. A CLASS III MITRAL STENOSIS HAS A VALVE CROSS SECTION
DIAMETER OF_____CM:
A. 4-6   D. 1
B. 2-2.5   E. 0.3-0.4
C. 1-2   Ref. p. 763

841. WHICH OF THE FOLLOWING PHYSIOLOGIC CHANGES OCCUR IN
SEVERE MITRAL STENOSIS?:
A. Increase in peripheral vascular resistance
B. Increase in cardiac output
C. Decrease in pulmonary vascular hypertension
D. Increase in left atrial pressure
E. Decrease in central venous pressure
                                    Ref. p. 763

842. A HEAVING LEFT VENTRICULAR IMPULSE ON PHYSICAL EXAMINA-
TION IN PATIENTS WITH MITRAL STENOSIS APPLIES TO WHICH OF
THE FOLLOWING?:
A. Is usual for stenotic lesions of 1 to 2 cm
B. Is indicative of associated cardiac disease
C. Is usual for all levels of the disease
D. Indicates severe decompensation
E. All of the above   Ref. p. 764

SELECT THE MOST APPROPRIATE ANSWER:

843. A GRADIENT OF 10 TO 20 mmHg BETWEEN THE LEFT ATRIUM AND
LEFT VENTRICLE IS INDICATIVE OF:
A. Cor triatriatum   D. Patent ductus arteriosus
B. Single ventricle   E. All of the above
C. Mitral stenosis   Ref. pp. 766-771

844. THE POST PERICARDIOTOMY SYNDROME DEVELOPS FOLLOWING
MITRAL VALVE REPLACEMENT IN_____PER CENT OF THE
CASES:
A. 5   D. 25-35
B. 10-15   E. 35-45
C. 15-25   Ref. pp. 766-771

ANSWER THE FOLLOWING QUESTION BY USING THE KEY
OUTLINED BELOW:
A. If both statement and reason are correct and related cause and effect
B. If both statement and reason are correct but not related cause and effect
C. If statement is true but reason is false
D. If statement is false but reason is true
E. If both statement and reason are false

845. In patients with mitral stenosis, the larger the left atrium, the greater the
chance of sudden decompensation BECAUSE there is direct correlation
between the size of the left atrium and the severity of the disease.
                              Ref. p. 768
SELECT THE MOST APPROPRIATE ANSWER:

846. THE DIFFERENCE BETWEEN MITRAL INSUFFICIENCY (MI) AND
MITRAL STENOSIS (MS) IS:
A. A diastolic gradient between left atrium and left ventricle in MS
B. A systolic spike, almost to ventricular levels in MI
C. No diastolic gradient in MI
D. All of the above   Ref. p. 772

847. IN MITRAL INSUFFICIENCY, THE INCIDENCE OF PROSTHETIC VALVE
THROMBOEMBOLISM IS_____WITHIN TWO YEARS:
A. 5-10%   D. 45-55%
B. 20-25%   E. 65-75%
C. 30-35%   Ref. p. 774

848. IN MITRAL INSUFFICIENCY, WHICH OF THE FOLLOWING IS THE
PREFERRED SURGICAL PROCEDURE?:
A. Prosthetic valve insertion
B. Annuloplasty
C. Both give equally favorable results   Ref. p. 774

849. DEVELOPMENT OF WHICH OF THE FOLLOWING IS THE MOST
OMINOUS SIGN IN AORTIC STENOSIS?:
A. Angina pectoris
B. Syncope
C. Left ventricular failure
D. Left ventricular hypertrophy   Ref. p. 775

850. INDICATIONS FOR SURGICAL INTERVENTION IN A PATIENT WITH
AORTIC STENOSIS INCLUDES ALL, EXCEPT:
A. Syncope
B. Angina pectoris
C. Congestive heart failure
D. Pressure gradient over 50 mmHg across the stenotic valve
E. Calcification of the stenotic valve   Ref. p. 776

851. WHICH HAS A LOWER MORTALITY RATE?:
    A. Mitral stenosis with prosthetic valve replacement
    B. Aortic stenosis with prosthetic valve replacement
    C. Equal   Ref. p. 779

ANSWER THE FOLLOWING STATEMENT T(RUE) OR F(ALSE):

852. In aortic insufficiency, the left ventricular end diastolic pressure does not
    become elevated until cardiac failure develops.
                                                Ref. p. 781

SELECT THE MOST APPROPRIATE ANSWER(S):

853. THE ETIOLOGY OF TRICUSPID VALVE DISEASE INCLUDES WHICH OF
    THE FOLLOWING:
    A. Rheumatic fever
    B. Syphilis
    C. Polyarteritis nodosum
    D. Annular dilatation secondary to pulmonary hypertension
    E. Bacterial endocarditis   Ref. p. 781

854. THE MAJOR PRINCIPLE FOR VENTRICULAR ANEURYSMIC RESECTION IS:
    A. To decrease asynchronous myocardial contractions and energy dissipation
    B. To prevent embolization of omnipresent mural thrombus
    C. Both of the above
                                                Ref. p. 799

855. THE MOST FREQUENT KNOWN CAUSE OF CONSTRICTIVE PERI-
    CARDITIS IS:
    A. Viral pericarditis
    B. Calcification of hemopericardium
    C. Leukemic infiltration with subsequent calcification
    D. Tuberculosis
    E. Unknown   Ref. p. 802

856. IN THE REMOVAL OF CALCIFIED PERICARDIAL SAC, WHICH PORTION
    IS EXCISED FIRST?:
    A. Over the right atrium   D. Over the left ventricle
    B. Over the right ventricle   E. It makes little difference
    C. Over the left atrium   Ref. p. 680 (1st Ed.)

857. CONSTRICTIVE PERICARDITIS PRESENTS WITH ALL OF THE
    FOLLOWING, EXCEPT:
    A. An increase in central venous pressure to 15-40 cm H_2O
    B. A decrease in cardiac output
    C. A decrease in diastolic filling
    D. Cyanosis
    E. Hepatomegaly, ascites and peripheral edema
                                                Ref. p. 802

858. THE MOST FREQUENT COMPLICATION OF PACEMAKER INSERTION IS:
    A. Perforation of the right ventricle
    B. Competition between fixed rate pacemaker and heart during vulnerable
       phase resulting
    C. Infection - bacterial endocarditis
    D. Power pack failure and return to patient's heartblock pattern
    E. Wire breakage following insertion   Ref. p. 807

859. MOST POWER UNITS HAVE TO BE CHANGED EVERY TWO YEARS. THE
     PRESENTING SYMPTOM(S) OF FAILURE IS (ARE):
     A. Increasing tachycardia
     B. Return to heartblock rhythm
     C. Both of the above   Ref. p. 807

860. THE HIGHEST MORTALITY IN ANIMAL CARDIAC TRANSPLANTATION
     RESULTS FROM:
     A. Acute rejection
     B. Pneumonitis due to immunosuppressive therapy
     C. Renal shut-down
     D. Carcinomatosis
     E. None of the above   Ref. p. 808

861. THE PRINCIPLE OF COUNTERPULSATION IN ASSISTED CIRCULATION
     SYNCHRONIZES THE PROSTHETIC DEVICE TO PUMP DURING DIASTOLE
     AND DECREASE THE VENTRICULAR WORK LOAD DURING SYSTOLE.
     AN EXAMPLE OF THIS IS:
     A. Venovenous by-pass
     B. Arteriovenous by-pass
     C. Intraaortic balloon pump
     D. The mechanical heart lung by-pass
     E. All of the above   Ref. p. 809

862. ANEURYSMS OF THE ASCENDING AORTA ARE DUE TO DEGENERATIVE
     CYSTIC MEDIAL NECROSIS. WHICH OF THE FOLLOWING DISEASE
     STATES ARE MOST OFTEN ASSOCIATED WITH THIS CONDITION?:
     A. Marfan's syndrome   D. All of the above
     B. Erdheim's disease   E. None of the above
     C. Syphilis   Ref. p. 815

863. THE PRIMARY DISABILITY WHICH LEADS TO DEATH IN PATIENTS
     WITH ANEURYSMS OF THE ASCENDING AORTA IS:
     A. Hemorrhage from acute rupture
     B. Vena cava compression from expanding saccular aneurysm
     C. Aortic valvular insufficiency
     D. Coronary artery compression from aneurysm
     E. Pulmonary artery obstruction   Ref. p. 815

864. TRAUMATIC THORACIC AORTIC ANEURYSMS OFTEN:
     A. Rupture early causing sudden death
     B. Rupture late
     C. Act as syphilitic aneurysms
     D. Progressively enlarge but do not rupture
     E. Require surgery within a week of their diagnosis
                                              Ref. p. 817

865. HOW LONG IS THE MINIMAL TIME FOR WHICH ISCHEMIA MAY BE
     TOLERATED BEFORE PARAPLEGIA WILL DEVELOP?:
     A. 6 minutes   D. 50 minutes
     B. 18 minutes   E. 120 minutes
     C. 30 minutes   Ref. p. 820

866. ANEURYSMS OF THE DESCENDING AORTA ARE:
     A. More often saccular
     B. More often fusiform
     C. Equal in incidence   Ref. p. 821

867. WHICH OF THE FOLLOWING HAVE A GREATER TENDENCY TO
     RUPTURE?:
     A. Saccular aneurysms
     B. Fusiform aneurysms
     C. Both A and B are equal   Ref. p. 821

868.   COMPLICATIONS FOLLOWING RESECTION FOR ANEURYSM OF THE
        DESCENDING THORACIC AORTA INCLUDE:
        A. Hemorrhage into the thoracic cavity
        B. Renal shut-down
        C. Paraplegia
        D. All of the above
        E. None of the above   Ref. p. 822

869.   THE MOST COMMON CAUSE OF HYPOTENSION DURING DESCENDING
        THORACIC AORTIC ANEURYSMIC DISSECTION IS:
        A. Acute myocardial infarction
        B. Hemorrhagic hypovolemia
        C. Decrease return on by-pass
        D. Peripheral vasodilatation due to neurologic damage
        E. None of the above   Ref. p. 823

870.   THE INCIDENCE OF DISSECTING AORTIC ANEURYSMS IS INCREASED
        IN WHICH OF THE FOLLOWING?:
        A. Pregnancy   D. Coarctation
        B. Marfan's syndrome   E. All of the above
        C. Idiopathic kyphoscoliosis   Ref. p. 825

871.   THE MOST FREQUENT DISSECTING ANEURYSM OF THE AORTA IS OF
        WHICH OF THE FOLLOWING TYPES?:
        A. A
        B. B
        C. C_1
        D. C_2 Ref. p. 826

872.   DISSECTING AORTIC ANEURYSMS TREATED BY THE FENESTRATION
        OPERATION:
        A. All improve
        B. Usually do not stop dissecting
        C. Develop a high incidence of left ventricular failure
        D. Continue to rupture with the same incidence as before the operation
        E. Have a high operative mortality   Ref. p. 827

        FILL IN THE MOST APPROPRIATE ANSWERS: (Questions 873-874)

        A. 40-50 per cent
        B. 50-60 per cent
        C. 60-70 per cent
        D. 70-80 per cent
        E. 80-90 per cent

        The mortality rate of a dissecting aortic aneurysm in the first two weeks
        is 873) _____ ; within the first year it is 874)_____ .
                                         Ref. p. 828

        SELECT THE MOST APPROPRIATE ANSWER:

875.   CONSERVATIVE TREATMENT OF DISSECTING AORTIC ANEURYSMS
        BY WHEAT et al. UTILIZES WHICH OF THE FOLLOWING?:
        A. Vasopressors
        B. Antihypertensives
        C. Plasmacentesis   Ref. p. 829

876.   CLAUDICATION INTERMITTENTS AT THE LEVEL OF THE HIP IS
        INDICATIVE OF:
        A. Common femoral artery occlusion
        B. Superficial femoral artery occlusion
        C. Bilateral iliac artery occlusion
        D. Popliteal artery occlusion
        E. Iliac vein occlusion   Ref. p. 840

877. IN VASCULAR DISEASE OF THE EXTREMITIES WHICH OF THE FOL-
      LOWING CARRIES GREATER VALUE ?:
      A. Physical examination
      B. Angiography
      C. Both are of equal value   Ref. p. 840

878. THE TIME PERIOD FROM THE DEVELOPMENT OF AN ACUTE OCCLU-
      SION TO THE ONSET OF TISSUE NECROSIS IS ABOUT:
      A. 2-4 hours   D. 16-32 hours
      B. 4-8 hours   E. 32-72 hours
      C. 8-16 hours   Ref. p. 841

879. THE MOST SENSITIVE PHYSICAL FINDING IN EVALUATING THE
      SEVERITY OF AN ARTERIAL OCCLUSION IS:
      A. Pain   D. Absent pulses
      B. Pallor   E. All are equal
      C. Paralysis and paresthesias Ref. p. 841

880. THE DISTINGUISHING CHARACTERISTICS OF CHRONIC ARTERIAL
      INSUFFICIENCY INCLUDE ALL EXCEPT:
      A. Loss of hair from digits
      B. Brittle opaque nails
      C. Skin atrophy
      D. Dependent rubor
      E. Claudication
      F. Cold susceptibility
      G. All of the above   Ref. p. 842

      FILL IN THE MOST APPROPRIATE ANSWERS: (Questions 881-882)

      A. Cervical rib
      B. Raynaud's disease
      C. Buerger's disease
      D. Atherosclerosis
      E. Embolization from the left atrium

      The most common cause of chronic arterial occlusion in the upper ex-
      tremity is 881)_____, in the lower extremity 882)_____.
                                         Ref. p. 842

      SELECT THE MOST APPROPRIATE ANSWER:

883. THE MOST COMMON POSTOPERATIVE COMPLICATION FOLLOWING A
      LUMBAR SYMPATHECTOMY IS:
      A. Impotence   D. Constipation
      B. Intestinal ileus   E. All of the above are common
      C. Acute bladder retention   Ref. p. 844

884. WITH FEMOROPOPLITEAL OBSTRUCTION PRODUCING CLAUDICA-
      TION AND NO EVIDENCE OF TROPHIC CHANGES:
      A. Surgery should be performed
      B. Surgery should be held off
      C. Surgeon's choice   Ref. p. 848

885. INTERMITTENT CLAUDICATION OF ONE BLOCK OR LESS IS MORE
      FREQUENTLY FOUND IN:
      A. Aorto-iliac obstruction
      B. Femoro-popliteal obstruction
      C. Occurs equally in both A and B   Ref. p. 848

886. WITH POPLITEAL ARTERY OBSTRUCTION, THE DECISION AS TO
     OPERABILITY IS MADE BY:
     A. Arteriography
     B. Physical examination and clinical estimation
     C. Neither   Ref. p. 848

887. LUMBAR SYMPATHECTOMY IS USEFUL PRIMARILY IN:
     A. Patients with claudication
     B. Patients with trophic changes
     C. Neither   Ref. p. 849

888. A SAPHENOUS VEIN BY-PASS GRAFT IN A FEMORO-POPLITEAL
     OPERATION SHOULD HAVE A MINIMUM DIAMETER OF:
     A. 3 mm   D. 10 mm
     B. 5 mm   E. 20 mm
     C. 8 mm   Ref. p. 849

889. THE FIVE YEAR PATENCY RATE WITH PROSTHETIC MATERIAL IS
     _____PER CENT:
     A. 10-20
     B. 20-30
     C. 30-40
     D. 40-50
     E. 50-60
     F. 60-70   Ref. p. 849

890. THE PATENCY RATE WITH A SAPHENOUS VEIN GRAFT IS:
     A. 10-20 per cent   D. 60-80 per cent
     B. 20-40 per cent   E. 80-100 per cent
     C. 40-60 per cent   Ref. p. 852

891. THE MOST FREQUENT CAUSE OF ARTERIAL EMBOLISM IS OF
     CARDIAC ORIGIN. WHICH OF THE FOLLOWING IS(ARE) MOST
     OFTEN RESPONSIBLE?:
     A. Mitral stenosis
     B. Atrial fibrillation
     C. Myocardial infarction
     D. Venous embolization in a patient with VSD or ASD
     E. All of the above are equally as common
                                              Ref. p. 857

892. THE INDICATION FOR AN ARTERIOGRAM IN ACUTE ARTERIAL
     THROMBOSIS IS:
     A. To confirm the diagnosis
     B. To localize the coagulum
     C. To evaluate patency of the distal vascular bed
     D. To visualize the adequacy of collateral circulation
     E. All of the above   Ref. p. 858

893. THE MOST RELIABLE SURGICAL FINDING TO INDICATE THE COM-
     PLETE REMOVAL OF PERIPHERAL EMBOLI IS:
     A. Back-bleeding
     B. Extraction of a long smooth solitary clot
     C. Extraction of primarily white coagulum
     D. There is no reliable clinical finding
                                              Ref. p. 859

894. SURGERY PERFORMED WITHIN A 4 TO 6 HOUR PERIOD AFTER AN
     ARTERIAL EMBOLUS CARRIES A SUCCESS RATE OF_____PER CENT:
     A. 15   D. 75
     B. 35   E. 95
     C. 55   Ref. p. 861

895. WITH BUERGER'S DISEASE, WHICH OF THE FOLLOWING IS NOT TRUE?:
A. Superficial migratory phlebitis is present
B. Most common symptom is claudication
C. Rest pain is a grave symptom
D. Increased sensitivity to cold is noted
E. Absence of posterior tibial and dorsal pedis vessels is noted
                                        Ref. p. 865

896. THE TISSUES WHICH RESPOND MOST RAPIDLY TO ISCHEMIC ANOXIA
ARE:
A. Skin   D. Striated muscle
B. Nerve   E. All respond equally
C. Tendon   Ref. p. 868

FILL IN THE MOST APPROPRIATE ANSWERS: (Questions 897-898)

A. 10
B. 30
C. 50
D. 70
E. 90

A vascular repair within 6 to 8 hours following trauma carries a success
rate of 897)_____per cent and after 12 hours the rate is 898)_____per cent.
                                        Ref. p. 868

SELECT THE MOST APPROPRIATE ANSWER(S):

899. IT IS PREFERABLE NOT TO USE AN ARTIFICIAL ARTERIAL GRAFT OF
LESS THAN_____MM DIAMETER BECAUSE OF THE HIGH INCI-
DENCE OF THROMBOSIS:
A. 2   D. 10
B. 4   E. 18
C. 8   Ref. p. 869

900. THE ANTERIOR COMPARTMENT SYNDROME IS A MANIFESTATION OF
INTRACOMPARTMENTAL PRESSURE. WHICH OF THE FOLLOWING
IS THE MOST OMNIOUS SIGN?:
A. Absence of pulsus dorsalis pedis
B. Loss of motor power of extensor digitorum brevis
C. Paralyzed extensor digitorum longus
D. Paralyzed extensor hallucis longus
E. None of the above   Ref. p. 870

901. WHICH OF THE FOLLOWING STRUCTURES ARE NOT WITHIN THE
ANTERIOR TIBIAL COMPARTMENT?:
A. Extensor hallis longus
B. Extensor digitorum longus
C. Extensor digitorum brevis
D. Anterior tibial artery
E. Peroneal nerve
F. All of the above   Ref. p. 870

902. THE MAJOR WAY TO DISTINGUISH BETWEEN THE TWO STATES IS BY:
A. Size   D. Pain
B. History   E. Pulsations
C. Auscultatory findings   Ref. pp. 871-872

903. WHICH OF THE FOLLOWING DOES NOT OCCUR AFTER AN ARTERIO-
VENOUS FISTULA IN THE FEMORAL AREA?:
A. Decreased peripheral resistance
B. Increased in cardiac output
C. Increase in venous pressure
D. Increase in diastolic pressure
E. Increase in heart size   Ref. p. 871

904.   IN WHICH OF THE FOLLOWING DOES A HEMATOMA PLAY A
       GREATER ROLE ?:
       A. True aneurysm
       B. False aneurysm
       C. Neither
       D. Both   Ref. p. 871

905.   A MASS IN THE FEMORAL AREA INCREASING IN SIZE, RED, TENDER
       AND WARM CAN BE:
       A. Abscess   D. False aneurysm
       B. Malignant degeneration   E. All of the above
       C. Tuberculosis   Ref. p. 872

906.   THE BRANHAM'S SIGN IS:
       A. A thrill felt over the A-V fistula
       B. The development of a bradycardia with digital compression of the
          fistula
       C. A machine murmur present over the A-V fistula
       D. Demonstration of unilateral varicosities
       E. Increase in pulse pressure   Ref. p. 872

907.   THE MOST FREQUENT SYMPTOM ASSOCIATED WITH THE THORACIC
       OUTLET SYNDROME IS:
       A. Pain with ulnar distribution
       B. Pain with radial nerve distribution
       C. Paresthesia
       D. Intermittent claudication with exercise
       E. Gangrene of the digits   Ref. p. 877

908.   THE ADSON TEST FOR THE THORACIC OUTLET SYNDROME IS
       POSITIVE WHEN:
       A. Numbness and tingling of the fingers develop
       B. Pallor of the hand is noted
       C. The development of acrocyanosis occurs
       D. The disappearance of the radial pulse occurs
       E. All of the above   Ref. p. 877

909.   WHICH OF THE FOLLOWING DOES NOT APPEAR IN THE DIFFEREN-
       TIAL DIAGNOSIS FOR THE THORACIC OUTLET SYNDROME ?:
       A. Cervical disc
       B. Cervical arthritis
       C. Carpal tunnel syndrome
       D. Raynaud's disease
       E. All of the above should be considered
                                                    Ref. p. 879

910.   WHICH OF THE FOLLOWING TESTS ESTABLISH THE PRESENCE OF
       CAROTID ARTERY OBSTRUCTION AND ARE OVER 80 PER CENT
       ACCURATE ?:
       A. Clinical finding of a bruit below the level of the jaw
       B. Electroencephalogram
       C. Ophthalmodynamometry
       D. All of the above
       E. None of the above   Ref. pp. 883-884

911.   A PARTIAL OBSTRUCTION OF THE SUBCLAVIAN ARTERY WITH
       RETROGRADE FLOW THROUGH THE VERTEBRAL ARTERY CAUSES
       WHICH OF THE FOLLOWING ?:
       A. Ischemic neurologic symptoms in the upper extremity
       B. Ischemic cerebral symptoms
       C. Both occur simultaneously   Ref. p. 883

912. THE SYNDROME DESCRIBED IN THE PREVIOUS QUESTION IS:
   A. Carotid steal syndrome
   B. Subclavian steal syndrome
   C. Vertebral steal syndrome   Ref. p. 883

913. INDICATIONS FOR CAROTID EXPLORATION FOR VASCULAR OCCLU-
   SION SHOULD INCLUDE:
   A. Acute cerebrovascular accident with loss of consciousness
   B. Chronic stroke with permanent neurologic damage
   C. Transient ischemic attacks
   D. The presence of a bruit at the angle of the jaw with no history of
      ischemic attacks
   E. All of the above   Ref. p. 883

914. THE INCIDENCE OF RUPTURE IN ABDOMINAL AORTIC ANEURYSMS
   WITHIN ONE YEAR IS_____PER CENT:
   A. 10   D. 60
   B. 20   E. 80
   C. 40   Ref. p. 887

915. THE MOST CONSISTENT ASSOCIATED FINDING IN PATIENTS WITH
   ATHEROSCLEROTIC AORTIC ANEURYSMS ARE:
   A. Coronary artery disease
   B. Hypertension
   C. Occlusive carotid artery disease
   D. Occlusive iliac artery disease
   E. Concomitant renal artery involvement
                                  Ref. p. 887

916. THE RESISTANCE OF THE KIDNEY TO TRAUMA IS GREATER IN WHICH
   OF THE FOLLOWING STATES?:
   A. Diuretic state
   B. Dehydrated state
   C. Equal response   Ref. p. 891

917. IF DIVISION OF THE INFERIOR MESENTERIC ARTERY IS ESSENTIAL
   BECAUSE OF ITS PROXIMITY TO THE ANEURYSM, WHICH VESSELS
   SHOULD BE MAINTAINED TO PREVENT ISCHEMIC CHANGES IN THE
   LEFT COLON?:
   A. Iliac artery   D. Inferior mesenteric vein
   B. Hypogastric artery   E. All of the above
   C. Femoral artery   Ref. p. 891

918. DECLAMPING HYPOTENSION FOLLOWING AORTIC ANEURYSMIC
   SURGERY IS MOST OFTEN CAUSED BY:
   A. Sudden hypovolemia
   B. Sudden release of ischemic products from distal vessels
   C. Both A and B contribute to the effect
                                  Ref. p. 891

919. THE MOST FREQUENT POSTOPERATIVE COMPLICATION FOLLOWING
   THE RESECTION OF AN ABDOMINAL AORTIC ANEURYSM IS:
   A. Declamping hypotension
   B. Renal shut-down
   C. Peripheral plaque embolization
   D. Paralytic ileus
   E. Development of a false aneurysm   Ref. p. 891

920. THE IDEAL POSITION FOR AORTIC PROXIMAL CONTROL IN A
     RUPTURED ABDOMINAL ANEURYSM IS:
     A. Distal to renal arteries   D. Intrathoracic
     B. Proximal to renal arteries   E. None are adequate
     C. Just below the diaphragm   Ref. p. 893

921. THE MOST COMMON PERIPHERAL VASCULAR ANEURYSMS ARE NOW
     OF ATHEROSCLEROTIC ORIGIN AND APPEAR IN WHICH OF THE
     FOLLOWING AREAS?:
     A. Radial   D. Axillary
     B. Femoral   E. Iliac
     C. Popliteal   Ref. p. 894

922. WHICH OF THE FOLLOWING OCCURS WITH A GREATER FREQUENCY
     AS A COMPLICATION OF PERIPHERAL ANEURYSMS?:
     A. Rupture
     B. Embolization
     C. Both are equal   Ref. p. 894

923. THE FREQUENCY OF ASSOCIATED ANEURYSMS IN PATIENTS WITH
     FEMORAL ANEURYSMS IS:
     A. 19 per cent
     B. 39 per cent
     C. 49 per cent
     D. 59 per cent
     E. 69 per cent
     F. 79 per cent   Ref. p. 894

924. WHICH OF THE FOLLOWING IS MORE LIKELY TO BE BILATERAL IN
     ITS PRESENTATION?:
     A. Raynaud's disease
     B. Raynaud's phenomenon
     C. Both
     D. Neither   Ref. p. 901

925. RAYNAUD'S PHENOMENON INCLUDES WHICH OF THE FOLLOWING?:
     A. Pallor   D. Nail opacity and skin atrophy
     B. Cyanosis   E. Pulseless extremity
     C. Rubor   Ref. p. 901

926. ONE CAN DISTINGUISH ACROCYANOSIS FROM RAYNAUD'S DISEASE
     BY THE ABSENCE OF:
     A. Rubor in the former
     B. Pallor in the former
     C. Bilateral cyanosis
     D. Chronic ischemic changes in the periphery in the latter
     E. All of the above   Ref. p. 903

927. THE USE OF SYMPATHECTOMY FOR HYPERHIDROSIS RESULTING
     FROM FROSTBITE IS:
     A. Considered to be of little value
     B. Is usually successful   Ref. p. 905

     ANSWER THE FOLLOWING QUESTION BY USING THE KEY
     OUTLINED BELOW:
     A. If both statement and reason are correct and related cause and effect
     B. If both statement and reason are correct but not related cause and effect
     C. If statement is true but reason is false
     D. If statement is false but reason is true
     E. If both statement and reason are false

928. Thrombophlebitis of the peripheral venous system will usually result in
     venous valvular destruction BECAUSE this leads to a chronic form of
     peripheral valvular insufficiency.   Ref. p. 913

SELECT THE MOST APPROPRIATE ANSWER:

929. THE TREATMENT OF SUPERFICIAL THROMBOPHLEBITIS SHOULD
INCLUDE:
    A. Antibiotics
    B. Clot dissolvers
    C. Butazoladine
    D. Walking with elastic support stockings
    E. Anticoagulants
    F. All of the above   Ref. p. 914

930. WHICH OF THE FOLLOWING ARE MOST USEFUL IN STRENGTHENING
A DIAGNOSIS OF DEEP VEIN THROMBOPHLEBITIS?:
    A. Swelling
    B. Tenderness
    C. Homans' sign
    D. Dilatation of superficial venous system
    E. All of the above   Ref. p. 915

931. THE PAGET-SCHROETTER SYNDROME REFERS TO:
    A. Ileofemoral vein thrombosis
    B. Axillary vein thrombosis
    C. Pelvic vein thrombosis
    D. Femoral vein thrombosis
    E. Calf vein thrombosis   Ref. p. 915

932. THE MOST USEFUL SCREENING TESTS TO ESTABLISH THE PRESENCE
OR ABSENCE OF THROMBOSIS ARE NON-INVASIVE. WHICH OF THE
FOLLOWING IS MOST EFFECTIVE FOR SMALL VESSEL OCCLUSION?:
    A. I^{125} labeled fibrinogen
    B. Doppler/Ultrasound Technique
    C. Electrical Impedance Test   Ref. p. 917

933. LOGICAL TREATMENT OF ACUTE DEEP VEIN THROMBOPHLEBITIS
SHOULD BE CONTINUED FOR A PERIOD OF TIME TO PERMIT THE
THROMBUS TO STRONGLY ADHERE TO THE VENOUS WALL. WHICH
OF THE FOLLOWING THERAPEUTIC MEASURES APPROPRIATELY
FOLLOWS THIS ASSUMPTION?:
    A. Complete bed rest with lower extremity elevation and heparinization
       for 7 days, followed by ambulation with elastic support and tapering of
       the heparin
    B. Complete bed rest with lower extremity elevation and heparinization
       for 14 days followed by ambulation with elastic support and tapering
       of heparin
    C. Complete bed rest with extremity elevation and heparinization for 7
       days followed by ambulation without elastic support and abrupt
       cessation of heparin   Ref. p. 918

934. WHICH OF THE FOLLOWING VENOUS CONDITIONS REQUIRES THE
LONGEST PERIOD OF ANTICOAGULATION?:
    A. Calf vein thrombosis
    B. Femoral vein thrombosis
    C. Ileofemoral vein thrombosis
    D. All are equal   Ref. p. 919

935. WHICH IS RESPONSIBLE FOR A GREATER NUMBER OF PULMONARY
EMBOLI?:
    A. Right atrium
    B. Pelvic vein
    C. Both are equally responsible   Ref. p. 920

936. THE MOST USEFUL AND ACCURATE WAY OF DIAGNOSING PULMONARY
EMBOLI IS BY:
   A. Angiography   D. Electrocardiogram
   B. Lung scan   E. All are of equal value
   C. Differential gas tensions   Ref. p. 920

937. A POSTIVE-POSITIVE TRENDELENBURG TEST IS INDICATIVE OF:
   A. Incompetent valves of perforating vessels
   B. Incompetent ileofemoral valve system
   C. Both of the above   Ref. p. 927

938. A TRENDELENBURG TEST WHICH IS POSITIVE-NEGATIVE IS INDICA-
TIVE OF:
   A. Competent perforators plus incompetent saphenous valves
   B. Incompetent perforators plus incompetent saphenous valves
   C. Incompetent perforators plus competent saphenous valves
   D. Competent perforators plus competent saphenous valves
   E. None of the above   Ref. p. 927

939. WHICH IS NOT AN INDICATION FOR OPERATIVE TREATMENT OF
LOWER EXTREMITY VARICOSITIES?:
   A. Moderate to severe symptomatic varicosities
   B. Severe varicosities without symptoms
   C. Severe venous insufficiency with recurrent ulcerations
   D. Recurrent subfacial ulcerations
   E. All are indications for surgery   Ref. p. 930

940. THE MOST FREQUENT SITE OF LYMPHANGIOSARCOMA IS:
   A. Lower extremities after venous stripping
   B. Upper extremities following radical mastectomy
   C. Neck, following radical neck dissection
   D. Thoracic duct following chest surgery
   E. None of the above   Ref. p. 933

SELECT THE MOST APPROPRIATE ANSWER:

941. SURGICAL HYPERTENSION IS_____PER CENT OF OVERALL
      HYPERTENSIVES:
      A. 1-5   D. 40-50
      B. 5-10   E. 60-70
      C. 20-30   Ref. p. 939

942. WHICH OF THE FOLLOWING FACTORS INFLUENCES SYSTEMIC
      BLOOD PRESSURE?:
      A. Blood viscosity   D. Vascular elasticity
      B. Blood volume   E. All of the above
      C. Cardiac output   Ref. p. 939

943. THE CHIEF DETERMINANT IN THE DEVELOPMENT OF DIASTOLIC
      HYPERTENSION IS:
      A. Blood viscosity   D. Cardiac output
      B. Blood volume   E. Vascular elasticity
      C. Peripheral resistance   Ref. p. 939

944. WHICH OF THE FOLLOWING ARE CHARACTERISTICS OF
      ANGIOTENSIN II?:
      A. Intense vasoconstriction
      B. Stimulation of renin secretion
      C. Stimulation of aldosterone production
      D. All of the above
      E. None of the above   Ref. p. 940

945. ALDOSTERONE PRODUCTION FROM THE ADRENAL CORTEX FOLLOW-
      ING SEVERE TRAUMA MAY BE STIMULATED BY:
      A. ACTH   D. None of the above
      B. GSH   E. All of the above
      C. TSH   Ref. p. 804 (1st Ed.)

MATCH THE FOLLOWING:

946. ___ Coarctation of the aorta   A. Flushing
947. ___ Renal fibromuscular hyperplasia   B. Abdominal stria, hirsutism
948. ___ Cushing's disease   C. Decreased femoral pulsus
949. ___ Pheochromocytoma   D. Hypokalemia, muscular
950. ___ Aldosteronism   weakness
                                            E. Abdominal bruit
                                            Ref. p. 940

CASE HISTORY: (Questions 951-952)

A 30 year-old obese white male presents with diastolic hypertension of
acute onset. A complete laboratory survey reveals a VMA of 10 mg/24
hours, potassium 2.5 mEq/l, sodium 144 mEq/l, chloride 103 mEq/l,
CO_2 35 mEq/l. The urinary potassium for 24 hours is 60 mEq/l and the
urine has a pH of 7.5.

951. THE MOST LIKELY DIAGNOSIS IS:
      A. Cushing's disease
      B. Pheochromocytoma
      C. Primary aldosteronism
      D. Coarctation of the aorta
      E. Renovascular hypertension   Ref. p. 941

952. WHICH OF THE FOLLOWING LABORATORY TESTS WOULD BE MOST
      USEFUL TO SUPPORT AND LOCATE THE DISEASE ENTITY?:
      A. Catecholamine levels (both epinephrine and norepinephrine)
      B. Selective angiography
      C. Renal scan
      D. Howard test
      E. All should be performed   Ref. p. 941

      SELECT THE MOST APPROPRIATE ANSWER(S):

953. THE MOST RELIABLE LABORATORY FINDING IN PRIMARY
      ALDOSTERONISM IS:
      A. Hypokalemia
      B. Serum hyponatremia
      C. Elevated CO_2
      D. Elevated urinary sodium levels
      E. Serum hypochloremia   Ref. p. 943

954. IN THE LABORATORY EXAMINATION PERFORMED IN THE PREVIOUS
      QUESTION, WHICH OF THE FOLLOWING IS USUALLY RESPONSIBLE
      FOR UNRELIABLE RESULTS?:
      A. Prior intravenous pyelogram
      B. Failure to obtain a catheterized urine specimen
      C. Failure to restrict the dietary intake of salt
      D. Failure to perform the test during a period of hyperventilation
      E. All are common errors   Ref. p. 943

955. WHICH OF THE FOLLOWING OFTEN DISTINGUISH PRIMARY FROM
      SECONDARY ALDOSTERONISM?:
      A. Serum hypokalemia   D. Low urinary sodium level
      B. Serum aldosterone level   E. Alkalosis
      C. Low serum renin level   Ref. p. 943

956. THE MOST COMMON CAUSE OF CUSHING'S DISEASE IS:
      A. Adrenocortical tumor
      B. Bilateral adrenocortical hyperplasia
      C. Adrenal carcinoma
      D. Adrenogenital syndrome   Ref. p. 943

957. CUSHING'S DISEASE DUE TO ECTOPIC ACTH SYNDROME IS MOST
      FREQUENTLY ASSOCIATED WITH WHICH OF THE FOLLOWING?:
      A. Lung   D. Pancreas
      B. Liver   E. Lymphatic system
      C. Kidney   Ref. p. 943

958. WITH BILATERAL ADRENAL HYPERPLASIA THE TREATMENT OF
      CHOICE IS:
      A. Bilateral adrenalectomy
      B. Bilateral subtotal adrenalectomy
      C. Pituitary irradiation followed by bilateral adrenalectomy if no remis-
          sion occurs
      D. Ortho para DDD administration
      E. Bilateral thoracic sympathectomy   Ref. p. 945

959. THE MORE COMMON FORM OF SURGICAL RENOVASCULAR HYPER-
      TENSION IS:
      A. Atherosclerosis
      B. Fibromuscular hyperplasia
      C. Renal carcinoma
      D. Embolus
      E. Single mural hyperplasia   Ref. p. 946

960. THE "STRING OF BEADS" SIGN IS DIAGNOSTIC OF:
   A. Urogram is subadventitial fibroplasia
   B. Single mural hyperplasia-arteriogram
   C. Fibromuscular hyperplasia-arteriogram
   D. Renal embolization-arteriogram   Ref. p. 947

961. THE BEST SCREENING TEST FOR RENOVASCULAR DISEASE IS THE:
   A. Renal angiogram
   B. Rapid sequence excretory urogram
   C. Intravenous pyelogram
   D. Renal scan
   E. Angiotensin II assay
   F. Renin level-following selective renal vein catheterization
                                          Ref. p. 951

962. THE MAJOR WEAKNESS IN USING THE RAPID SEQUENCE UROGRAM IS:
   A. 10 per cent false positives
   B. Bilateral disease is not picked up
   C. It is only 80 per cent accurate
   D. There is a risk involved because of frequent reaction to the injected dye
   E. It does not demonstrate curable lesions
                                          Ref. p. 951

963. THE HOWARD TEST IS BASED ON:
   A. Selective reduction of urine volume of 50 per cent and increase of urine
      sodium concentration of at least 15 per cent in the involved kidney
   B. Selective reduction of urine volume of 50 per cent and in the involved
      kidney and decreased sodium concentration on the opposite
   C. Selective reduction of urine creatinine of 15 per cent on the involved
      side with a urine volume reduction of at least 50 per cent
   D. Selective reduction of urine volume of 50 per cent and decrease of
      urine sodium concentration by at least 15 per cent in the involved kid-
      ney or increase in urinary creatinine by 15 per cent
                                          Ref. p. 954

964. THE LAST TEST TO BE PERFORMED IN A RENAL STUDY FOR
   RENOVASCULAR OCCLUSION IS:
   A. Renal scan   D. Renal biopsy
   B. Selective renal arteriograms E. Creatinine clearance
   C. Split renal function studies Ref. p. 954

965. WHICH OF THE FOLLOWING IS OF MORE VALUE?:
   A. Serum renin level from peripheral blood
   B. Renin level from renal vein specimen
   C. Both are equal   Ref. p. 955

966. ALL OF THE FOLLOWING SHOULD BE INCLUDED IN THE SURGICAL
   PROCEDURE FOR RENOVASCULAR HYPERTENSION, EXCEPT:
   A. Wedge biopsy of both kidneys and frozen section
   B. Record the pressure gradient on either side of stenotic areas
   C. Try to demonstrate renal artery gradient if not obvious, with vaso-
      pressors or vasodilators
   D. Administration of reserpine during the procedure for hypertensive
      crisis
   E. Mannitol administration to promote osmotic diuresis
                                          Ref. pp. 956-958

SELECT THE MOST APPROPRIATE ANSWER:

967. IN APPENDICITIS WHICH USUALLY PRESENTS FIRST?:
     A. Pain
     B. Vomiting
     C. Both together   Ref. p. 972

968. VOMITING WITHOUT PRIOR NAUSEA IS SUGGESTIVE OF WHICH OF
     THE FOLLOWING?:
     A. Small bowel obstruction
     B. Pyloric obstruction
     C. Increased intracranial pressure
     D. Peritonitis associated with appendicitis
     E. All of the above   Ref. p. 976

969. CHRONIC EMESIS IS OFTEN REPRESENTED BY WHICH OF THE
     FOLLOWING ELECTROLYTE IMBALANCES?:
     A. Hypochloremic hypokalemic acidosis
     B. Hypochloremic hyponatremic alkalosis
     C. Hyperchloremic hypernatremic alkalosis
     D. Hypochloremic hypokalemic alkalosis
     E. Hyperchloremic hypernatremic acidosis
                                         Ref. p. 976

970. IN A COMPENSATED STATE RESULTING FROM SEVERE VOMITING
     WHICH OF THE FOLLOWING EXISTS?:
     A. Alkaline urine
     B. Plasma bicarbonate is increased
     C. Decrease in rate and depth of respiration
     D. Serum pH is within normal limits
     E. All of the above   Ref. p. 976

971. BARIUM TAKEN BY MOUTH SHOULD REACH THE CECUM BY_____
     HOURS IN UNOBSTRUCTED PATIENTS WITH AN ADYNAMIC ILEUS:
     A. 2 to 4   D. 12 to 15
     B. 6 to 8   E. Over 24
     C. 9 to 11   Ref. p. 976

972. WHICH OF THE FOLLOWING ANAL SPHINCTERS IS UNDER INVOLUN-
     TARY CONTROL AND THEREFORE IMPORTANT FOR CONTINENCE?:
     A. External anal sphincter
     B. Internal anal sphincter
     C. Both   Ref. p. 977

973. AN ILEUS WHICH DEVELOPS FOLLOWING RETROPERITONEAL
     DISSECTION PROBABLY RESULTS FROM:
     A. Parasympathetic nerve stimulation
     B. Sympathetic nerve stimulation
     C. A combination of both   Ref. p. 977

     FILL IN THE MOST APPROPRIATE ANSWERS: (Questions 974-976)

     A. Incarcerated hernias
     B. Gallstone ileus
     C. Neoplastic
     D. Adhesive bands
     E. Intussusception

     The most frequent cause of intestinal obstruction is 974)_____; in
     children 975) _____; and in adults 976)_____.
                                         Ref. p. 980

SELECT THE MOST APPROPRIATE ANSWER:

977. WHICH OF THE FOLLOWING GASES CONTRIBUTES THE <u>LEAST</u> TO
       INTESTINAL DISTENTION WHEN OBSTRUCTION IS PRESENT?:
       A. Nitrogen   D. Hydrogen sulfide
       B. Carbon dioxide   E. All are equally responsible
       C. Oxygen   Ref. p. 982

978. THE GREATEST CAUSE OF ABDOMINAL DISTENTION WHEN AN ILEUS
       IS PRESENT IS:
       A. Aerophagia
       B. Gas manufactured in colon by E. coli
       C. Gas diffusion from blood into intestine
       D. None of the above   Ref. p. 982

979. THE BEST AVAILABLE METHOD FOR FOLLOWING FLUID REPLACE-
       MENT IN SEVERELY DEPLETED PATIENTS IS:
       A. Urine output   D. CVP
       B. Hematocrit (serial)   E. All of the above
       C. Pulse rate   Ref. p. 986

980. POSTOPERATIVE INTRAVENOUS THERAPY MAY BE COMPLICATED BY
       REVERSAL IN DIRECTION OF THIRD SPACE FLUIDS. THIS AUTO-
       TRANSFUSION OCCURS ABOUT THE_____DAY:
       A. 1st   D. 4th
       B. 2nd   E. 5th
       C. 3rd   Ref. p. 990

981. WHICH OF THE FOLLOWING IS AN EXAMPLE OF "SPASTIC ILEUS?":
       A. Pancreatitis   D. Hypokalemia
       B. Porphyria   E. Basal pneumonia
       C. Retroperitoneal hematoma   Ref. p. 990

982. PROLONGED POSTOPERATIVE ILEUS IS BEST TREATED WITH:
       A. Reoperation   D. Gastrointestinal pacing
       B. Levine tube   E. Alpha-pantothenyl alcohol
       C. Passage of a long tube   Ref. p. 990

FILL IN THE MOST APPROPRIATE ANSWERS: (Questions 983-984)

       A. 1
       B. 5
       C. 13
       D. 21
       E. 29

The presence of 1000 cc of blood in the gastrointestinal tract on a single
bleed will maintain melanotic stools up to 983)_____ days and guaiac
positive stools for 984)_____ days.   Ref. p. 991

SELECT THE MOST APPROPRIATE ANSWER:

985. THE HEMATOCRIT AS A GUIDE TO BLOOD LOSS DEPENDS ON HOMEO-
       STATIC EQUILIBRIUM. IF INTRAVENOUS STABILIZATION IS NOT ES-
       TABLISHED, HOW LONG WILL THIS GENERALLY LAST?:
       A. To 4 hours
       B. 6 to 48 hours
       C. 48 to 72 hours
       D. 72 to 96 hours   Ref. p. 991

986. AFTER GASTROINTESTINAL BLEEDING OF 1000 CC ON A SINGLE
      OCCASION, HOW LONG MAY THE STOOL REMAIN GUAIAC POSITIVE?:
      A. 3 days   D. 14 days
      B. 7 days   E. 21 days
      C. 9 days   Ref. p. 991

987. IN PATIENTS WITH CURLING ULCERS, THE GASTRIC ACIDITY:
      A. Increases
      B. Decreases
      C. Remains unchanged   Ref. p. 993

      FILL IN THE MOST APPROPRIATE ANSWERS: (Questions 988-989)

      A. Duodenal ulcer   A. Extrahepatic portal vein ob-
      B. Acute gastritis   struction
      C. Esophageal varices   B. Intrahepatic obstruction
      D. Mallory-Weiss syndrome   C. Pyloric stenosis
      E. Gastric ulcer   D. Foreign body trauma

      Massive hematemesis in children is usually (95%) 988)_____due to
      989) _____ .   Ref. p. 993

      SELECT THE MOST APPROPRIATE ANSWER:

990. IN CIRRHOTIC PATIENTS, THE MOST COMMON CAUSE OF GASTRO-
      INTESTINAL BLEEDING IS (53%):
      A. Esophageal varices   D. Gastric ulcer
      B. Gastritis   E. None of the above
      C. Duodenal ulcer   Ref. p. 993

991. THE INCIDENCE OF UPPER GASTROINTESTINAL BLEEDING IS
      GREATEST IN WHICH OF THE FOLLOWING?:
      A. Para-esophageal hiatus hernia
      B. Esophageal hiatus hernia
      C. Equal   Ref. p. 993

992. IN WHICH OF THE FOLLOWING GROUPS IS THE MALLORY-WEISS
      SYNDROME MOST APT TO APPEAR?:
      A. Patients with hiatus hernia   D. Pregnant females
      B. Obese patients   E. Children
      C. Patients with high salicylate intake   Ref. p. 994

993. IN WHICH OF THE FOLLOWING STATES MAY BSP RETENTION BE
      ABNORMAL?:
      A. Primary biliary cirrhosis
      B. Osler-Weber-Rendu disease
      C. Hemorrhagic shock
      D. All of the above   Ref. p. 994

994. THE ULCERATIONS FOUND IN RELATION TO ECTOPIC GASTRIC
      MUCOSA IN A PATIENT WITH MECKEL'S DIVERTICULUM LIE:
      A. Adjacent to the diverticulum
      B. In the diverticulum
      C. Neither   Ref. p. 996

995. WHICH OF THE FOLLOWING RESULTS IN A BLACK LIVER BECAUSE OF
      AN INABILITY TO CONDUCT CONJUGATED BILIRUBIN DUE TO
      CANALICULAR DAMAGE?:
      A. Gilbert's disease   D. Neonatal hepatitis
      B. Crigler-Najjar   E. Physiologic jaundice of infancy
      C. Dubin-Johnson   Ref. p. 1001

996. THE VASCULAR SUPPLY TO THE ESOPHAGUS INCLUDES ALL OF THE
     FOLLOWING, EXCEPT:
     A. Inferior thyroid artery   D. Inferior phrenic artery
     B. Bronchial artery   E. All of the above
     C. Aorta   Ref. p. 1010

997. THE DIAPHRAGMATIC NOOSE ABOUT THE ESOPHAGUS CONSISTS OF:
     A. Left crus
     B. Right crus
     C. Both   Ref. p. 1011

998. METASTATIC SPREAD FROM ESOPHAGEAL CARCINOMA OF THE
     UPPER AND MIDDLE THIRDS IS TO THE:
     A. Cervical nodes   D. Supraclavicular nodes
     B. Gastric and celiac nodes   E. All of the above
     C. Pretracheal nodes   Ref. p. 1011

999. THE PREDOMINANT MUSCLES OF THE UPPER PORTION OF THE
     ESOPHAGUS CONSIST OF:
     A. Smooth involuntary muscle
     B. Striated voluntary muscle
     C. Both   Ref. p. 1011

     FILL IN THE MOST APPROPRIATE ANSWERS: (Questions 1000-1001)

     A. Hiatal hernia
     B. Esophageal spasm   A. Auerbach's plexus
     C. Achalasia   B. Meissner's plexus
     D. Zenker's diverticulum   C. Both A and B
     E. All of these
     Which of the following disease states is most likely of neurogenic origin?
     1000)_____ What is the involvement? 1001)_____
                                         Ref. p. 1013

     SELECT THE MOST APPROPRIATE ANSWER:

1002. THE COMPLICATION OF PERFORATION IN BOUGIEING FOR PATIENTS
      WITH ACHALASIA IS ABOUT_____%:
      A. 2   D. 20
      B. 5   E. 30
      C. 10   Ref. p. 1015

1003. THE SUCCESS RATE OF CONSERVATIVE DILATATION TREATMENT IN
      ACHALASIA ON THE FIRST ATTEMPT IS_____%:
      A. 20   D. 80
      B. 40   E. 100
      C. 60   Ref. p. 1015

1004. THE SUCCESS RATE OF SURGICAL INTERVENTION WITH THE "HELLER
      OPERATION" IS_____%:
      A. 10   D. 90
      B. 30   E. 100
      C. 60   Ref. p. 1016

1005. IN CHILDREN WITH CARDIOSPASM, WHICH OF THE FOLLOWING
      SHOULD BE ATTEMPTED FIRST?:
      A. Bougieing
      B. Resection
      C. By-pass
      D. Esophagomyotomy
      E. None of the above   Ref. p. 1016

1006.   WHICH OF THE FOLLOWING IS THE WORST POSTOPERATIVE COMPLI-
        CATION FOLLOWING AN ESOPHAGEAL REPAIR IN ACHALASIA?:
        A. Hiatal hernia
        B. Reflux esophagitis
        C. Esophageal stricture   Ref. p. 1016

ANSWER THE FOLLOWING STATEMENT T(RUE) OR F(ALSE):

1007.   In the Heller procedure a vagotomy and drainage procedure is indicated
        over 70 per cent of the time.   Ref. p. 1016

SELECT THE MOST APPROPRIATE ANSWER(S):

1008.   THE SYMPTOMATOLOGY IN ACHALASIA VS. HYPERMOTILITY VARIES.
        WHICH IS GREATER IN THE LATTER?:
        A. Pain
        B. Dysphagia
        C. Equal   Ref. p. 1017

1009.   WHICH OF THE FOLLOWING ARE MOST COMMONLY ASSOCIATED WITH
        ESOPHAGEAL HYPERMOTILITY?:
        A. Hiatus hernia   D. Epiphrenic diverticulum
        B. Achalasia   E. All of the above
        C. Zenker's diverticulum   Ref. p. 1017

1010.   THE MOST COMMON SYMPTOM OF PATIENTS WITH ZENKER'S
        DIVERTICULI LOCATED ABOVE THE SUPERIOR ESOPHAGEAL
        SPHINCTER OFTEN PRESENTS WITH:
        A. Recurrent aspiration pneumonitis   D. Reflux esophagitis
        B. Regurgitation   E. All of the above
        C. Obstruction   Ref. p. 1018

1011.   A NECK EXPLORATION FOR A ZENKER'S DIVERTICULUM SHOULD
        FIRST BE PERFORMED BY:
        A. Transverse incision through the midline
        B. A vertical incision in the neck midline
        C. A right-sided oblique incision
        D. A left-sided oblique incision
        E. All of the above   Ref. p. 1019

1012.   THE MOST FREQUENT CAUSE OF REFLUX ESOPHAGITIS IS:
        A. Sliding hiatus hernia
        B. Paraesophageal hiatus hernia
        C. Carcinoma of the esophagus
        D. Achalasia
        E. Ectopic gastric mucosa in the esophagus
                                              Ref. p. 1023

1013.   THE HILL REPAIR OF A HIATAL HERNIA BASICALLY UTILIZES
        WHICH PORTIONS OF THE LOCAL ANATOMY?:
        A. Gastric fundus and esophagus
        B. The esophagus and right crus of the diaphragm
        C. The pre-aortic fascia and esophagus
        D. None of the above   Ref. p. 1025

1014. THE BASIC THEORY BEHIND HIATAL HERNIA REPAIR IS TO PREVENT
      REFLUX ESOPHAGITIS. THIS IS PERFORMED BY:
      A. Repairing the defect in the diaphragm
      B. Reconstituting the angle of His
      C. Bringing the stomach below the level of the diaphragm
      D. None of the above
      E. All of the above   Ref. p. 1025

1015. THE MOST IMPORTANT DIAGNOSTIC TEST TO ESTABLISH REFLUX
      ESOPHAGITIS IS:
      A. Barium swallow   D. Esophageal motility
      B. Esophagoscopy   E. All are equally important
      C. Bernstein test   Ref. p. 1026

1016. THE MOST COMMON CAUSE OF ESOPHAGEAL PERFORATIONS IS:
      A. Stress
      B. Hyperemesis (post-emetic)
      C. Instrumentation
      D. Chemical ingestion (i.e. lye)   Ref. p. 1029

1017. WHICH OF THE FOLLOWING HAS A MORE FAVORABLE PROGNOSIS
      SURGICALLY TREATED?:
      A. Cervical esophageal perforation
      B. Thoracic and subphrenic esophageal perforation
      C. Equal   Ref. p. 1032

1018. CARCINOMA OF THE ESOPHAGUS IS CHARACTERISTICALLY OF WHICH
      CELL TYPE?:
      A. Adenocarcinoma   D. Leiomyosarcoma
      B. Carcino-sarcoma   E. Melanoma
      C. Squamous cell carcinoma   Ref. p. 1033

1019. THE MOST FREQUENT SITE OF ESOPHAGEAL CARCINOMA IS:
      A. Upper one-third
      B. Middle one-third
      C. Lower one-third   Ref. p. 1034

1020. IN WHICH OF THE FOLLOWING DO WE FIND THE BEST RESULTS FOR
      ESOPHAGEAL CARCINOMA?:
      A. Radiation
      B. Surgical excision
      C. Surgical excision and postoperative radiation
      D. Pre-operative radiation and surgical excision
      E. All are equally poor   Ref. p. 1034

1021. IN ESOPHAGEAL SURGERY WHICH APPROACH IS CONSIDERED APPRO-
      PRIATE IF THE LESION EXTENDS ABOVE THE LOWER ONE-THIRD?:
      A. Right thoracoabdominal incision
      B. Left thoracoabdominal incision
      C. No difference in approach   Ref. p. 1035

1022. PALLIATION OF PATIENTS WITH OBSTRUCTING ESOPHAGEAL CAR-
      CINOMA CONSISTS OF:
      A. Establishing a means of feeding
      B. Establishing a route for saliva evacuation
      C. Both, A the more important of the two
      D. Both, B the more important of the two
                                      Ref. p. 1036

1023. AT THE GASTROESOPHAGEAL JUNCTION, WHICH OF THE FOLLOW-
       ING HAS THE GREATEST FIVE YEAR SURVIVAL?:
       A. Squamous carcinoma with negative lymph nodes
       B. Squamous carcinoma with positive lymph nodes
       C. Adenocarcinoma with negative lymph nodes
       D. Adenocarcinoma with positive lymph nodes
                                                    Ref. p. 1037

1024. THE BARRET ULCER IS DUE TO:
       A. Congenital ectopic gastric mucosa
       B. Gastric mucosa cephalad growth
       C. Both   Ref. p. 1038

1025. WHICH OF THE FOLLOWING ARE TRUE CONCERNING THE FORAMEN
       OF BOCHDALEK HERNIA?:
       A. More frequently left-sided
       B. Most common diaphragmatic hiatal hernia in infants
       C. May or may not have a peritoneal sac
       D. A gastrostomy should be included with the surgical repair
       E. All of the above   Ref. p. 1040

1026. THE BLOOD GROUP ANTIGENS A, B AND H ARE NOT OFTEN PRESENT
       IN PATIENTS WITH:
       A. Gastric ulcers
       B. Duodenal ulcers
       C. Both of the above   Ref. p. 1053

1027. GASTRIC RELEASE IS STIMULATED BY:
       A. Antral distention   D. Peptones (secretagogues)
       B. Cholecystokinin   E. All of the above
       C. pH of gastric material below 2   Ref. p. 1054

1028. THE SECRETION OF GASTRIN BY THE GASTRIC ANTRUM IS
       INHIBITED BY:
       A. Enterogastrone   D. Serotonin
       B. Secretin   E. Bile (reflux)
       C. Antral pH below 2   Ref. p. 1055

1029. WHICH OF THE FOLLOWING IS NOT RESPONSIBLE FOR INCREASED
       GASTRIC ACIDITY?:
       A. Vagal stimulus
       B. Antral distention
       C. Alkaline secretions in antrum
       D. Peptones in small intestine
       E. All of the above are responsible   Ref. p. 1055

1030. BLOOD GROUPS HAVE BEEN IMPLICATED IN "PEPTIC ULCER
       DISEASE." THE INABILITY TO SECRETE BLOOD GROUP ANTIGENS
       A, B AND H IN SALIVA AND GASTRIC JUICE ARE ASSOCIATED WITH:
       A. Gastric ulcers   D. Zollinger-Ellison syndrome
       B. Duodenal ulcers   E. Gastric polyposis
       C. Gastric carcinoma   Ref. p. 1057

1031. WHICH DISEASE STATES ARE NOT ASSOCIATED WITH AN INCREASE
       IN INCIDENCE OF PEPTIC ULCERATION?:
       A. Chronic pulmonary emphysema
       B. Laennec's cirrhosis
       C. Chronic pancreatitis
       D. Parathyroid hyperplasia
       E. Zollinger-Ellison tumor   Ref. p. 1058

1032. ZOLLINGER-ELLISON SYNDROME IS CHARACTERIZED BY ALL OF THE
FOLLOWING, EXCEPT:
A. Postbulbar or jejunal ulceration
B. Gastric secretion over 100 mEq HCl/12 hours
C. Histamine stimulation test producing excessively high HCl secretion
rate
D. Rapid recurrence of peptic ulcers
E. Severe diarrhea plus hypokalemia   Ref. p. 1058

1033. STEROID-INITIATED ULCERS AS WELL AS THOSE ASSOCIATED WITH
ASPIRIN INTAKE AND PHENYLBUTAZONE HAVE WHICH OF THE
FOLLOWING IN COMMON?:
A. The development of peptic duodenal ulceration
B. Defective or diminished gastric mucous secretion
C. Frequent perforations
D. Local necrotizing effects with oral intake
E. High gastric acidity   Ref. pp. 1059, 1071

1034. WHICH OF THE FOLLOWING TESTS WOULD MOST LIKELY HELP CON-
FIRM A DIAGNOSIS OF ZOLLINGER-ELLISON SYNDROME?:
A. Upper G. I. series   D. Hollander insulin test
B. 12 hour overnight gastric analysis   E. Urinary and serum amylase
C. Augmented histamine test   Ref. p. 1061

1035. IN LONG-TERM ULCER MANAGEMENT THE USE OF CREAM IS
FROWNED UPON BECAUSE OF ITS FAT CONTENT. THE REASON FOR
THIS IS ITS:
A. Secretagogue effect
B. Vagal effect
C. Stimulation of enterogastrone
D. Antral phase effect and retardation of gastric emptying
E. Frequency as a stimulus for accompanying acute cholecystitis
Ref. p. 1061

1036. IN CHRONIC PYLORIC OBSTRUCTION, WHICH OF THE FOLLOWING
IS NOT TRUE?:
A. Alkaline urine   D. Hypochloremia
B. Hypokalemia   E. All of the above
C. Alkalosis   Ref. p. 1062

1037. A SUBTOTAL GASTRIC RESECTION ALONG WITH GASTROJEJUNOSTOMY
BETWEEN THE COMPLETE BORDER OF THE STOMACH AND JEJUNUM
IS CALLED:
A. Billroth I   D. Polya
B. Billroth II   E. Schoemaker
C. Hofmeister   Ref. p. 1064

1038. THE DUMPING SYNDROME INCLUDES ALL OF THE FOLLOWING,
EXCEPT:
A. Nausea and/or vomiting
B. Weakness, sweating and pallor
C. Electrocardiogram T wave and S-T segment change
D. Hypoglycemia
E. Decrease in blood volume   Ref. p. 1065

1039. WHICH OF THE FOLLOWING APPEARS MORE FREQUENTLY POST-
OPERATIVELY AFTER A GASTRECTOMY?:
A. B_{12} deficiency
B. Iron deficiency anemia
C. Both are equal   Ref. p. 1065

1040. IN A GASTROJEJUNOCOLIC FISTULA THE CAUSE OF THE DIARRHEA
IS:
A. Gastric HCl stimulating colon
B. Gastric pepsin stimulating the colon
C. Reflux of feces in small bowel
D. A result of the frequency accompanying vagotomy
E. None of the above   Ref. p. 1065

1041. THE INCIDENCE OF POSTVAGOTOMY DIARRHEA IS_____BY A
SELECTIVE VAGOTOMY:
A. Decreased
B. Increased
C. Unchanged   Ref. p. 1065

1042. THE MORTALITY RATE ASSOCIATED WITH A VAGOTOMY AND
PYLOROPLASTY IS_____PER CENT:
A. 10   D. 3
B. 8   E. Less than 1
C. 6   Ref. p. 1067

1043. THE TREATMENT OF A PYLORIC "CHANNEL ULCER" WHICH IS
ACTIVELY BLEEDING SHOULD INCLUDE:
A. Subtotal gastrectomy
B. Vagotomy, pyloroplasty
C. Vagotomy, pyloroplasty-suture ligation of ulcer base
D. Vagotomy, hemigastrectomy
E. Surgeon's discretion   Ref. p. 1068

1044. A PATIENT WITH A PERFORATED DUODENAL ULCER OF 12 HOURS
DURATION SHOULD HAVE:
A. Subtotal gastrectomy
B. Vagotomy + hemigastrectomy
C. Vagotomy + pyloroplasty
D. Plication of ulcer with omental reinforcement
E. Surgeon's discretion   Ref. p. 1068

1045. WHICH OF THE FOLLOWING SHOULD BE INCLUDED IN THE DIAGNOSIS
AND TREATMENT OF "MARGINAL ULCER"?:
A. Hollander test
B. Augmented histamine test
C. Transthoracic vagotomy if indicated
D. Reconstruction of anastomosis
E. All of the above   Ref. p. 1069

1046. THE ETIOLOGY OF GASTRIC ULCERS IS LIKENED TO A STATE OF:
A. Hyperacidity
B. Decreased mucosal resistance
C. Both   Ref. p. 1070

1047. "STEROID ULCERS":
A. Do not have an increase in HCl
B. Have a decrease in HCl secretion
C. HCl secretion is not altered   Ref. p. 1071

1048. GASTRIC CARCINOMA MAY BE DIAGNOSED WITH THE HELP OF
RADIOGRAPHIC TECHNIQUES. THE ACCURACY APPROACHES
_____PER CENT:
A. 25   D. 75
B. 40   E. 90
C. 60   Ref. pp. 1072-1073

1049. ANTICHOLINERGICS ARE:
   A. Contraindicated in most gastric ulcers
   B. Indicated in the treatment of both gastric and duodenal ulcers
   C. Of no value in either disease   Ref. p. 1074

1050. THE BEST OPERATIVE TREATMENT OF GASTRIC ULCERATION IS:
   A. Vagotomy plus pyloroplasty and biopsy of ulcer
   B. Gastrectomy plus Billroth I
   C. Gastrectomy plus Billroth II anastomosis
   D. Vagotomy plus gastroenterostomy
   E. All are equal in results   Ref. p. 1076

1051. WHICH OF THE FOLLOWING LEAST APPLIES TO ATROPHIC
   GASTRITIS?:
   A. Found in alcoholics
   B. Associated with achlorhydria
   C. Diagnosed by gastroscopy
   D. Frequently associated with Zollinger-Ellison syndrome
   E. Associated with gastric carcinoma   Ref. p. 1078

1052. CORROSIVE GASTRITIS DUE TO ACID INGESTION MAY RESULT IN
   WHICH OF THE FOLLOWING?:
   A. Atrophic gastritis   D. Gastric mucosal prolapse
   B. Hypertrophic gastric reaction   E. Gastric volvulus
   C. Pyloric obstruction   Ref. p. 1078

1053. THE MOST FREQUENT SITE OF GASTRIC CARCINOMA IS:
   A. Gastric fundus
   B. Lesser curvature
   C. Greater curvature
   D. Antrum   Ref. p. 1079

1054. WHEN A DIAGNOSIS OF A GASTRIC ULCER IS MADE AND IS HIGHLY
   SUSPICIOUS OF BEING MALIGNANT, THE COURSE OF ACTION TO
   TAKE IS:
   A. Therapeutic trial for two weeks followed by upper G. I. series and
      evaluation of ulcer for decrease in size
   B. Therapeutic trial for six weeks followed by upper G. I. series and
      evaluation of ulcer for decrease in size
   C. Immediate surgical intervention after upper G. I. series
   D. None of the above   Ref. p. 1080

1055. WHICH IS GREATER: THE SUBMUCOSAL SPREAD OF GASTRIC
   CARCINOMA INTO THE:
   A. Duodenum
   B. Esophagus
   C. Equal   Ref. p. 1080

   FILL IN THE MOST APPROPRIATE ANSWERS: (Questions 1056-1057)

   A. Gastric carcinoma
   B. Gastric leiomyosarcoma
   C. Gastric lymphoma

   Which of these has the greatest five year survival? 1056) _____
   Which has the least? 1057) _____
                                   Ref. p. 1083

SELECT THE MOST APPROPRIATE ANSWER(S):

1058. THE MOST FREQUENT COMPLICATION OF REGIONAL ILEITIS IS:
A. Hemorrhage
B. Perforation
C. Intestinal obstruction
D. Internal fistula
E. Abscess formation
Ref. p. 1090

1059. WHICH IS MORE EFFECTIVE IN REGIONAL ILEITIS?:
A. Salicylazosulfapyridine
B. Corticotropin or corticosteroids
C. Equal   Ref. p. 1092

1060. THE OVERALL RECURRENCE RATE AFTER SURGERY IN REGIONAL
ILEITIS IS:
A. 5-10%
B. 10-30%
C. 35-50%
D. 55-70%
E. 75-100%
Ref. p. 1094

1061. THE MOST COMMON CAUSE OF BLEEDING FROM SMALL BOWEL
LESIONS ARE:
A. Leiomyomas
B. Fibromas
C. Myxomas
D. Hemangiomas
E. Adenomas
Ref. p. 1095

1062. THE MALIGNANT POTENTIAL OF_____IS LOWER:
A. Gardner's syndrome
B. Peutz-Jegher syndrome
C. Equal   Ref. p. 1096

1063. KULCHITSKY CELLS ARE COMMONLY FOUND IN:
A. Peutz-Jegher's syndrome
B. Gardner's syndrome
C. Meckel's diverticulum
D. Carcinoid
E. All of the above   Ref. p. 1097

1064. THE MOST FREQUENT NEOPLASTIC LESION OF THE APPENDIX IS:
A. Adenocarcinoma
B. Carcinoid
C. Lymphosarcoma
D. Hemangiosarcoma
E. Metastatic
Ref. p. 1097

1065. APPENDICEAL CARCINOIDS HAVE A METASTATIC RATE OF:
A. 0-3%
B. 10-20%
C. 20-30%
D. 30-40%
E. 40-50%
Ref. p. 1097

1066. A CARCINOID TUMOR OF 1-2 CM CONSTITUTES 20% OF PRIMARY CAR-
CINOID TUMORS AT THE TIME OF DISCOVERY. WHAT IS THE META-
STATIC POTENTIAL?:
A. 10%
B. 30%
C. 50%
D. 70%
E. 90%
Ref. p. 1097

1067. WHICH OF THE FOLLOWING TUMORS DO NOT HAVE MULTICENTRIC
TENDENCIES?:
A. Hepatoma
B. Papillary carcinoma of thyroid
C. Carcinoid
D. Adenocarcinoma of rectum   Ref. p. 1098

1068.   THE FOLLOWING SYMPTOMATOLOGY IS FOUND WITH CARCINOID
        LOCALIZED TO THE INTESTINE, EXCEPT:
        A. Diarrhea
        B. Cutaneous flushing
        C. Vasomotor collapse
        D. Asthma
        E. Tricuspid stenosis and insufficiency
                                        Ref. p. 1098

1069.   WHICH OF THE FOLLOWING VITAMIN DEFICIENT DISEASE STATES
        CAN BE FOUND WITH CARCINOID?:
        A. Pellagra
        B. Scurvy
        C. Prothrombin deficiency
        D. Pernicious anemia   Ref. p. 1099

1070.   THE FIVE YEAR SURVIVAL RATE FOLLOWING SURGERY FOR SMALL
        BOWEL CARCINOID IS_____PER CENT:
        A. 20   D. 70
        B. 40   E. 90
        C. 50   Ref. p. 1100

1071.   SMALL BOWEL ULCERATION AND ULTIMATE PERFORATION CAN
        BE CAUSED BY:
        A. Increased intraluminal pressure due to large umbilical hernia
        B. Potassium chloride tablets in concentrations greater than 10%
        C. Foreign body migration and hang-up
        D. Meckel's diverticulae with gastric mucosa
        E. Pneumatosis cystoides intestinales
                                        Ref. p. 1101

1072.   IN THE SHORT BOWEL SYNDROME, THE MOST DIFFICULT PROBLEM
        RELATES TO:
        A. B_{12} absorption
        B. Fat absorption
        C. Water and electrolyte balance   Ref. p. 1104

1073.   THE MOST FREQUENTLY INVOLVED AREA OF THE COLON IN
        ULCERATIVE COLITIS IS:
        A. Terminal ileum   D. Sigmoid colon
        B. Cecum   E. Rectum
        C. Transverse colon   Ref. p. 1111

1074.   THE "PSEUDOPOLYPS" IN ULCERATIVE COLITIS ARE:
        A. Ulcerations surrounded by normal mucosa
        B. Edematous mucosa surrounded by ulcers
        C. Polypoid projections from the colon
        D. None of the above   Ref. p. 1112

1075.   THE USE OF CORTICOSTEROIDS IN THE ACUTE FULMINATING STAGE
        OF ULCERATIVE COLITIS_____THE CONDITION:
        A. Improves
        B. Masks
        C. Does not change   Ref. p. 1113

1076.   MALIGNANT POTENTIAL OF_____IS GREATER:
        A. Pseudopolyps
        B. Villous adenoma
        C. Equal   Ref. p. 1113

1077.   THE FIVE YEAR SURVIVAL RATE FOR COLONIC CARCINOMA IS
        GREATER IF:
        A. Associated with ulcerative colitis
        B. Idiopathic type
        C. Equal   Ref. p. 1114

1078.   THE TREATMENT OF CHOICE FOR PATIENTS WITH ULCERATIVE
        COLITIS IS:
        A. Surgical
        B. Medical
        C. Equal   Ref. p. 1114

1079.   WHAT PERCENTAGE OF PATIENTS WITH IDIOPATHIC ULCERATIVE
        COLITIS RESPOND TO MEDICAL THERAPY?:
        A. 10-20   D. 75-80
        B. 20-40   E. 85-95
        C. 45-65   Ref. p. 1115

1080.   WHAT PERCENTAGE OF PATIENTS WITH IDIOPATHIC ULCERATIVE
        COLITIS ARE CURED WITH SURGERY?:
        A. 15-25   D. 75-85
        B. 25-45   E. 95-100
        C. 55-65   Ref. p. 1115

1081.   THE DIAGNOSIS OF IDIOPATHIC ULCERATIVE COLITIS IN CHILDREN
        USUALLY NECESSITATES A SURGICAL APPROACH BECAUSE OF:
        A. Retardation of growth
        B. High incidence of cancer development.at an early age
        C. High frequency of toxic megacolon
        D. Child can tolerate ileostomy better than an adult
        E. More frequent development of intestinal obstructions
                                               Ref. p. 1115

1082.   THE SURGICAL TREATMENT OF CHOICE IN IDIOPATHIC ULCERA-
        TIVE COLITIS IS:
        A. Subtotal colectomy and ileostomy
        B. By-pass ileostomy for colon dysfunction
        C. Total proctocolectomy and ileostomy
        D. None of the above
        E. All of the above   Ref. p.1115

1083.   WHICH OF THE FOLLOWING IS NOT CORRECT ABOUT GRANULOMA-
        TOUS COLITIS?:
        A. Lower frequency of carcinoma development than idiopathic ulcera-
            tive colitis
        B. Presenting symptoms often are diarrhea with grossly bloody stools
        C. Recurrence rate after surgery is about 50%
        D. The disease often presents with multiple internal fistulas
        E. Affects the right colon more often and ulcerative colitis
            left   Ref. p. 1116

1084.   THE TREATMENT OF PSEUDOMEMBRANOUS ENTEROCOLITIS IN-
        CLUDES ALL OF THE FOLLOWING, EXCEPT:
        A. ACTH
        B. Discontinuation of all antibiotics
        C. Retention enemas of saline with fecal suspension
        D. Azulfidine
        E. If pseudomonas is the cause, sodium colistimethate is used
                                               Ref. p. 1119

1085. THE ETIOLOGY OF DIVERTICULOSIS APPEARS TO BE RELATED TO:
A. Weakened muscularis mucosa
B. Chronic colonic inflammation
C. Irritable toxins produced by enteric bacteria
D. Increased intraluminal pressure
E. All of the above   Ref. p. 1121

1086. THE MOST COMMON CAUSE OF <u>MASSIVE</u> LOWER GASTROINTESTINAL
BLEEDING IS:
A. Carcinoma of the colon   D. Gardner's syndrome
B. Diverticulitis   E. Intussusception
C. Diverticulosis   Ref. p. 1122

1087. THE MOST FREQUENT CAUSE OF RECTAL BLEEDING IS:
A. Colorectal carcinoma
B. Diverticulosis
C. Equal   Ref. p. 1122

1088. THE MOST CHARACTERISTIC FINDING IN ACUTE DIVERTICULITIS IS:
A. Nausea and vomiting
B. Urinary frequency
C. Inability to pass a sigmoidoscope beyond 15 cm
D. Colonic strictures
E. Left lower quadrant colic   Ref. p. 1123

1089. A LOCALIZED PERFORATED TRUE DIVERTICULUM OF THE CECUM
SHOULD BE TREATED BY:
A. Right hemi-colectomy
B. Ileostomy and drainage
C. Local diverticulectomy and inversion of stump
D. Antibiotics and observation
E. None of the above   Ref. p. 1125

1090. WHICH OF THE FOLLOWING IS THE MOST COMMON SITE OF FISTULI-
ZATION OF THE SIGMOID DIVERTICULITIS,?:
A. Bladder   D. Skin
B. Uterus   E. Vagina
C. Ileum   Ref. p. 1125

1091. IN SIGMOIDOVESICULAR FISTULA WHICH WOULD BE OF GREATER
DIAGNOSTIC VALUE WITH FECALURIA AND PNEUMATURIA:
A. Sigmoidoscopy
B. Cystoscopy
C. Both are equal   Ref. p. 1125

1092. WHICH OF THE FOLLOWING HAVE THE LEAST MALIGNANT
POTENTIAL?:
A. Pedunculated polyps   D. Juvenile polyps
B. Familial polyposis   E. Gardner's syndrome
C. Villous adenoma   Ref. pp. 1125-1129

1093. WHAT PERCENTAGE OF VILLOUS ADENOMAS ARE WITHIN
SIGMOIDOSCOPIC RANGE?:
A. 20-30
B. 40-50
C. 50-60
D. 60-70
E. 80-90   Ref. p. 1126

1094. WHAT TYPE OF ELECTROLYTE DISTURBANCE CAN BE ATTRIBUTED
      TO VILLOUS ADENOMA?:
      A. Hyponatremia   D. Dehydration
      B. Hypokalemia   E. All of the above
      C. Hypochloremia   Ref. p. 1127

1095. THE POLYP OF FAMILIAL POLYPOSIS IS OF WHICH TYPE?:
      A. Villous adenoma
      B. Adenomatous polyps
      C. Juvenile polyps   Ref. p. 1128

1096. WHICH OF THE FOLLOWING STATEMENTS ABOUT ADENOMATOUS
      POLYPS IS TRUE?:
      A. They frequently degenerate to carcinoma
      B. Polyps under 1.2 cm rarely degenerate to carcinoma
      C. Should be observed when found and not immediately removed
      D. Pedunculated lesions rarely metastasize
      E. None of the above   Ref. p. 1128

1097. WITH THE NEW FIBER COLONOSCOPE, IT IS POSSIBLE TO
      VISUALIZE AND BIOPSY POLYPS OF THE COLON UP TO THE LEVEL
      OF THE SPLENIC FLEXURE. WHAT PERCENTAGE OF TOTAL
      COLONIC POLYPS WOULD BE INVOLVED?:
      A. 20-30   D. 50-60
      B. 80-90   E. 70-80
      C. 40-50   Ref. p. 1128

1098. THE GARDNER'S SYNDROME CONSISTS OF:
      A. Polyposis coli and melanous coli
      B. Polyposis coli and oral pigmentation
      C. Polyposis, osteomas (exostoses)
      D. Pseudopolyposis coli and pancreatitis
      E. Diverticulosis, hiatus hernia, cholelithiasis
                                   Ref. p. 1129

      FILL IN THE MOST APPROPRIATE ANSWERS: (Questions 1099-1100)

      A. 4 cm
      B. 10 cm
      C. 1 cm
      D. 7 cm
      E. 12 cm

      Because of intramural extension of tumors, a resection should extend
      beyond 1099)_____ proximal to the tumor, and 1100)_____
      distal.   Ref. p. 1132

      SELECT THE MOST APPROPRIATE ANSWER(S):

1101. DUKE'S CLASSIFICATION OF B-2 INDICATES:
      A. Wall involvement including muscularis
      B. Node involvement
      C. Distant metastasis to liver
      D. Local pericolic fat invasion   Ref. p. 1132

1102. OBSTRUCTING LESIONS OF THE TRANSVERSE COLON HAVE A
      _____PROGNOSIS THAN NON-OBSTRUCTING LESIONS:
      A. Better
      B. Worse
      C. No different   Ref. p. 1133

1103. THE TURNBALL NO-TOUCH TECHNIQUE FOR SIGMOID COLON
RESECTION REQUIRES THE FIRST MANEUVER TO BE:
A. Isolation of the proximal and distal loops
B. Retroperitoneal dissection and ureter localization
C. Isolation and ligation of the A-V complex in the colon area to be
resected
D. Lymph node dissection in mesentery
E. Intraluminal instillation of 40% alcohol
                                        Ref. p. 1135

1104. A PALLIATIVE COLON OPERATION_____SURVIVAL:
A. Increases
B. Decreases
C. Does not alter   Ref. p. 1136

1105. FIVE YEAR SURVIVAL RATE IN DUKE'S A + B IS_____PER CENT:
A. 30   D. 70
B. 40   E. 80
C. 60   Ref. p. 1140

1106. CARCINOID TUMOR IS PRESENT MOST FREQUENTLY IN WHICH
OF THE FOLLOWING?:
A. Rectum   D. Descending colon
B. Sigmoid   E. Cecum
C. Transverse colon   Ref. p. 1141

1107. IN WHICH OF THE FOLLOWING CAN A VOLVULUS BE FOUND?:
A. Transverse colon   D. Ascending colon
B. Sigmoid colon   E. Descending colon
C. Cecum   Ref. p. 1143

1108. WHICH OF THE FOLLOWING DISEASE STATES MAY A VOLVULUS
BE FOUND MORE OFTEN THAN NORMAL?:
A. Congenital megacolon (Hirschsprung's disease)
B. Ulcerative colitis
C. Granulomatous colitis
D. Situs inversus
E. Malrotation   Ref. p. 1143

1109. WHICH OF THE FOLLOWING IS (ARE) RESPONSIBLE FOR AN
ACQUIRED MEGACOLON?:
A. Chagas' disease   D. Radiation proctitis
B. Lymphogranuloma venereum E. All of the above
C. Endometriosis   Ref. p. 1145

ANSWER THE FOLLOWING STATEMENT T(RUE) OR F(ALSE):

1110. Congenital megacolon is due to a dysfunction at Auerbach's plexus in the
bowel.   Ref. p. 1145

SELECT THE MOST APPROPRIATE ANSWER:

1111. THE MOST IMPORTANT MUSCLE TO PRESERVE FECAL CONTINENCE
IS:
A. Internal sphincter
B. External sphincter
C. Pelvic diaphragm
D. Pubo rectalis
E. None of the above   Ref. p. 1146

1112. WHICH OF THE FOLLOWING ANATOMICAL AREAS ARE (IS)
      PENETRATED TO DRAIN AN ANORECTAL ABSCESS OF THE PELVI-
      RECTAL GROUP?:
      A. Levator ani   D. Obturator internus
      B. Ischio rectal space   E. Infra-levator fascia
      C. Perianal space   Ref. p. 1153

      ANSWER THE FOLLOWING STATEMENT T(RUE) OR F(ALSE):

1113. In the treatment of anal fistula, the external sphincter should be care-
      fully avoided.   Ref. p. 1156

      SELECT THE MOST APPROPRIATE ANSWER(S):

1114. WHICH IS MORE MALIGNANT?:
      A. Squamous cell carcinoma of the anus
      B. Malignant melanoma of the anus
      C. Equal   Ref. p. 1159

1115. ANAL CARCINOMA CARRIES A FIVE YEAR SURVIVAL RATE OF 40%.
      THE MODE OF METASTASIS IS TO:
      A. Primarily pelvic nodes
      B. Primarily inguinal nodes
      C. Both inguinal and pelvic nodes   Ref. p. 1160

1116. THE APPENDIX ALONG WITH THE TONSILS AND PEYER'S PATCHES
      MAY BE RELATED TO THE AVIAN BURSA OF FABRICIUS AND PLAY
      A STRONG ROLE IN:
      A. Calcium regulation   D. Adrenal cortical regulation
      B. Cellular immunity   E. Lubrication of the colon
      C. Humeral immunity   Ref. p. 1167

1117. WHICH OF THE FOLLOWING SHOULD MAKE ONE QUESTION THE
      CLINICAL DIAGNOSIS OF ACUTE APPENDICITIS?:
      A. A patient who remains hungry
      B. Temperature above 101 degrees
      C. Cutaneous hyperesthesia in the levels of T_{10} T_{11} T_{12}
      D. A history of vomiting preceding pain
      E. A normal sedimentation rate   Ref. p. 1169

1118. A SURGEON WHO IS OPERATING ON PATIENTS WITH ACUTE APPEN-
      DICITIS AND FINDS THAT 90% OF HIS PATIENTS DO IN FACT HAVE
      THE DISEASE SHOULD:
      A. Be concerned that he is missing the diagnosis in some patients pre-
         senting with symptomatology similar to that of appendicitis
      B. Be confident that he is correct in judgment
      C. Be concerned that he is doing too many unnecessary operations
      D. None of the above   Ref. p. 1170

1119. A MAJOR COMPLICATION OF GANGRENOUS APPENDICITIS, RESULT-
      ING IN CHILLS, SPIKING FEVER AND JAUNDICE IS:
      A. Hemolytic crisis
      B. Pyelophlebitis
      C. Subphrenic abscess
      D. Subhepatic abscess
      E. All of the above   Ref. p. 1170

1120.   WHICH OF THE FOLLOWING ARE NOT TRUE CONCERNING APPEN-
        DICITIS IN CHILDREN UNDER TWO YEARS OF AGE?:
        A. Diagnostic accuracy is poor
        B. The rupture rate approaches 50%
        C. Progression of the disease is more rapid
        D. Fever is often higher
        E. Vomiting is more frequent   Ref. p. 1174

        FILL IN THE MOST APPROPRIATE ANSWERS: (Questions 1121-1123)

        A. Appendectomy
        B. Appendectomy plus right hemicolectomy
        C. Subtotal colectomy

        The procedure of choice for adenocarcinoma of the appendix is
        1121) _____ , for carcinoid of the appendix it is 1122) _____ , and
        for a mucocele of the appendix 1123) _____
                                          Ref. p. 1176

        SELECT THE MOST APPROPRIATE ANSWER(S):

1124.   THE ANATOMIC DIVISION OF THE RIGHT AND LEFT LOBE OF THE
        LIVER DEPENDS ON THE BILIOUS AND VASCULAR DRAINAGE.
        WHICH OF THE FOLLOWING CORRESPONDS TO THIS DIVISION?:
        A. Falciform ligament
        B. A line with the inferior vena cava and the gall bladder fossa
        C. Both
        D. Neither   Ref. p. 1177

1125.   THE "TRIANGLE OF CALOT" IS FORMED BY WHICH STRUCTURES?:
        A. Cystic artery, cystic duct and common duct
        B. Liver, cystic artery, common duct
        C. Liver, cystic duct and common duct
        D. Hepatic artery, cystic duct and common duct
        E. Liver, portal vein, common duct   Ref. p. 1178

1126.   WHICH OF THE FOLLOWING ORGANS HAVE A DUAL BLOOD SUPPLY?:
        A. Lung   D. Liver
        B. Kidney   E. All of the above
        C. Spleen   Ref. p. 1178

1127.   PATHOLOGIC SPONTANEOUS LIVER RUPTURE OCCURS WITH WHICH
        OF THE FOLLOWING DISEASE STATES?:
        A. Spherocytosis   D. Primary biliary atresia
        B. Portal hypertension   E. All of the above
        C. Primary carcinoma of the liver   Ref. p. 1181

1128.   THE TREATMENT OF A RIGHT LOBE LIVER RUPTURE MAY INCLUDE
        ALL, EXCEPT:
        A. Resection of devitalized segments
        B. Packing with gauze
        C. Interlocking through and through mattress sutures
        D. Direct clamping of exposed blood vessels and biliary radicals
        E. External drainage of wound   Ref. p. 1182

1129.   WHICH CARRIES THE MOST GRAVE PROGNOSIS?:
        A. Stab wound to the liver
        B. Gunshot wound of the liver
        C. Blunt trauma to the liver   Ref. pp. 1182-1183

FILL IN THE MOST APPROPRIATE ANSWERS: (Questions 1130-1131)

A. Cholangitis   A. Staphylococcus aureus
B. Septicemia   B. Hemolytic streptococcus
C. Direct extension from intra-   C. Escherichia coli
   peritoneal infection   D. Endamoeba histolytica

The most frequent cause of an hepatic abscess is said to be 1130)_____
and the organism most often responsible is 1131)_____.
                                Ref. p. 1184

SELECT THE MOST APPROPRIATE ANSWER(S):

1132.   THE MOST COMMON PRESENTING FEATURE IN HEPATIC AMOEBIC
        ABSCESS IS:
        A. Hepatic pain
        B. Fever and chills
        C. Antecedent diarrhea
        D. Bloody bowel movements   Ref. p. 1186

1133.   HEPATIC ABSCESS RUPTURE IS MOST COMMONLY INTO THE:
        A. Peritoneal cavity   D. Pleuropulmonary area
        B. Intra-abdominal viscus   E. All are of equal incidence
        C. Pericardial cavity   Ref. p. 1186

1134.   ECHINOCOCCUS CYST ABSCESSES ARE OFTEN COMPLICATED BY:
        A. Intrabiliary rupture   D. Suppuration
        B. Hemorrhage   E. All of the above
        C. Neoplastic changes   Ref. p. 1188

1135.   THE MOST COMMON NODULE FOUND IN THE LIVER IS:
        A. Hemangioma
        B. Hamartoma
        C. Hepatoadenoma
        D. Cholangioadenoma   Ref. p. 1189

1136.   THE SYMPTOMS MOST FREQUENTLY ASSOCIATED WITH HEPATIC
        CARCINOMA ARE:
        A. Pain   D. Jaundice
        B. Weight loss   E. All of the above
        C. Ascites   Ref. p. 1191

1137.   UP TO HOW MUCH OF THE LIVER MAY BE RESECTED BEFORE A
        MAJOR CHANGE IN THE LIVER FUNCTION TAKES PLACE ?:
        A. 90 per cent   D. 40 per cent
        B. 80 per cent   E. 20 per cent
        C. 60 per cent   Ref. p. 1193

1138.   THE GREATEST INCIDENCE OF PATIENTS WITH PORTAL HYPER-
        TENSION FALL INTO WHICH CATEGORY ?:
        A. Increased hepatopetal flow
        B. Extrahepatic outflow obstruction
        C. Extrahepatic portal venous obstruction
        D. Intrahepatic obstruction   Ref. p. 1197

1139.   THE TERM "POSTSINUSOIDAL OBSTRUCTION" CAN BE APPLIED
        TO ALL, EXCEPT:
        A. Wilson's disease   D. Postnecrotic cirrhosis
        B. Nutritional cirrhosis   E. Infiltrative lesions
        C. Schistosomiasis   Ref. p. 1197

1140. WHICH OF THE FOLLOWING IS CONSISTENTLY ELEVATED IN
PORTAL HYPERTENSION?:
A. OHVP (Occlusive catheterization of hepatic venule)
B. Splenic pulp pressure
C. Both   Ref. p. 1197

1141. COLLATERAL CIRCULATION IN THE FACE OF PORTAL HYPERTEN-
SION INCLUDES ALL, EXCEPT:
A. Coronary veins   D. Veins of Retzius
B. Superior hemorrhoidal veins   E. Arcade of Drummond
C. Paraumbilical veins   Ref. p. 1199

1142. WHICH OF THE FOLLOWING GROUPS HAVE A GREATER INCIDENCE
OF EXTRAHEPATIC PORTAL HYPERTENSION?:
A. Adults
B. Children
C. Equal incidence   Ref. pp. 1198-1199

1143. OF A GROUP OF PATIENTS WITH LAENNEC'S CIRRHOSIS AND
ESOPHAGEAL VARICES, WHAT PERCENT WILL BLEED WITHIN
TWO YEARS OF THE DIAGNOSIS?:
A. 10
B. 20
C. 30
D. 40
E. 60
F. 90   Ref. p. 1199

1144. ·FOR PATIENTS WITH ESOPHAGEAL VARICES, WHAT PERCENT WILL
EXPIRE FROM THE FIRST BLEEDING EPISODE?:
A. 0-9
B. 9-19
C. 19-29
D. 29-39
E. 39-49
F. 49-59   Ref. p. 1199

1145. WHICH OF THE FOLLOWING STATEMENTS BEST EXPRESSES THE
RATIONALE AGAINST PROPHYLACTIC PORTACAVAL SHUNTS?:
A. 70 per cent of the patients who bleed die within one year
B. 25 per cent of those patients shunted have severe chronic neurologic
disease and 5 per cent die at surgery
C. 30 per cent of cirrhotic patients with esophageal varices bleed
D. 60 per cent of cirrhotic patients who have hemorrhaged, rebleed
within one year   Ref. p. 1199

1146. CHILDREN WITH BLEEDING VARICES:
A. Usually stop spontaneously
B. Usually require at least a Sengstaken-Blakemore tube
C. Require immediate surgical intervention
D. Respond to drug therapy rapidly   Ref. p. 1200

1147. FOR PRESINUSOIDAL OBSTRUCTION, WHICH OF THE FOLLOWING
SHUNT PROCEDURES IS OF LEAST VALUE?:
A. Splenorenal
B. Mesocaval
C. End to side
D. None are helpful   Ref. p. 1201

1148. THE MOST SUCCESSFUL TREATMENT OF ASCITES CONSISTS OF:
       A. Side to side portacaval shunt
       B. Omentopexy
       C. Diuretics, i.e. chlorothiazide, spironolactone
       D. Strict dietary control of sodium and protein
                                            Ref. p. 1202

1149. WHICH CAUSES A GREATER MORTALITY IN A CIRRHOTIC WITH
       GASTROINTESTINAL VARICES?:
       A. Exsanguination
       B. Coma
       C. Both are equal   Ref. p. 1203

1150. WHICH OF THE FOLLOWING IS RESPONSIBLE FOR A GREATER IN-
       CIDENCE OF HEPATIC ENCEPHALOPATHY?:
       A. Splenorenal anastomosis
       B. Portacaval anastomosis
       C. Both are equal   Ref. p. 1203

1151. IF UPON DIRECT PRESSURE OF THE PORTAL VEIN AT SURGERY,
       THERE IS NO DECREASE IN THE MANOMETRIC PRESSURE, WHICH
       PROCEDURE WOULD BE INDICATED?:
       A. End to side portacaval anastomosis
       B. Side to side portacaval anastomosis
       C. Splenorenal shunt
       D. Transesophageal ligation of the varices
                                            Ref. pp. 1206-1207

1152. WHICH OF THE FOLLOWING BEST EXPRESSES THE RATIONALE FOR
       POSTOPERATIVE DRAINAGE AFTER CHOLECYSTECTOMY?:
       A. Collecting area for blood
       B. Impending infection following bile leakage from the gall bladder
       C. Accessory hepatic ducts leak
       D. Prevent duodenal adhesions to the gall bladder bed
       E. All of the above   Ref. p. 1223

1153. THE MOST COMMON VASCULAR ANOMALY OF THE CYSTIC
       ARTERY IS:
       A. Origin from left hepatic artery
       B. Origin from superior mesenteric artery
       C. Origin from common hepatic artery
       D. Double cystic artery
       E. None of the above   Ref. p. 1224

1154. THE DIFFERENTIAL DIAGNOSIS FOR NEONATAL JAUNDICE SHOULD
       INCLUDE WHICH OF THE FOLLOWING?:
       A. Neonatal hepatitis   D. Inspissated bile syndrome
       B. Choledochal cyst   E. All of the above
       C. Biliary atresia   Ref. p. 1224

1155. THE BEST DIAGNOSTIC METHOD TO DISTINGUISH PRIMARY BILIARY
       ATRESIA (PBA) FROM NEONATAL HEPATITIS (NH) IS:
       A. Liver biopsy
       B. The difference in alkaline phosphatase values
       C. Liver scan
       D. Coomb's test
       E. SGOT, SGPT, LDH difference Ref. p. 1225

1156. WHICH OF THE FOLLOWING STIMULATES GALL BLADDER
CONTRACTION?:
A. Bile salts   D. Enterogastrone
B. Secretin   E. All of the above
C. Cholecystokinin   Ref. p. 1228

1157. AN INTRAVENOUS CHOLANGIOGRAM IS OF NO VALUE IN JAUNDICED
PATIENTS WITH THE BILIRUBIN GREATER THAN:
A. 2 mg/100 ml   D. 10.5 mg/100 ml
B. 3.5 mg/100 ml   E. 15.0 mg/100 ml
C. 5.5 mg/100 ml   Ref. p. 1230

1158. WHICH CAUSES A GREATER REACTION IN THE PERITONEAL
CAVITY?:
A. Non-infected bile
B. infected bile
C. Both are equally irritating   Ref. p. 1232

1159. DEMONSTRATION OF POSTOPERATIVE STRICTURE OF THE COMMON
DUCT IS BEST DEMONSTRATED WITH:
A. Oral cholecystogram
B. Intravenous cholangiogram
C. Percutaneous transhepatic cholangiogram
D. All are of equal value
E. None of the above   Ref. p. 1232

1160. WHICH OF THE FOLLOWING DISEASE STATES FAVORS THE ONSET
OF GALL BLADDER SYMPTOMATOLOGY?:
A. Cirrhosis   D. Thrombophlebitis
B. Uremia   E. All of the above
C. Pregnancy   Ref. p. 1233

1161. ASCENDING CHOLANGITIS IS MORE COMMONLY CAUSED BY:
A. Escherichia coli
B. Staphylococcus aureus
C. Both with equal frequency   Ref. p. 1235

1162. ALL OF THE FOLLOWING ARE INDICATIONS FOR COMMON DUCT
EXPLORATION, EXCEPT:
A. Dilated common duct
B. Cystic duct greater than 12 mm
C. Intermittent jaundice
D. Multiple large faceted stones
E. Palpable stones in the common duct
                                 Ref. p. 1235

1163. THE INCIDENCE OF COMMON DUCT STONES BEING PRESENT AT
EXPLORATION FOR ACUTE CHOLECYSTITIS IS:
A. 0-5 per cent   D. 20-30 per cent
B. 7-10 per cent   E. 30-40 per cent
C. 10-20 per cent   Ref. p. 1236

1164. WHICH OF THE FOLLOWING HAS A GREATER INCIDENCE OF
PERFORATION?:
A. Emphysematous cholecystitis
B. Hydrops of the gall bladder
C. Both A and B are equal   Ref. p. 1238

1165.   THE POST-CHOLECYSTECTOMY SYNDROME OCCURS MORE OFTEN
        FOLLOWING:
        A. Simple cholecystectomy
        B. Cholecystectomy plus common duct exploration
        C. Both are equal   Ref. p. 1239

1166.   ACALCULOUS CHOLECYSTITIS DEVELOPS IN_____PER CENT OF
        THE AMERICAN POPULATION WITH GALL BLADDER DISEASE:
        A. 0-5   D. 15-20
        B. 5-10   E. 20-30
        C. 10-15   Ref. p. 1240

1167.   PATIENTS WITH ACUTE SUPPURATIVE CHOLANGITIS IN SHOCK
        SHOULD:
        A. Be placed on broad spectrum antibiotics, intravenous fluids and an
            interval cholecystectomy be performed
        B. Have an attempt at reversal of shock and immediate surgical decom-
            pression of the common duct
        C. Under no circumstances have surgical intervention
        D. All of the above   Ref. p. 1241

1168.   CHOLANGIOHEPATITIS IS ASSOCIATED WITH WHICH OF THE
        FOLLOWING ?:
        A. Ascariasis   D. Intrahepatic stones
        B. Clonorchiasis   E. All of the above
        C. Malaria   Ref. p. 1241

1169.   PRIMARY SCLEROSING CHOLANGITIS IS OFTEN ASSOCIATED WITH:
        A. Ulcerative colitis   D. No biliary tract stones
        B. Riedel's struma   E. All of the above
        C. Retroperitoneal fibrosis   Ref. p. 1242

1170.   _____PER CENT OF THE PATIENTS OVER THE AGE OF 65 YEARS
        WITH SYMPTOMATIC CHOLELITHIASIS HAVE CARCINOMA OF THE
        GALL BLADDER:
        A. 0-2   D. 10-15
        B. 2-5   E. 15-20
        C. 5-10   Ref. p. 1244

1171.   IF AT SURGERY FOR CHOLELITHIASIS, THE CYSTIC ARTERY IS
        DIVIDED AND SLIPS FREE, THE CORRECT PROCEDURE IS:
        A. Insertion of pressure packing into the area and wait 10 minutes be-
            fore careful examination of the area and then ligation of the artery
        B. The obvious source of hemorrhage is immeidately clamped and
            ligated
        C. Pressure is placed on the hepatic artery at the Foramen of Winslow
            and the cystic artery is then searched for, clamped and ligated
        D. Pressure is placed on the portal vein at the level of the Foramen of
            Winslow and the cystic artery is then searched for, clamped and
            ligated
        E. None of the above   Ref. p. 1247

        ANSWER THE FOLLOWING STATEMENT T(RUE) OR F(ALSE):

1172.   The most proximal pancreatic duct entering the duodenum is the duct of
        Wirsung, which enters about 7 cm beyond the pylorus.
                                                    Ref. p. 1255

SELECT THE MOST APPROPRIATE ANSWER:

1173.   THE VASCULAR ARCADE TO THE ANTERIOR PORTION OF THE
        PANCREAS ARISES FROM:
        A. Gastroduodenal artery
        B. Superior mesenteric artery
        C. Inferior mesenteric artery
        D. Gastroduodenal and superior mesenteric artery
        E. Superior and inferior mesenteric artery
                                        Ref. p. 1256

1174.   THE ANATOMIC POSITION OF THE SPLENIC ARTERY IS USUALLY:
        A. The superior border of the pancreas
        B. The inferior border of the pancreas
        C. Not related to the pancreas
        D. Covered by the pancreas   Ref. p. 1256

ANSWER THE FOLLOWING STATEMENT T(RUE) OR F(ALSE):

1175.   The superior mesenteric vein receives three major veins at the anterior
        border of the pancreatic neck. They are the right gastroepiploic, the
        anterior superior pancreaticoduodenal and the middle colic vein.
                                        Ref. p. 1256

SELECT THE MOST APPROPRIATE ANSWER(S):

1176.   PAIN RELIEF IN CHRONIC PANCREATITIS AND CARCINOMA OF THE
        HEAD OF THE PANCREAS MAY BE RELIEVED BY DESTRUCTION OF
        WHICH OF THE FOLLOWING?:
        A. Vagus nerve
        B. Splenic plexus
        C. Celiac ganglia and plexus   Ref. p. 1257

1177.   ANNULAR PANCREAS IS BEST TREATED BY:
        A. Local resection of obstructing pancreas
        B. Whipple procedure
        C. Duodenojejunostomy
        D. Gastrojejunostomy
        E. All of the above   Ref. p. 1257

1178.   ACTIVE TRANSPORT MECHANISMS ARE PRESENT FOR WHICH OF
        THE FOLLOWING PANCREATIC IONS?:
        A. Bicarbonate   D. Potassium
        B. Sodium   E. All of the above
        C. Chloride   Ref. p. 1258

1179.   ACTIVATION OF PANCREATIC TRYPSINOGEN AND CHYMOTRYPSIN
        IS PRODUCED BY:
        A. Trypsin   D. Carbonic anhydrase
        B. pH above 7   E. Secretin
        C. Enterokinase   Ref. p. 1258

1180.   THE FACTORS WHICH STIMULATE PANCREATIC SECRETION
        INCLUDE:
        A. Vagus nerve stimulation
        B. Secretin
        C. Gastrin
        D. Pancreozymin
        E. All of the above   Ref. p. 1259

ANSWER THE FOLLOWING STATEMENT T(RUE) OR F(ALSE):

1181. Pancreozymin has a primarily vagal-like effect in stimulating enzyme
       production whereas secretin stimulates the flow of H_2O and electrolytes.
                                         Ref. p. 1259

SELECT THE MOST APPROPRIATE ANSWER(S):

1182. WHICH OF THE FOLLOWING OCCURS AFTER PANCREATIC
       EXTIRPATION?:
       A. Decrease in B_{12} absorption   D. Iron deficiency anemia
       B. Gastric hyperacidity   E. All of the above
       C. Fatty infiltration of the liver   Ref. p. 1259

1183. GLUCAGON CORRESPONDS TO WHICH OF THE FOLLOWING?:
       A. Is produced in alpha cells
       B. Increases the cardiac output
       C. Initiates glycogenolysis in the liver
       D. Is composed of 20 amino acids
       E. All of the above   Ref. p. 1259

1184. A COMMON POSTOPERATIVE COMPLICATION RESULTING FROM RE-
       SECTION OF THE HEAD OF THE PANCREAS IS GASTRIC HYPER-
       SECRETION. TO PREVENT THIS, AND TO DECREASE THE CHANCE
       OF MARGINAL ULCERATION ONE SHOULD:
       A. Anastomose the distal pancreas to the GI tract
       B. Close off the distal pancreatic remnant
       C. Administer pancreatic extracts
       D. Administer atropine postoperatively
                                         Ref. pp. 1259-1260

1185. WHICH OF THE FOLLOWING INCREASES PANCREATIC DUCT
       PRESSURE?:
       A. Secretin   D. Alcohol
       B. Sodium dehydrocholate   E. All of the above
       C. Atropine   Ref. p. 1259

1186. THE PRIMARY STIMULUS TO THE SECRETION OF INSULIN IS:
       A. Secretin   D. High blood sugar
       B. HCl   E. Epinephrine
       C. GSH   Ref. p. 1259

1187. THE COMMON CHANNEL THEORY AS A STIMULUS FOR PANCREATITIS
       IS AT QUESTION BECAUSE OF WHICH OF THE FOLLOWING?:
       A. Normal pancreatic secretory pressure is higher than that of the liver
       B. Sphincter of Oddi contraction frequently occludes both the pancreatic
           and biliary ducts and separates them from one another
       C. Reflux into pancreatic duct with T-tube cholangiogram is frequent
           and rarely stimulates pancreatitis
       D. Only about 18% of the patients with gallstone pancreatitis have
           choledocholithiasis
       E. All of the above   Ref. pp. 1259-1260

1188. THE PRIMARY STIMULUS FOR INSULIN SECRETION IS:
       A. Duodenal pH below 5   D. Glucocorticoid
       B. An increase in blood sugar   E. Epinephrine
       C. Vagal   Ref. p. 1260

1189. PANCREATIC PAIN IS MOST OFTEN:
   A. Midepigastric and radiates to the back
   B. Back pain with radiation to the flanks
   C. A colic developing in the right or left upper quadrants and radiating
      to the midline   Ref. p. 1261

1190. THE HIGHEST MORTALITY IN PANCREATITIS OCCURS IN WHICH OF
   THE FOLLOWING TYPES?:
   A. Alcoholic   D. Metabolic
   B. Postoperative   E. Vascular, toxic or allergic
   C. Gallstone-associated   Ref. p. 1261

1191. IN_____PER CENT OF PATIENTS WITH PANCREATITIS, A
   MILD JAUNDICE IS PRESENT:
   A. 0-10   D. 30-40
   B. 10-20   E. 40-50
   C. 20-30   Ref. p. 1262

1192. THE BEST DIAGNOSTIC TEST FOR PANCREATITIS IS_____LEVELS:
   A. Serum amylase   D. Serum calcium
   B. Serum lipase   E. None of the above
   C. 2 hour urine amylase   Ref. p. 1262

   FILL IN THE MOST APPROPRIATE ANSWERS: (Questions 1193-1194)

   A. Immediately
   B. 3 weeks
   C. 6 weeks
   D. 9 weeks
   E. 12 weeks

   Nonvisualization of the biliary tract with an oral cholecystogram in contrast to an intravenous cholangiogram, pancreatitis will occur (up to)
   1193)_____ whereas in the latter, it will occur (up to) 1194)_____.
                                        Ref. p. 1262

   SELECT THE MOST APPROPRIATE ANSWER:

1195. THE USUAL TREATMENT OF PANCREATITIS CONSISTING OF
   ELIMINATING PANCREATIC SECRETORY STIMULATION CAN BEST
   BE INSTITUTED BY:
   A. Constant gastric suction
   B. Parasympatholytic drugs
   C. Withholding diet
   D. All of the above   Ref. p. 1263

1196. THE MOST COMMON COMPLICATION OF PANCREATITIS IS:
   A. Pseudocyst   D. Diabetes
   B. Pancreatic abscess   E. Pancreatic calcification
   C. Pancreatic hemorrhage   Ref. p. 1263

1197. PANCREATIC PSEUDOCYST DEVELOPMENT IS MORE COMMON IN
   PANCREATITIS OF_____ETIOLOGY:
   A. Gallstone   D. Alcoholic
   B. Vascular   E. Metabolic
   C. Postoperative   Ref. p. 1263

   ANSWER THE FOLLOWING STATEMENTS T(RUE) OR F(ALSE):

1198. In chronic pancreatitis, the bicarbonate level is below 90 mEq/l.
                                        Ref. p. 1264

1199. The best therapy for alcoholic-stimulated chronic pancreatitis is abstinence.   Ref. p. 1264

SELECT THE MOST APPROPRIATE ANSWER:

1200. CLINICAL FINDINGS INDICATIVE OF CHRONIC PANCREATITIS INCLUDE ALL, EXCEPT:
A. History of heavy prolonged alcoholic intake
B. Multiple calcification viewed on X-ray
C. Diabetes mellitus
D. Recurrent bouts of cholecystitis
E. Steatorrhea   Ref. p. 1264

ANSWER THE FOLLOWING STATEMENT T(RUE) OR F(ALSE):

1201. The rationale for the Puestow-Gillesby procedure for chronic pancreatitis results from multiple pancreatic ductal strictures and therefore poor drainage.   Ref. p. 1264

SELECT THE MOST APPROPRIATE ANSWER(S):

1202. CONTINUED ELEVATIONS IN SERUM AMYLASE ARE INDICATIVE OF:
A. Pseudocyst formation in the pancreas
B. Acute pancreatitis
C. Trauma to the pancreas with resulting inadequate drainage
D. Recurrent chronic pancreatitis
E. All of the above   Ref. p. 1265-1266

1203. THOROUGH EXAMINATION OF THE PANCREAS SHOULD INCLUDE:
A. Subcolic evaluation
B. Kocher procedure of duodenum
C. Entrance into omental bursa
D. Dissection of splenic attachments to tail
E. All of the above   Ref. p. 1266

1204. PANCREATIC CYSTADENOMA AND CYSTADENOCARCINOMA MAY BE DIFFICULT TO DISTINGUISH FROM PSEUDOCYSTS. THE CORRECT SURGICAL PROCEDURE FOR CORRECTION OF THE CYSTADENOMA IS:
A. Marsupialization
B. Excision or resection
C. Internal drainage   Ref. p. 1268

1205. THE MOST COMMON CAUSE OF PANCREATIC PSEUDOCYST FORMATION IS:
A. Trauma 60% of the time
B. Neoplastic 25% of the time
C. Pancreatitis 75% of the time
D. Pancreatitis 40% of the time   Ref. p. 1269

1206. THE MOST COMMON CLINICAL FINDING WITH A PANCREATIC PSEUDOCYST IS:
A. Jaundice   D. Anorexia
B. Epigastric pain   E. Nausea and vomiting
C. Epigastric mass   Ref. p. 1269

1207. PANCREATIC CARCINOMA MOST OFTEN ARISES IN THE_____ WITHIN THE PANCREAS:
A. Acini
B. Duct   Ref. p. 1270

1208. AN I.V. CHOLANGIOGRAM IS OF NO VALUE FOR BILIARY TRACT
       VISUALIZATION IF THE BILIRUBIN EXCEEDS:
       A. 1 mg   D. 12 mg
       B. 3.5 mg   E. 16 mg
       C. 8 mg   Ref. p. 1271

1209. SURVIVAL FOLLOWING THE DIAGNOSIS OF NON-RESECTABLE
       PANCREATIC CARCINOMA IS ABOUT:
       A. 6 months   D. 24 months
       B. 12 months   E. 72 months
       C. 18 months   Ref. p. 1272

1210. THE FIVE YEAR SURVIVAL RATE FOLLOWING A PANCREATIC
       DUODENOTOMY FOR PANCREATIC CARCINOMA IS:
       A. Less than 5%   D. Less than 20%
       B. Less than 10%   E. Less than 25%
       C. Less than 15%   Ref. p. 1272

1211. A "REVERSE 3 SIGN" IN THE DUODENUM IS USUALLY INDICATIVE OF:
       A. Ampullary carcinoma   D. Relapsing pancreatitis
       B. Pancreatic carcinoma   E. All of the above
       C. Common bile duct carcinoma   Ref. p. 1272

1212. THE WHIPPLE OPERATION FOR PANCREATIC CARCINOMA HAS A
       CURRENT MORTALITY RATE OF ABOUT:
       A. 10%   D. 40%
       B. 20%   E. 50%
       C. 30%   Ref. p. 1273

1213. COMPLIMENTARY DUODENAL OBSTRUCTION IN PANCREATIC CAR-
       CINOMA PATIENTS DEVELOPS IN_____PER CENT OF THE CASES
       REQUIRING GASTROJEJUNOSTOMY ALONG WITH THE BILIARY
       TRACT BY-PASS:
       A. 10   D. 40
       B. 20   E. 50
       C. 30   Ref. p. 1273

1214. IN A WHIPPLE PROCEDURE, THE BILIARY TRACT AND PANCREATIC
       DUCTS SHOULD BE ANASTOMOSED TO THE JEJUNUM IN WHICH OF
       THE FOLLOWING WAYS TO PREVENT MARGINAL ULCER FORMATION?:
       A. Proximal to the gastrojejunostomy
       B. Distal to the gastrojejunostomy
       C. It makes little difference   Ref. p. 1273

1215. THE MAJORITY OF PANCREATIC HYPERINSULINOMAS ARE:
       A. Benign
       B. Malignant   Ref. p. 1275

1216. WHIPPLE'S TRIAD CONSISTS OF ALL OF THE FOLLOWING, EXCEPT:
       A. Hypoglycemia initiated by rest or exertion
       B. FBS below 50 mg%
       C. Hyperinsulinism
       D. Symptomatic relief by oral or intravenous glucose
       E. All are correct   Ref. p. 1275

ANSWER THE FOLLOWING QUESTION BY USING THE KEY
OUTLINED BELOW:
A. If both statement and reason are correct and related cause and effect
B. If both statement and reason are correct but not related cause and
    effect
C. If statement is true but reason is false
D. If statement is false but reason is true
E. If both statement and reason are false

1217.   There is a relationship between the absolute blood glucose level and
        severity and character of symptoms BECAUSE with a rapid glucose fall
        the symptoms are due to epinephrine release.
                                                        Ref. p. 1275

SELECT THE MOST APPROPRIATE ANSWER(S):

1218.   SPONTANEOUS HYPOGLYCEMIA IN 80% OF CASES IS DUE TO:
        A. Functional hyperinsulinism   D. Functional hypoglycemia
        B. Organic hyperinsulinism   E. Alimentary hypoglycemia
        C. Hepatogenic hypoglycemia   Ref. p. 1275

1219.   IN THE ABOVE QUESTION WHICH IS THE MOST DIFFICULT TO DIS-
        TINGUISH FROM AN INSULINOMA?:
        A. Functional hyperinsulinism   D. Functional hypoglycemia
        B. Organic hyperinsulinism   E. Alimentary hypoglycemia
        C. Hepatogenic hypoglycemia   Ref. p. 1275

1220.   INSULIN RELEASE BY TUMOR TISSUE IS STIMULATED BY:
        A. Tolbutamide
        B. Leucine
        C. Both   Ref. p. 1275

1221.   A FUNCTION OF THE SPLEEN IS FILTRATION. WHICH OF THE
        FOLLOWING ARE NOT REMOVED FROM THE BLOOD STREAM?:
        A. Cells with Howell-Jolly bodies
        B. Cells with Heinz bodies
        C. Siderocytes
        D. Target cells
        E. Platelets coated with antibody from ITP
                                                        Ref. p. 1283

1222.   RADIOISOTOPE SCANNING OF THE SPLEEN IS PERFORMED USING:
        A. Normal erythrocytes tagged with Cr^{51}
        B. Spheroid erythrocytes tagged with Cr^{51}
        C. Selenium
        D. Albumin tagged with I ^{125}
        E. All of the above   Ref. p. 1284

1223.   ASSUMING THAT A PATIENT IS SPHEROCYTIC AND DESTROYING HIS
        OWN RBD'S, HE WEIGHS 70 Kg WITH A BLOOD VOLUME OF 5000 CC,
        A Cr^{51} TAGGED CELL STUDY INDICATES THE RBC LIFE SPAN TO BE
        20 DAYS. HIS HEMATOCRIT IS 30 PER CENT. HOW LONG WILL IT
        TAKE HIM TO DESTROY ONE UNIT OF HIS OWN BLOOD?:
        A. 1 day
        B. 3 days
        C. 5 days
        D. 7 days
        E. 11 days   Ref. p. 1142 (1st Ed.)

1224. THE FREQUENCY OF DELAYED SPLENIC RUPTURE FOLLOWING
      BLUNT TRAUMA APPROACHES:
      A. 5 per cent   D. 50 per cent
      B. 15 per cent   E. 75 per cent
      C. 30 per cent   Ref. p. 1286

1225. SPONTANEOUS SPLENIC RUPTURE OCCURS IN WHICH OF THE
      FOLLOWING?:
      A. Histoplasmosis   D. Infectious mononucleosis
      B. Cirrhosis with portal hypertension E. Gastric carcinoma
      C. Polyarteritis nodosa   Ref. p. 1286

1226. IN WHICH OF THE FOLLOWING IS AN ELECTIVE CHOLECYSTECTOMY
      FREQUENTLY INDICATED?:
      A. Hereditary spherocytosis   D. Thalassemia
      B. Sickle cell anemia   E. All of the above
      C. Hereditary elliptocytosis   Ref. pp. 1287-1288

1227. IN WHICH OF THE FOLLOWING DISEASE STATES IS "AUTO-
      SPLENECTOMY" FREQUENT?:
      A. Hereditary spherocytosis   D. Sickle cell anemia
      B. Hereditary elliptocytosis   E. Thalassemia major
      C. Pyruvate kinase (P-K) deficiency Ref. p. 1288

1228. INDICATIONS FOR SPLENECTOMY IN IDIOPATHIC THROMBOCYTO-
      PENIC PURPURA (ITP) ARE:
      A. A diagnosis of I.T.P.
      B. Prolonged purpura
      C. Platelet count under 50,000
      D. No response to steroid therapy
      E. All of the above   Ref. p. 1289

1229. POST-SPLENECTOMY, ONE SHOULD NOT CONSIDER PATIENT ANTI-
      COAGULATION WITH PLATELET ELEVATIONS BELOW:
      A. 50,000   D. 1,000,000
      B. 250,000   E. 2,000,000
      C. 500,000   Ref. p. 1151 (1st Ed.)

1230. X-RAY FINDINGS WHICH ARE INDICATIVE OF SPLENIC ARTERY
      ANEURYSM ARE (IS):
      A. Gastric serrations on the greater curvature
      B. Ballance's sign
      C. Egg shell sign
      D. Kehr's sign
      E. Wandering spleen   Ref. p. 1293

1231. THE MOST COMMON POSTOPERATIVE COMPLICATION FROM
      SPLENECTOMY IS:
      A. Left lower lobe atelectasis
      B. Pleural effusion
      C. Subphrenic abscess
      D. Perforation of the stomach
      E. Pancreatic fistula or pseudocyst   Ref. p. 1294

SECTION VIII -MECHANISMS OF ABDOMINAL PROTECTION
                       AND SUPPORT

SELECT THE MOST APPROPRIATE ANSWER(S):

1232. WHICH OF THE FOLLOWING IS CORRECT CONCERNING INTRA-
       PERITONEAL BLOOD TRANSFUSIONS?:
       A. They are usually responsible for elevations in the BUN and renal
           failure
       B. They are of no value since only hemolyzed blood is absorbed
       C. The blood is absorbed into the blood stream within 48 to 96 hours
       D. None of the above   Ref. p. 1297

1233. PRIMARY PERITONITIS OF THE PNEUMOCOCCAL VARIETY IS OFTEN
       ASSOCIATED WITH:
       A. Hodgkin's disease   D. Nephrosis
       B. Cirrhosis   E. Carcinomatosis
       C. Gonorrhea   Ref. p. 1298

1234. A PERITONEAL TAP IN THE FACE OF PERITONITIS WHICH YIELDS
       ASCITIC FLUID WITH EXUDATE CHARACTERISTICS WOULD MOST
       LIKELY BE:
       A. Hemolytic streptococcus   D. Gonococcal
       B. Pneumococcal   E. None of the above
       C. Mycobacterium tuberculosis   Ref. p. 1299

1235. THE MOST COMMON CAUSE OF SECONDARY PERITONITIS IS:
       A. Acute appendicitis
       B. Perforated peptic ulcer
       C. Strangulation of the small bowel due to incarcerated hernia
       D. Mesenteric vascular accident
       E. Gonococcal salpingitis   Ref. p. 1299

1236. THE PRESENCE OF HEMOGLOBIN WITHIN THE PERITONEAL CAVITY
       IN ASSOCIATION WITH ESCHERICHIA COLI DOES WHICH OF THE
       FOLLOWING TO THE VIRULENCE OF THE ORGANISM?:
       A. Increases
       B. Decreases
       C. Has no effect   Ref. p. 1300

1237. THIRD SPACE SEQUESTRATION OF FLUIDS IN THE PRESENCE OF
       PERITONITIS IS FACILITATED BY:
       A. ACTH increase   D. ADH secretion
       B. Aldosterone secretion   E. All of the above
       C. Catecholamine secretion   Ref. p. 1300

1238. WHICH OF THE FOLLOWING PRODUCES A MORE SEVERE REFLEX
       ABDOMINAL MUSCULAR SPASM?:
       A. Bacterial peritonitis
       B. Chemical peritonitis
       C. They are equal in severity   Ref. p. 1303

1239. WHICH OF THE FOLLOWING IS INDICATIVE OF PROGRESSIVE
       RESPIRATORY DECOMPENSATION?:
       A. Increase A-V O_2 difference   D. Decreased pCO_2
       B. Bradycardia   E. All of the above
       C. Metabolic alkalosis   Ref. p. 1304

1240. MASSIVE PERITONEAL IRRIGATION OF A CONTAMINATED ABDOMINAL
       CAVITY_____MORBIDITY AND MORTALITY:
       A. Increases
       B. Decreases
       C. Does not alter   Ref. p. 1304

1241. WHICH DISEASE STATE IS MORE VIRULENT?:
       A. Ruptured duodenal ulcer with spillage
       B. Ruptured sigmoid diverticulitis with spillage
       C. Both are equal   Ref. p. 1304

1242. THE LAYER OF TISSUE IN THE ABDOMINAL WALL WHICH PROVIDES
       THE GREATEST STRENGTH IS THE:
       A. External rectus fascia   D. Peritoneum
       B. Internal rectus fascia   E. Epidermis
       C. Transversalis fascia   Ref. p. 1313

1243. THE ABDOMINAL VEIN MOST EASILY REACHED WHICH MAY UPON
       DILATATION PERMIT A CATHETER ENTRANCE INTO THE PORTAL
       VEIN (PORTA HEPATIS) IS THE:
       A. Superficial epigastric vein   D. Vena paraumbilicalis
       B. Inferior deep epigastric vein E. Lower intercostal veins
       C. Obliterated umbilical vein   Ref. p. 1313

1244. THE DEEP EPIGASTRIC ARTERY AND VEIN MAY OCCASIONALLY BE
       RESPONSIBLE FOR A RECTUS SHEATH HEMATOMA. THEY
       ANATOMICALLY RUN:
       A. Superior to the rectus sheath
       B. Beneath the rectus muscle and above the posterior rectus sheath
       C. Above the rectus muscle and beneath the anterior rectus sheath
       D. Lateral to the rectus sheath
       E. None of the above   Ref. p. 1314

       FILL IN THE MOST APPROPRIATE ANSWERS: (Questions 1245-1246)

       A. Fascia of the external oblique
       B. Fascia of the internal oblique
       C. Fascia of the transverse abdominus
       D. Fascia of the latissimus dorsi   Ref. p. 1314

       Which of these tissues are responsible for the formation of the anterior
       rectus sheath? 1245) _____
       Which of these tissues are responsible for the posterior rectus sheath
       above the level of the umbilicus? 1246)_____

       SELECT THE MOST APPROPRIATE ANSWER(S):

1247. TO DIFFERENTIATE A RECTUS SHEATH HEMATOMA FROM AN ACUTE
       ABDOMEN ONE DEPENDS UPON:
       A. The absence of associated rebound
       B. The absence of a localizing mass
       C. The presence of a mass which does not cross the midline
       D. The presence of voluntary guarding and the absence of involuntary
           guarding
       E. The absence of bowel sounds   Ref. p. 1315

1248. DESMOID TUMORS OF THE ABDOMEN ARE CHARACTERIZED BY ALL
       OF THE FOLLOWING, EXCEPT:
       A. Found deep to the anterior abdominal muscles
       B. Are locally invasive
       C. May transform to a low grade fibrosarcoma
       D. Are unencapsulated
       E. Frequently metastasize   Ref. p. 1315

1249. THE TREATMENT OF CHOICE FOR DESMOID TUMORS OF THE
ABDOMEN IS:
A. Radiation   D. Radiation and wide excision
B. Local excision   E. None of the above
C. Wide excision   Ref. p. 1316

1250. THE OMENTUM IS AN APRON LIKE STRUCTURE OF TWO ENDOTHELI-
AL CELL LAYERS WHICH DERIVES ITS MAJOR BLOOD SUPPLY FROM:
A. The greater curvature of the stomach
B. The tinea libra of the colon
C. The anterior abdominal wall
D. The structures to which it becomes adherent
E. None of the above   Ref. p. 1316

1251. IN WHICH OF THE FOLLOWING PATIENTS IS THE OMENTUM LEAST
LIKELY TO BE OF VALUE AS THE "POLICEMENT OF THE ABDOMEN"?:
A. Perforated duodenal ulcer in a 45 year-old male
B. Perforated diverticulosis of a 60 year-old male
C. Traumatically perforated jejunum in a 45 year-old female
D. Intraabdominal abscess in a 3 month-old male
E. Intraabdominal abscess in an 8 year-old male
Ref. p. 1316

1252. SECONDARY OMENTAL TORSION IS MORE COMMON THAN PRIMARY;
IT MOST FREQUENTLY OCCURS IN PATIENTS WITH:
A. Metastatic carcinoma   D. Prostatic carcinoma
B. Inguinal hernias   E. Obesity
C. Severe emphysema   Ref. p. 1316

1253. THE RATIONALE FOR OMENTECTOMY AS A CANCER PALLIATION
ONCE THE TUMOR METASTASIZES IS TO PREVENT AND CONTROL:
A. The tendency toward omental torsion
B. The development of an internal hernia
C. The onset of hemorrhage from eroded vessels
D. The development of ascites
E. The local invasion of adjacent organs
Ref. p. 1318

1254. THE MESENTERIC ROOT OF THE SMALL INTESTINE EXTENDS FOR
ABOUT 6 TO 7 INCHES AND CONTAINS WHICH OF THE FOLLOWING
BLOOD VESSELS?:
A. Superior mesenteric artery   D. Inferior mesenteric vein
B. Inferior mesenteric artery   E. Hypogastric artery
C. Superior mesenteric vein   Ref. p. 1318

1255. THE MESENTERIC ATTACHMENTS BETWEEN THE ASCENDING AND
DESCENDING COLON AND THE LATERAL PERITONEUM ARE:
A. Free from vascular pedicles and provide excellent surgical cleavage
planes
B. The primary source of arterial blood supply and should be carefully
dissected
C. A frequent route of metastatic spread in colonic carcinoma and there-
fore should be divided first in a cancer operation
D. None of the above
E. All of the above   Ref. p. 1318

1256. THE MOST FREQUENT VOLVULUS ENCOUNTERED IS A_____
       VOLVULUS AND IS DEPENDENT UPON THE LENGTH OF THE
       MESOCOLONIC ATTACHMENT:
       A. Cecum   D. Descending colon
       B. Ascending colon   E. Sigmoid colon
       C. Transverse colon   Ref. p. 1319

1257. THE SIGNIFICANCE OF THE SPACE OF RIOLAN IS:
       A. The anatomic proximity to the inferior mesenteric vein
       B. The occasional defect encouraging the formation of internal hernias
       C. The topographic relationship to the pancreas
       D. The availability of the stomach for a retrocolic gastrojejunostomy
       E. None of the above   Ref. p. 1320

1258. WHICH OF THE FOLLOWING VESSELS IS RESPONSIBLE FOR THE
       MESENTERIC ARTERY SYNDROME?:
       A. Compression of the duodenum between the superior mesenteric
           artery and the inferior mesenteric artery
       B. Compression of the superior mesenteric artery by the duodenum
       C. Compression of the duodenum between the superior mesenteric
           artery and the aorta
       D. Compression of the duodenum between the superior mesenteric
           artery and the superior mesenteric vein
                                            Ref. p. 1321

1259. A COLLATERAL VENOUS PATHWAY BETWEEN THE PORTAL AND
       CAVAL CIRCULATION IS DEPENDENT ON:
       A. Superior mesenteric vein
       B. Left colic vein
       C. Superior hemorrhoidal vein (middle and inferior)
       D. Sigmoid vein
       E. Middle sacral vein   Ref. p. 1323

1260. THE PORTAL VENOUS PRESSURE IS NORMALLY:
       A. 3-5 cm H_2O D. 16-20 cm H_2O
       B. 7-11 cm H_2O E. 20-30 cm H_2O
       C. 12-15 cm H_2O Ref. p. 1324

1261. MESENTERIC VASCULAR OCCLUSION IS MORE COMMONLY DUE TO
       OBSTRUCTION OF:
       A. Venous system
       B. Arterial system
       C. Both are of equal incidence   Ref. p. 1324

1262. ARTERIAL OCCLUSION OF THE SUPERIOR MESENTERIC ARTERY AT
       ITS ORIGIN WILL PRODUCE ISCHEMIA OF THE:
       A. Small bowel beginning at the pylorus
       B. Small bowel beginning at the ligament of Treitz
       C. Small bowel beginning at the ligament of Treitz and including the
           ascending colon
       D. Ascending and transverse colon
       E. Entire small and large bowel up to the recto-sigmoidal junction
                                            Ref. p. 1324

1263. THE RELATIVELY FREQUENT COMPLICATION OF MESENTERIC
INFARCTION IN AN ELDERLY PATIENT WHO IS HOSPITALIZED FOR
AN ACUTE MYOCARDIAL INFARCTION IS DUE TO:
A. Obstruction from an atherosclerotic plaque
B. Obstruction due to embolization of an auricular thrombus
C. Low cardiac output and resulting thrombosis
D. Associated aortic aneurysmal development with thrombus deposition
E. None of the above   Ref. p. 1325

1264. AN ACUTE MESENTERIC INFARCTION MAY BE SUSPECTED WHEN:
A. Severe abdominal pain is present which is out of proportion to the
clinical findings
B. Severe abdominal pain is noted in association with voluntary and in-
voluntary guarding
C. Abdominal colic in association with a sudden mass
D. Nausea and vomiting precede the onset of abdominal pain
Ref. p. 1325

1265. IN A PATIENT SUSPECTED OF HAVING A MESENTERIC INFARCTION,
WHICH OF THE FOLLOWING WOULD BE OF GREATEST DIAGNOSTIC
VALUE ?:
A. Leukocyte count
B. Abdominal paracentesis
C. Emergency upper G. I. series
D. Emergency barium enema
E. Flat plate and upright X-ray of the abdomen
Ref. p. 1325

1266. WHAT PERCENTAGE OF SMALL INTESTINE MAY BE REMOVED IN AN
ADULT WITHOUT CAUSING EXTENSIVE DIGESTIVE DISABILITIES ?:
A. 20 per cent   D. 90 per cent
B. 50 per cent   E. 100 per cent
C. 70 per cent   Ref. p. 1326

1267. NON-OCCLUSIVE MESENTERIC INFARCTION MAY BE CONTRIBUTED
TO BY ALL, EXCEPT:
A. Myocardial infarction
B. Severe dehydration
C. Vasopressor therapy
D. Massive anticoagulation
E. Septicemia with associated hypoxia
Ref. p. 1326

FILL IN THE MOST APPROPRIATE ANSWERS: (Questions 1268-1269)

A. Colostomy
B. Systemic treatment, permit the questionable bowel to remain in situ
and perform a second look procedure in 24 to 36 hours
C. Resection of the ischemic segments to remove gangrenous and po-
tentially gangrenous tissue
D. Local instillation of vasodilators

In patients with a mesenteric vascular occlusion and bowel which is
questionably viable, the correct surgical procedure for completely involved small intestine is 1268)_____, and that for a segmental
ischemic bowel is 1269)_____.
Ref. p. 1326

SELECT THE MOST APPROPRIATE ANSWER(S):

1270. WHICH OF THE FOLLOWING MAY BE USED TO EXPLAIN NON-
OCCLUSIVE MESENTERIC INFARCTION?:
A. Decrease in cardiac output
B. Splanchnic vasoconstriction
C. Erythrocyte sludging
D. Critical closing pressure of the splanchnic bed is reached
E. All of the above   Ref. p. 1326

1271. IN WHICH OF THE FOLLOWING DISEASE STATES IS PAIN ON FOOD
CONSUMPTION AN IMPORTANT DIAGNOSTIC POINT?:
A. Neoplasm   D. Pancreatitis
B. Intestinal angina   E. Cholecystitis
C. Peptic ulcer   Ref. p. 1327

1272. WHICH OF THE FOLLOWING HAS A PROLONGED INSIDIOUS ONSET?:
A. Mesenteric infarction involving the small bowel and ascending colon
B. Mesenteric infarction involving the descending colon
C. Both have similar presenting patterns
                                Ref. p. 1328

1273. WHICH OF THE FOLLOWING MAY PROVE TO BE DIAGNOSTIC FOR
INFERIOR MESENTERIC ARTERY INFARCTION?:
A. Flat plate and upright of the abdomen
B. Leukocyte count
C. Sigmoidoscopy
D. Barium enema
E. Upper gastrointestinal series   Ref. p. 1329

1274. CAUSES OF VENOUS MESENTERIC OCCLUSION MAY INCLUDE:
A. Hypercoagulability
B. Shock
C. Cirrhosis with portal hypertension
D. Pyelophlebitis
E. All of the above   Ref. p. 1329

1275. BLOODY DIARRHEA IS MORE FREQUENT IN WHICH OF THE FOLLOW-
ING STATES?:
A. Mesenteric arterial occlusion
B. Mesenteric venous occlusion
C. Equal incidence   Ref. p. 1330

1276. SPONTANEOUS ARTERIAL RUPTURE MAY DEVELOP MORE OFTEN IN
PREGNANT FEMALES FROM WHICH VESSEL?:
A. Superior mesenteric artery   D. Inferior vena cava
B. Inferior mesenteric artery   E. Hypogastric artery
C. Splenic artery   Ref. p. 1331

1277. MESENTERIC ADENITIS IS MOST OFTEN DUE TO:
A. Viral infection
B. Hemolytic streptococcus infection
C. Escherichia coli infection
D. Ascariasis   Ref. p. 1333

1278.   IT IS MOST DIFFICULT TO DISTINGUISH BETWEEN MESENTERIC
        ADENITIS AND APPENDICITIS. WHICH OF THE FOLLOWING MAY
        NOT BE UTILIZED?:
        A. The patient's inability to pinpoint the site of pain in the former
        B. Facial flush in the former
        C. Rhinorrhea in the former
        D. Minimal rebound tenderness in the former
                                        Ref. p. 1333

        FILL IN THE MOST APPROPRIATE ANSWERS: (Questions 1279-1280)

        A. Cystic
        B. Solid
        C. Malignant
        D. Benign

        Tumors of the mesentery are more frequently of the 1279)_____
        variety and tend to be 1280)_____.
                                        Ref. p. 1334

        SELECT THE MOST APPROPRIATE ANSWER:

1281.   THE MESENTERIC ATTACHMENTS MOST OFTEN AFFECTED WITH
        TUMOR DEVELOPMENT IS:
        A. Jejunal   D. Transverse colon
        B. Ileal   E. Sigmoid colon
        C. Ascending colon   Ref. p. 1335

1282.   THE SYMPTOMATOLOGY OF MESENTERIC TUMORS IS DEPENDENT
        ON THEIR LOCATION. WHICH OF THE FOLLOWING WILL MOST
        LIKELY PRESENT EARLIER?:
        A. Leiomyosarcoma at the root of the mesentery of the small bowel
        B. Lipoma present at the vasa recta of the small bowel
        C. Malignant teratoma in the transverse mesocolon
        D. Malignant teratoma in the sigmoid mesocolon
                                        Ref. p. 1335

1283.   WHICH OF THE FOLLOWING TUMORS WILL HAVE A TENDENCY TO
        BECOME EXCEPTIONALLY LARGE BEFORE PRESENTING WITH
        SYMPTOMS?:
        A. Lipoma at the vasa recti of the small bowel
        B. Malignant teratoma in the transverse mesocolon
        C. Lymphangiosarcoma of the small bowel
                                        Ref. p. 1335

1284.   ORMOND'S SYNDROME (IDIOPATHIC FIBROUS RETROPERITONITIS)
        IS OFTEN CONSIDERED AN AUTOIMMUNE REACTION WHICH
        PRESENTS WITH:
        A. Hemorrhage
        B. Malignant degeneration
        C. Perforation of the abdominal viscera
        D. Obstruction of the retroperitoneal tubular channels
        E. Anaphylactic shock   Ref. p. 1337

1285.   IN PATIENTS WITH IDIOPATHIC RETROPERITONEAL FIBROSIS,
        WHICH OF THE FOLLOWING STRUCTURES IS USUALLY INVOLVED
        FIRST?:
        A. Aorta   D. Duodenum
        B. Vena cava   E. Urethra
        C. Ureter   Ref. p. 1337

1286. WHICH OF THE FOLLOWING MEDICATIONS HAVE BEEN SUSPECTED
AS A CAUSE OF RETROPERITONEAL FIBROSIS?:
A. Thorazine (Chlorpromazine)   D. Ariminol
B. Methylsergide   E. None of the above
C. Chlordiazepoxide   Ref. p. 1337

1287. OF THE FOLLOWING SYMPTOMS, WHICH WOULD LEAST LIKELY BE
FOUND RELATED TO RETROPERITONEAL TUMORS?:
A. Rectal tenesmus
B. Ascites
C. Scrotal varicosities
D. Hemorrhoids
E. Dilated superficial abdominal veins
F. All are related   Ref. p. 1338

1288. THE MOST FREQUENT RETROPERITONEAL TUMOR IS:
A. Sarcoma   D. Pheochromocytoma
B. Lymphoma   E. Teratoma
C. Neuroblastoma   Ref. p. 1339-1340

1289. THE CREMESTERIC MUSCLE CONTAINS MUSCLE FIBERS FROM
WHICH OF THE FOLLOWING?:
A. Internal oblique muscle, external oblique muscle, transverse ab-
dominal muscle
B. Internal oblique muscle, external oblique muscle
C. Internal oblique muscle, transverse abdominal muscle
D. External oblique muscle, transverse abdominal muscle
E. Transverse abdominal muscle   Ref. p. 1346

1290. THE ABDOMINAL WALL DEFECT WHICH BOTH A FEMORAL AND
INGUINAL HERNIA HAVE IN COMMON IS:
A. Scarpa's fascia   D. None of the above
B. Hesselbach's triangle   E. All of the above
C. Transversalis fascia   Ref. p. 1347

1291. THE ANATOMIC POSITION OF A FEMORAL HERNIA IN RELATION TO
THE INGUINAL LIGAMENT AND FEMORAL VEIN IS THAT IT:
A. Travels above the inguinal ligament and medial to the vein
B. Travels below the inguinal ligament and medial to the vein
C. Travels below the inguinal ligament and lateral to the vein
D. Travels above the inguinal ligament and lateral to the vein
Ref. p. 1347

FILL IN THE MOST APPROPRIATE ANSWERS: (Questions 1292-1293)

A. Obturator hernia   A. Rectus sheath, Cooper's ligament
B. Direct inguinal hernia   B. Epigastric vessels, inguinal liga-
C. Indirect inguinal hernia   ment, rectus sheath
D. Femoral hernia   C. None of the above
E. Spigelian hernia

The anatomic interest in Hasselbach's triangle derives from it as a bound-
ary within which lies 1292) _____ . It consists of 1293) _____ .
Ref. p. 1347

SELECT THE MOST APPROPRIATE ANSWER:

1294. NEONATAL UMBILICAL HERNIAS:
A. Usually require surgery by the age of three
B. Spontaneously close by the age of three
C. Should be operated on at birth because of the high incidence of
incarceration   Ref. p. 1348, 1350

1295. OF LEAST IMPORTANCE IN THE DIAGNOSIS OF AN INGUINAL HERNIA
      IS:
      A. The size of the external ring
      B. The protrusion of abdominal viscera into the scrotum
      C. A pulsation felt by digital examination of the inguinal canal
      D. A history of an inguinal mass developing following severe abdominal
         stress
      E. All are important to the diagnosis
                                              Ref. p. 1349

1296. A HERNIA WHICH INCARCERATES ONLY A PORTION OF THE IN-
      TESTINAL LUMEN IS CALLED A_____HERNIA:
      A. Littre
      B. Richter
      C. Petit
      D. Obturator   Ref. p. 1350

1297. IN UNCOMPLICATED INCARCERATED HERNIAS WHERE THERE IS NO
      EVIDENCE OF INTESTINAL COMPROMISE THE PROCEDURE OF
      CHOICE IN CHILDREN SHOULD BE:
      A. Immediate surgery, to prevent the imminent ischemic bowel changes
      B. Sedation and elevation of the lower end of the bed to permit muscular
         relaxation and autoreduction, followed by surgery in several days
      C. Sedation and elevation of the lower end of the bed to permit muscular
         relaxation and autoreduction, and a future surgical procedure if a
         recurrence develops or at the age of 6 years
                                              Ref. p. 1350

1298. FOLLOWING AN INGUINAL HERNIORRHAPHY HOW LONG SHOULD A
      PATIENT AVOID STRENUOUS ACTIVITY ?:
      A. Two weeks   D. Twelve weeks
      B. Four weeks   E. Sixteen weeks
      C. Six weeks   Ref. p. 1351

      FILL IN THE MOST APPROPRIATE ANSWERS: (Questions 1299-1300)

      A. Femorogenital   A. External ring
      B. Ileohypogastric   B. Internal ring
      C. Ileoinguinal   C. Adjacent to the cord beneath the
      D. Lateral femoral cutaneous   external oblique aponeurosis
      E. Obturator

      During an inguinal herniorrhaphy, 1299)_____ nerves are most likely
      to be injured and at 1300)_____ position.
                                              Ref. p. 1354

      SELECT THE MOST APPROPRIATE ANSWER(S):

1301. FOLLOWING MOBILIZATION OF THE CORD AND ITS CONTENTS DUR-
      ING A HERNIORRHAPHY FOR AN INDIRECT INGUINAL HERNIA THE
      SAC IS USUALLY FOUND:
      A. Posteriomedial to the cord structures
      B. Anteriomedial to the cord structures
      C. Posteriolateral to the cord structures
      D. Anteriolateral to the cord structures
                                              Ref. p. 1354

1302.   WHICH OF THE FOLLOWING IS NOT A BENEFIT DERIVED FROM
        OPENING THE PERITONEAL SAC AND INSERTING A FINGER DURING
        A SURGICAL REPAIR OF AN INGUINAL HERNIA?:
        A. Palpate the femoral ring
        B. Palpate the direct wall for an additional weakness
        C. Palpate the obturator membrane
        D. Palpate the median lobe of the prostate
        E. Examine local peritoneum for possible metastatic implants
        F. All of the above   Ref. p. 1354

1303.   A SLIDING HERNIA PRESENT IN THE LEFT INGUINAL AREA USUALLY
        CONTAINS_____AS PART OF ITS SAC:
        A. Bladder   D. Cecum
        B. Sigmoid colon   E. Ovary
        C. Mesosigmoid   Ref. p. 1355

1304.   WHICH OF THE FOLLOWING IS THE WEAKEST ANATOMICAL PLANE
        FOLLOWING A MCVAY (COOPER LIGAMENT) REPAIR?:
        A. Transversalis fascia to the femoral sheath
        B. Transversalis fascia to Cooper's ligament
        C. Transversalis fascia to Poupart's ligament
                                            Ref. p. 1356

1305.   IN CHILDREN, THE INCIDENCE OF AN INGUINAL HERNIA BEING
        BILATERAL ONCE ONE PRESENTS IS:
        A. 5 per cent   D. 50 per cent
        B. 20 per cent   E. 80 per cent
        C. 30 per cent   Ref. p. 1358

1306.   IN THE FOLLOWING LISTING, POSITION THE HERNIA REPAIRS IN
        ORDER OF THEIR RECURRENCE RATE. THE HIGHEST FIRST:
        A. ___ Femoral herniorrhaphy
        B. ___ Inguinal herniorrhaphy for an indirect inguinal hernia
        C. ___ Ventral herniorrhaphy
        D. ___ Inguinal herniorrhaphy for a sliding inguinal hernia
                                            Ref. p. 1359

SELECT THE MOST APPROPRIATE ANSWER:

1307.   WHICH OF THE FOLLOWING IS NOT TRUE ABOUT ACTH?:
A. Derived from both basophilic and chromophobic cells
B. Can be controlled by hypothalamic hormone
C. Is increased in trauma
D. Is secreted at a constant rate responsive only to feed back
    mechanisms
E. Mostly influences zona fasciculata of the adrenal gland
                                            Ref. p. 1365

1308.   FOLLOWING TOTAL HYPOPHYSECTOMY, (SURGICAL) WHICH OF
THE HORMONES IS AFFECTED LAST?:
A. GTH   D. ACTH
B. GH   E. ADH
C. TSH   Ref. p. 1368

1309.   A DEFICIENCY IN WHICH HORMONE PRODUCES THE MOST
SERIOUS EFFECTS?:
A. GTH   D. ACTH
B. GH   E. ADH
C. TSH   Ref. p. 1368

1310.   THE TESTING OF HYPOPITUITARISM IS CONDUCTED WITH:
A. Pitressin   D. ACTH
B. Metyrapone   E. Cortisone
C. Dexamethasone   Ref. p. 1368

1311.   WHICH IS THE MOST COMMON TYPE OF PITUITARY TUMOR?:
A. Chromophobe adenoma
B. Basophilic adenoma
C. Eosinophilic adenoma   Ref. p. 1372

1312.   WHICH OF THE FOLLOWING IS NOT AN INDICATION FOR HYPO-
PHYSECTOMY?:
A. Severe diabetic retinopathy
B. Metastatic carcinoma of the breast
C. Enlarging pituitary adenoma
D. Metastatic carcinoma of the prostate
E. None of the above   Ref. p. 1373

1313.   THE MOST COMMON ECTOPIC PITUITARY TUMOR PRODUCING
ACTH IS:
A. Pancreatic   D. Liver
B. Oat cell carcinoma of the lung   E. Thymus
C. Parotid   Ref. p. 1373

1314.   WHICH HAS A GREATER OCCURRENCE?:
A. Extra-adrenal medullary tissue
B. Extra-adrenal cortical tissue
C. Equal   Ref. p. 1376

FILL IN THE MOST APPROPRIATE ANSWERS: (Questions 1315-1316)

A. Entoderm
B. Mesoderm
C. Ectoderm

The adrenal gland embryologically develops from two separate cell types:
the medulla from 1315) _____ and the cortex from 1316) _____ .
                        Ref. p. 1376

FILL IN THE MOST APPROPRIATE ANSWERS: (Questions 1317-1318)

A. Inferior vena cava
B. Portal vein
C. Renal vein
D. Hemi azygous vein
E. Superior mesenteric vein

The major venous return in the right adrenal is to 1317)_____ and
that of the left to 1318)_____.   Ref. p. 1376

FILL IN THE MOST APPROPRIATE ANSWERS: (Questions 1319-1320)

A. Corticosterone
B. Cortisol
C. 11-desoxycortisol
D. Aldosterone
E. Androstenedione

The two most important adrenal corticosteroids are 1319)_____ and
1320)_____.   Ref. p. 1377

SELECT THE MOST APPROPRIATE ANSWER:

1321. THE EFFECT OF METYRAPONE (METOPIRONE) IS TO PREVENT 11-B
       HYDROXYLATION. IT IS USED TO DIRECTLY DEPRESS WHICH OF
       THE FOLLOWING?:
       A. ACTH   D. 11-desoxycortisol
       B. CRF   E. 18-oxidase
       C. Cortisol   Ref. p. 1378, 1385

1322. THE PRESENCE OF 17 HYDROXYLATING ENZYMES IN THE ADRENAL
       GLAND IS LIMITED TO:
       A. Zona glomerulosa
       B. Zona fasciculata
       C. Zona reticularis   Ref. p. 1378

1323. WHICH OF THE FOLLOWING FEEDBACK MECHANISMS IS NOT DE-
       TERMINED BY CONCENTRATION OF HORMONES?:
       A. Cortisol
       B. Aldosterone
       C. Both   Ref. p. 1379

1324. THE MOST COMMON FORM OF CUSHING'S SYNDROME IS RELATED TO:
       A. Adrenal adenoma   D. Adrenal hyperplasia
       B. Pituitary adenoma   E. Ectopic ACTH source
       C. Adrenal carcinoma   Ref. p. 1381

A PATIENT PRESENTING WITH CUSHING'S SYNDROME CAN HAVE
THREE POSSIBLE VARIATIONS IN ACTH AND CORTISOL WHEN GIVEN
THE DEXAMETHASONE SUPPRESSION TEST (2 mg). MATCH THESE
CHANGES WITH THE DISEASE THAT CAUSES THEM:

1325. ___ Decreased cortisol, normal ACTH   A. Ectopic ACTH tumor
1326. ___ Increased cortisol, normal ACTH   B. Adrenal hyperplasia
1327. ___ Increased cortisol, increased   C. Adrenal carcinoma or
          ACTH   adenoma
                                                D. Normal gland
                                                Ref. p. 1382-1383

SELECT THE MOST APPROPRIATE ANSWER(S):

1328. IN WHICH OF THE FOLLOWING STATES IS ACTH NOT FUNCTIONAL?:
   A. Adrenal nodular hyperplasia
   B. Adrenal hyperplasia
   C. Ectopic pituitary tumor
   D. Adrenal adenoma
   E. Pituitary basophilic adenoma   Ref. p. 1384

1329. WHICH OF THE FOLLOWING ANTI-TUMOR MEDICATIONS IS DE-
   STRUCTIVE TO ADRENOCORTICAL CELLS?:
   A. Metyrapone   D. Ortho-paraprime DDD
   B. SU-9055   E. Diphenylhydantoin
   C. Aminoglutethimide   Ref. p. 1386

1330. WHICH OF THE FOLLOWING DISEASE STATES DOES NOT REQUIRE
   IMMEDIATE SURGICAL EXTIRPATION OF THE ADRENALS?:
   A. Adrenocortical carcinoma
   B. Adrenocortical hyperplasia
   C. Non-resectable ectopic ACTH-secreting tumors
   D. Adrenocortical hyperplasia with hypotension and rapidly progressing
      Cushing's syndrome
   E. None of the above   Ref. p. 1387

1331. DEFICIENCY IN WHICH OF THE FOLLOWING WILL LEAD TO NO
   ALDOSTERONE PRODUCTION AND THEREFORE, SEVERE SALT
   LOSING?:
   A. C21 hydroxylation block   D. C17 hydroxylation block
   B. C20 hydroxylation block   E. C11 hydroxylation block
   C. C18 hydroxylation block   Ref. p. 1390

1332. THE ADRENOGENITAL SYNDROME IS MORE OFTEN OF_____
   ORIGIN:
   A. Neoplastic
   B. Hyperplastic   Ref. p. 1390

   FILL IN THE MOST APPROPRIATE ANSWERS: (Questions 1333-1334)

   A. Increases
   B. Suppresses
   C. Does not alter

   To distinguish between hyperplasia and tumor, several tests are performed. In hyperplasia ACTH stimulation 1333)_____17 ketosteroid
   excretion in contrast to a tumor, and in the adenoma, cortisol, ACTH
   stimulation 1334)_____17 ketosteroid production.
                                    Ref. p. 1392

SELECT THE MOST APPROPRIATE ANSWER(S):

1335. WHICH OF THE FOLLOWING ARE CHROMATIN POSITIVE?:
   A. Klinefelter's syndrome
   B. Turner's syndrome
   C. Mixed gonadal dysgenesis gonadogenesis disorder
   D. Female pseudohermaphroditism due to congenital adrenal hyperplasia
   E. Male pseudohermaphroditism gonadogenesis disorder
                                    Ref. p. 1393-1394

1336. THE BEST RESULTS WITH ADRENALECTOMY FOR METASTATIC
BREAST CARCINOMA OCCUR IN:
A. Lesions which involve less than 30% of the liver
B. Lesions of bone and skin
C. Lesions of bone, skin and lung
D. Lesions with liver spread over 30%
E. None of the above   Ref. p. 1394

1337. THE REMISSION RATE OF METASTATIC BREAST CARCINOMA AFTER
BILATERAL ADRENALECTOMY IS_____PER CENT:
A. 10-20   D. 70-90
B. 30-50   E. None
C. 50-70   Ref. p. 1394

1338. THE PRINCIPLE OF "TUMOR AUTONOMY" IS EXEMPLIFIED IN
MOST ENDOCRINE ADENOMAS AND CARCINOMAS. WHICH OF THE
FOLLOWING BEST DEMONSTRATES THIS PRINCIPLE ?:
A. In adrenocortical hyperplasia, the administration of 1 mg dexametha-
sone suppresses secretion of 17-hydroxycortico-steroids
B. In primary aldosteronism, desoxycortico-sterone will not diminish
the urinary aldosterone output
C. Neither   Ref. p. 1395

1339. IN PRIMARY ALDOSTERONISM, THE MOST SIMPLE EFFECTIVE AND
CONSISTENT LABORATORY TEST IS:
A. Depression of plasma potassium with chlorothiazide therapy
B. Increase in urinary potassium as long as patient is on a normal salt
diet
C. Salivary sodium/potassium ratio
D. Aldosterone excretion in urine
E. Spironolactone test   Ref. p. 1397

1340. THE DIFFERENTIAL DIAGNOSIS OF ALDOSTERONISM INCLUDES A
"POTASSIUM-LOSING NEPHRITIS." HOW MAY ONE DISTINGUISH THE
TWO?:
A. In the former, there is alkalosis and in the latter, acidosis
B. In the former, there is hypernatremia and in the latter, hyponatremia
C. In the former, there is hypervolemia and in the latter, hypovolemia
D. All of the above
E. None of the above   Ref. p. 1397

1341. THE PRIME REASON FOR SURGICAL TREATMENT IN PRIMARY
ALDOSTERONISM IS:
A. Frequency of metastatic spread
B. Local adrenocortico compression with resulting atrophy
C. To correct hypokalemia
D. To prevent recurrent alkalosis
E. All of the above   Ref. p. 1401

1342. WHICH OF THE FOLLOWING MAY CAUSE ADDISON'S DISEASE ?:
A. Orthopara prime DDD   D. Patients with burn sepsis
B. Tuberculosis   E. All of the above
C. Meningococcal infection   Ref. p. 1402

1343. PATIENTS WITH ADDISON'S DISEASE ARE HYPERSENSITIVE TO
SEVERAL EXTERNAL STIMULI, AMONG THEM ARE:
A. Salt at 1 mm/liter
B. Heat applied to skin
C. Hypersensitivity to skin to pain
D. Galvanic current applied to tongue
E. All of the above   Ref. p. 1403

1344. IN PITUITARY INSUFFICIENCY CAUSING ADRENAL INSUFFICIENCY,
WHICH OF THE FOLLOWING IS LEAST AFFECTED?:
A. Cortisol secretion   D. Androstenedione
B. Aldosterone secretion   E. Estradiol
C. Dihydrocortisol   Ref. p. 1403

1345. THE MOST COMMON CAUSE OF ADRENAL INSUFFICIENCY IS:
A. TBC
B. Disuse atrophy due to steroid administration
C. Waterhouse-Friderichsen's syndrome
D. Sepsis
E. Pneumococcal sepsis   Ref. p. 1403

1346. THE MOST FREQUENT COMPLICATIONS RESULTING FROM CORTICO-
STEROID TREATMENT ARE:
A. Activation of tuberculosis   D. Acute pancreatitis
B. Gastric and duodenal ulcers   E. Adrenocortical insufficiency
C. Small bowel ulcers   Ref. p. 1404

1347. AN AWARENESS OF ADRENAL INSUFFICIENCY IS ESSENTIAL IN PA-
TIENT CARE. THE MOST USEFUL TEST WHICH INDICATES THE
PROBABLE PATHOLOGICAL STATE IS:
A. ACTH stimulation test   D. Urinary sodium/24 hours
B. Serum hyponatremia   E. Eosinopenia
C. Serum hyperkalemia   Ref. p. 1404

1348. WHICH OF THE FOLLOWING TUMORS ARE FOUND IN THE ADRENAL
MEDULLA?:
A. Pheochromocytoma   D. Neuroblastoma
B. Adenocarcinoma   E. Sarcoma
C. Carcinoid   Ref. p. 1405

1349. IN PHEOCHROMOCYTOMA, BILATERAL INVOLVEMENT MOST OFTEN
APPEARS IN:
A. Children
B. Adults
C. Equal   Ref. p. 1407

1350. WHICH IS MORE FREQUENT? IN PHEOCHROMOCYTOMA, HYPER-
TENSION IS:
A. Paroxysmal
B. Persistent
C. Equal   Ref. p. 1408

1351. TO DIFFERENTIATE A MALIGNANT PHEOCHROMOCYTOMA FROM
BENIGN PHEOCHROMOCYTOMA IN THE FORMER, THERE IS:
A. Dopamine metabolism increased D. Epinephrine increased
B. VMA over 10 mgm/24 hours   E. No way to distinguish
C. Norepinephrine increased   Ref. p. 1408

1352. WHICH IS GREATER? RETINOPATHY IN:
A. Pheochromocytoma
B. Primary aldosteronism
C. Equal   Ref. p. 1409

1353. WHICH IS GREATER IN A PHEOCHROMOCYTOMA OF THE ADRENAL
MEDULLARY ORIGIN VS. EXTRAMEDULLARY ORIGIN?:
A. Norepinephrine
B. Epinephrine
C. Equal   Ref. p. 1409

1354. WHICH OF THE FOLLOWING WILL INITIATE AN INCREASE IN VMA?:
A. Ganglioneuroma   D. Carotid body tumor
B. Ganglioneuroblastoma   E. All of the above
C. Retinoblastoma   Ref. p. 1410

1355. WHICH OF THE FOLLOWING WILL INITIATE INCREASES IN HVA?:
A. Ganglioneuroma
B. Melanoma
C. Parkinson's disease
D. Wilson's disease
E. All of the above   Ref. p. 1411

1356. WHICH OF THE FOLLOWING STATEMENTS ARE TRUE OF FAMILIAL
PHEOCHROMOCYTOMA?:
A. Increase in bilateral incidence
B. More apt to be on right side
C. Low incidence of associated polyglandular involvement
D. High frequency in organs of Zuckerlandl than others
E. All of the above   Ref. p. 1412

ANSWER THE FOLLOWING STATEMENT T(RUE) OR F(ALSE):

1357. Pregnant patients with toxemia, preeclampsia and headaches should all
have screening for presence of pheochromocytoma.
                                 Ref. p. 1412

SELECT THE MOST APPROPRIATE ANSWER(S):

1358. THE GREATEST PROBLEM IN SURGERY FOR NEUROBLASTOMA IS:
A. Sudden hypertension
B. Spread of tumor
C. Hemorrhage
D. Inability to resist whole tumor
E. All of the above   Ref. p. 1417

1359. LIGATION OF WHICH OF THE FOLLOWING VESSELS CARRIES THE
GREATEST CHANCE OF SUPERIOR LARYNGEAL NERVE INJURY?:
A. Superior thyroid artery
B. Inferior thyroid artery
C. Thyroidea ima   Ref. p. 1430

1360. LIGATION OF WHICH OF THE FOLLOWING VESSELS CARRIES THE
GREATEST CHANCE OF RECURRENT LARYNGEAL NERVE INJURY?:
A. Superior thyroid artery
B. Inferior thyroid artery
C. Thyroidea ima   Ref. p. 1430

1361. EMBRYOLOGICAL DEVELOPMENT OF THE THYROID IS MOSTLY
FROM THE:
A. 2nd and 3rd bronchial pouch
B. 4th and 5th bronchial pouch
C. 6th and 7th bronchial pouch
D. Foramen cecum
E. None of the above   Ref. p. 1430

1362. WHICH OF THE FOLLOWING STATES MAY BE REPRESENTED BY
SYMPTOMS OF HYPOTHYROIDISM?:
A. Nephrotic syndrome   D. Ether anesthesia
B. Cirrhosis   E. All of the above
C. Pregnancy   Ref. p. 1432-1434

1363. WHICH OF THE FOLLOWING IS MOST POTENT?:
A. Thyroxine
B. Triiodothyronine
C. Equal   Ref. p. 1432

1364. THE NORMAL THYROXINE CONCENTRATION IN THE HUMAN GLAND
PERMITS NORMAL FUNCTION FOR_____WEEKS BEFORE
DEPLETION:
A. 2   D. 8
B. 4   E. 10
C. 6   Ref. p. 1432

1365. WHICH OF THE FOLLOWING IS NOT CHARACTERISTIC OF T3?:
A. 4x more active than T4
B. Lower concentration than T4 in ratio of 10-20:1
C. Less firmly bound to protein than T4
D. Half-life 6-11 days
E. Conjugated in liver   Ref. p. 1432

1366. WHICH OF THE FOLLOWING ANTITHYROID MEDICATIONS IS USED TO
PREVENT CONCENTRATION OF IODINE?:
A. Thiourea   D. Thiocyanate
B. Perchlorate   E. All of the above
C. Sulfonamides   Ref. p. 1433

1367. WHICH ANTITHYROID MEDICATION PREVENTS BINDING OF IODINE
TO TYROSINE?:
A. Thiourea   D. Thiocyanate
B. Pechlorate   E. All of the above
C. Sulfonamides   Ref. p. 1433

1368. WHICH OF THE FOLLOWING FACTORS DIRECTLY AFFECT TSH
SECRETION?:
A. TRF   D. Thyroxine
B. Plasma iodide   E. Thiourea
C. Intrathyroidal iodide   Ref. p. 1433

1369. THE ENLARGED DELPHIAN NODE WHICH APPEARS IN THE MIDLINE
PRETHYROIDEAL AREA ABOVE THE ISTHMUS OFTEN IS INDICATIVE
OF WHICH DISEASE?:
A. Thyroiditis   D. Carcinoma of thyroid
B. Graves' disease   E. Parathyroid carcinoma
C. Myxedema   Ref. p. 1434

1370. A RADIOACTIVE THYROID UPTAKE TESTED AT 24 HOURS NORMALLY
FALLS IN WHICH RANGE?:
A. 0-10%   D. 40-70%
B. 10-15%   E. 70-95%
C. 15-40%   Ref. p. 1434

ANSWER THE FOLLOWING STATEMENT T(RUE) OR F(ALSE):

1371. The thyroid uptake studies vary with renal excretion.
Ref. p. 1434

SELECT THE MOST APPROPRIATE ANSWER:

1372. ALL OF THE FOLLOWING WILL INCREASE THE PBI,EXCEPT:
A. Hyperthyroidism   D. Hashimoto's disease
B. Thyroid suppression   E. Thyroid carcinoma
C. Subacute thyroiditis   Ref. p. 1435

1373. WHICH PLAYS A GREATER PART IN THE ETIOLOGY OF GRAVES'
DISEASE?:
A. TSH
B. Long-acting thyroid stimulation (LATS)
C. Equal   Ref. p. 1437

1374. ATRIAL FIBRILLATION OCCURS WITH GREATER FREQUENCY IN:
A. Graves' disease (Hyperthyroidism)
B. Toxic adenoma
C. Both equally   Ref. p. 1438

1375. OBSTRUCTIVE SYMPTOMS ARE RELATED TO:
A. Graves' disease
B. Toxic multinodular goiter
C. Equal   Ref. p. 1439

1376. EXOPHTHALMOS SYMPTOMS ARE RELATED TO:
A. Graves' disease
B. Multinodular goiter
C. Equal   Ref. p. 1439

1377. GRAVES' DISEASE PRESENTS WITH PERNICIOUS ANEMIA IN 1% OF
THE CASES. WHICH OF THE FOLLOWING REPRESENTS THE MOST
LIKELY ETIOLOGY?:
A. Decrease in terminal ileum absorption of B_{12}
B. Destruction of extrinsic factor in stomach
C. Production of anti-gastric parietal cell antibodies
                                      Ref. p. 1439

CASE HISTORY:

A 45 year-old female presents with a history of intolerance to heat,
exophthalmos, a loss of appetite and weight. A diffusely enlarged
thyroid gland is palpated.

1378. THE MOST LIKELY DIAGNOSIS IS:
A. Graves' disease
B. Toxic multinodular goiter
C. Toxic adenoma   Ref. p. 1439

1379. THE PATIENT WOULD MOST LIKELY PRESENT WITH ALL OF THE
FOLLOWING, EXCEPT:
A. PBI elevated over 10 mg%   D. Atrial fibrillation
B. BMR elevated over +35   E. All of the above
C. Exophthalmos   Ref. p. 1439

1380. IN THE ABOVE CASE HISTORY, THE PREOPERATIVE TREATMENT
OF HYPERACTIVE THYROID GLANDS WITH ANTITHYROID DRUGS
OFTEN:
A. Increases glandular vascularity while creating a normal metabolic
state
B. Decreases glandular vascularity
C. Does not alter glandular vascularity
                                      Ref. p. 1440

1381. TREATMENT OF THYROID DISEASE WITH RADIOACTIVE I^{131} IS OF
QUESTIONABLE USE BECAUSE OF ALL OF THE FOLLOWING, EXCEPT:
A. The time necessary to control the disease is so long
B. The incidence of myxedema is high
C. Potential development of carcinoma or leukemia
D. Frequent accompanying hypoparathyroidism
E. Transplacental migration to fetus during pregnancy
                                      Ref. p. 1440

1382. JUVENILE HYPOTHYROIDISM PRESENTS WITH WHICH ASSOCIATED
      STATES?:
      A. Abdominal distension   C. Prolapse of rectum
      B. Umbilical hernia   D. All of these   Ref. p. 1442

ANSWER THE FOLLOWING STATEMENT T(RUE) OR F(ALSE):

1383. Cretinism often manifests itself at birth.   Ref. p. 1442

SELECT THE MOST APPROPRIATE ANSWER(S):

1384. WHICH OF THE FOLLOWING STATES IS CONSIDERED TO BE AN
      AUTOIMMUNE PHENOMENON?:
      A. Quervain's disease   D. Riedel's struma
      B. Hashimoto's disease   E. All of these
      C. Granulomatous thyroiditis   Ref. p. 1443

1385. THE TYPE OF THYROID CARCINOMA FOUND IN HASHIMOTO'S
      DISEASE IS:
      A. Papillary carcinoma
      B. Follicular carcinoma
      C. Both are equal   Ref. p. 1443

1386. TREATMENT OF CHOICE IN HASHIMOTO'S DISEASE IS:
      A. Suppressive thyroid hormone therapy   D. Propylthiouracil
      B. Subtotal thyroidectomy   E. Perchlorate
      C. Radioactive I^{131} Ref. p. 1444

1387. QUERVAIN'S DISEASE (ACUTE NONSUPPURATIVE THYROIDITIS) IS
      TREATED WITH:
      A. Surgical excision   D. Propylthiouracil
      B. Radioactive I^{131} E. Lugol's solution
      C. Aspirin and glucocorticoids   Ref. p. 1445

1388. WHICH OF THE FOLLOWING DOES NOT HELP TO DISTINGUISH A
      MULTINODULAR GOITER FROM THYROID CARCINOMA?:
      A. Scan indicating cold nodule
      B. Presence of Horner's syndrome in the former
      C. Male patients less than 40 years old
      D. X-rays with psammoma bodies
      E. All of the above distinguishes   Ref. pp. 1446, 1448

1389. THE ABILITY TO RETAIN THE CAPACITY TO ACCUMULATE IODIDE
      IS PRESENT IN:
      A. Follicular carcinoma
      B. Medullary carcinoma
      C. Neither   Ref. p. 1449

1390. WHICH OF THE FOLLOWING HAVE A HIGH ASSOCIATION WITH
      PHEOCHROMOCYTOMA?:
      A. Follicular carcinoma of thyroid
      B. Papillary carcinoma of thyroid
      C. Medullary carcinoma of thyroid
      D. Anaplastic carcinoma of thyroid
      E. Nontoxic multinodular goiter   Ref. p. 1449

1391. WHICH OF THE FOLLOWING IS NOT APPLICABLE TO FOLLICULAR
      CARCINOMA OF THE THYROID?:
      A. Often is TSH dependent
      B. Represents 25% of the thyroid carcinomas
      C. The bone lesions are usually osteolytic
      D. Calcified psammoma bodies are often seen on X-ray
      E. Hematogenous spread is more frequent than lymph node metastasis
                                           Ref. p. 1451

1392. PREOPERATIVE PREPARATION FOR THYROID SURGERY SHOULD MAKE THE PATIENT EUTHYROID. THIS IS OFTEN ACCOMPLISHED WITH:
A. Lugol's solution
B. Propylthiouracil
C. Thyroid extract
D. Prednisone
E. Perchlorate
Ref. p. 1453

1393. THYROID STORM CARRIES A MORTALITY RATE OF:
A. 10%
B. 20%
C. 30%
D. 40%
E. 50%
Ref. p. 1455

1394. THYROID STORM PRESENTS WITH ALL, EXCEPT:
A. Hyperthermia
B. Massive diuresis
C. Profuse sweating
D. Tachycardia
E. Nausea, vomiting, abdominal pain
Ref. p. 1455

1395. THE MAJOR PROBLEM ASSOCIATED WITH BILATERAL LARYNGEAL NERVE DAMAGE IS:
A. Hoarseness
B. Tracheomalacia
C. Airway obstruction
Ref. p. 1455

1396. THE TREATMENT OF HYPOPARATHYROIDISM SHOULD BE INITIATED PROMPTLY AND MAY CONSIST OF:
A. Calcium lactate 5-15 gm
B. Vitamin D_2 50,000-200,000
C. Parathormone dihydrotachysterol
D. Calcium gluconate 5-15 gm
E. Parathyroid transplantation
Ref. p. 1456

1397. THE PARATHYROID GLANDS DEVELOP FROM WHICH OF THE FOLLOWING BRONCHIAL POUCHES?:
A. 4th and 3rd bronchial pouch
B. 2nd and 3rd bronchial pouch
C. 4th and 5th bronchial pouch
D. 5th and 6th bronchial pouch
Ref. p. 1457

1398. THE NORMAL DAILY CALCIUM EXCRETION IN URINE IS ABOUT:
A. 30 mg
B. 100 mg
C. 300 mg
D. 400 mg
E. 600 mg
Ref. p. 1459

1399. WHICH OF THE FOLLOWING IS AFFECTED BY PARATHORMONE (PTH)?:
A. Renal excretion of calcium
B. Phosphate absorption in GI tract
C. Increase bone resorption
D. Magnesium reabsorption in kidneys
E. All of the above
Ref. p. 1460

1400. WHICH OF THE FOLLOWING DOES NOT INCREASE PHOSPHATE URINARY EXCRETION?:
A. Hyperparathyroidism
B. Hypervitaminosis D
C. Vitamin D deficiency with secondary hyperparathyroidism
D. Addison's disease
E. Osteoporosis
Ref. p. 1460

1401. WHICH OF THE FOLLOWING HORMONES DOES NOT ALTER HYDROXYPROLINE EXCRETION IN THE URINE?:
A. Parathormone
B. Thyroxin
C. Cortisol
D. Growth hormone
Ref. p. 1461

1402. IN HYPERPARATHYROIDISM, BONE RESORPTION IS:
A. Increased
B. Decreased
C. Remains the same
Ref. p. 1462

1403. IN CHRONIC RENAL FAILURE AND SECONDARY HYPERPARATHY-
      ROIDISM, INSENSITIVITY TO PTH IS DEMONSTRATED BY BONE AND
      A RESULTING HYPOCALCEMIC STATE. THIS MOST LIKELY REFLECTS:
      A. Increase in PTH breakdown   D. Inactivation of Vitamin D
      B. Accumulation of thyrocalcitonin E. None of the above
      C. More rapid protein-calcium binding   Ref. p. 1465

      ANSWER THE FOLLOWING STATEMENT T(RUE) OR F(ALSE):

1404. The renal effects of parathormone are accelerated and decreased by
      vitamin D and thyrocalcitonin.   Ref. p. 1465

      SELECT THE MOST APPROPRIATE ANSWER:

1405. THE PRODUCTION OF PTH IS PRIMARILY FROM _____ CELLS:
      A. Oxyphilic
      B. Water clear cells
      C. Chief cells   Ref. p. 1467

      ANSWER THE FOLLOWING STATEMENTS T(RUE) OR F(ALSE):

1406. Parathyroid hyperplasia frequently involves only a solitary gland making
      excision a relatively simple procedure.   Ref. p. 1468

1407. The major differentiating factor in parathyroid adenoma vs. hyperplasia
      is that the former is primarily a chief cell type.   Ref. p. 1468

1408. A patient found to have one normal parathyroid gland usually indicates
      that the enlarged gland is adenomatous rather than hyperplastic.
                                                    Ref. p. 1469

      SELECT THE MOST APPROPRIATE ANSWER:

1409. WHICH IS GREATER IN SIZE?:
      A. Chief cell hyperplasia
      B. Clear cell hyperplasia
      C. Both are equal   Ref. p. 1468

1410. THE MOST FREQUENT CAUSE OF HYPERCALCEMIC CRISIS IS:
      A. Parathyroid disease
      B. Carcinoma of breast
      C. Equal   Ref. p. 1469

1411. PRESENTING SYMPTOMS OF HYPERPARATHYROIDISM ARE MORE
      OFTEN:
      A. Renal symptoms
      B. Skeletal symptoms
      C. Equal   Ref. p. 1472

1412. HYPERPARATHYROID CRISIS USUALLY HAS ALL OF THE FOLLOWING,
      EXCEPT:
      A. Serum calcium over 16 mg%   D. A mortality of 100% without surgery
      B. High degree of renal failure E. A 60% mortality with surgery
      C. Low serum phosphate level   Ref. p. 1473

1413. WHICH HAS A GREATER RELATIONSHIP TO IONIZED CALCIUM IN
      HYPERPARATHYROIDISM?:
      A. Pancreatitis
      B. Duodenal ulcer
      C. Equal   Ref. p. 1475

1414. ULCER DISEASE IN HYPERPARATHYROIDISM PRESENTS WITH:
      A. Gastric symptoms
      B. Duodenal symptoms
      C. Equal   Ref. p. 1475

1415. WHICH OF THE FOLLOWING ARE NOT THE RESULT OF THE DIRECT
       EFFECT OF PARATHORMONE?:
       A. Renal stone formation   D. Demineralization of skeleton
       B. Hypertension   E. None of the above
       C. Pancreatitis   Ref. p. 1476

1416. METASTATIC CALCIFICATION IS PRESENT IN:
       A. Primary hyperparathyroidism
       B. Secondary hyperparathyroidism
       C. Equal   Ref. pp. 1477, 1482

1417. METASTATIC CALCIFICATION IN:
       A. Secondary hyperparathyroidism
       B. Vitamin D intoxication
       C. Equal   Ref. p. 1477

1418. IN WHICH OF THE FOLLOWING TESTS FOR HYPERPARATHYROIDISM IS
       THE (TRP) TUBULAR REABSORPTION OF PHOSPHATE NOT UTILIZED?:
       A. Phosphate deprivation test   D. Cortisone administration (Dent test)
       B. PTH infusion test   E. Calcium infusion test
       C. EDTA test   Ref. p. 1479

1419. THE EFFECT OF AN INCREASE OF (PARATHORMONE) PTH ON THE
       TRP IS TO _____ IT:
       A. Increase
       B. Decrease
       C. Show no change in   Ref. p. 1479

1420. WHICH OF THE FOLLOWING POLYGLANDULAR SYNDROMES MOST
       FREQUENTLY ACCOMPANIES HYPERPARATHYROIDISM?:
       A. Acromegaly   C. Zollinger-Ellison syndrome
       B. Hypercalcemia   D. Pancreatic beta cell tumor
                                          Ref. pp. 1486, 1487

1421. WHICH OF THE FOLLOWING IS NOT AN INDICATION FOR PARA-
       THYROIDECTOMY?:
       A. Development of severe bone pain in the presence of secondary hyper-
           parathyroidism
       B. Following renal transplantation
       C. Development of cellular autonomy as chief cell hyperplasia or adenoma
       D. Along with thyroid if resecting thyroid carcinoma
                                          Ref. p. 1490

1422. WHICH IS GREATER? CALCIUM LEVELS IN:
       A. Primary hyperparathyroidism
       B. Secondary hyperparathyroidism
       C. Equal   Ref. p. 1497

1423. THE MOST COMMON CAUSE OF DEATH FOLLOWING PARATHYROID-
       ECTOMY IS:
       A. Tracheal compression   D. Liver failure
       B. Cardiac arrhythmias associated with low CO_2 E. None of the above
       C. Renal failure   Ref. p. 1497

1424. THE MOST SIGNIFICANT DIFFERENCE(S) BETWEEN PRIMARY AND
       SECONDARY HYPERPARATHYROIDISM IS (ARE):
       A. Normal serum calcium in the former and elevated in the latter
       B. A low total protein in the latter
       C. A low phosphorus level in the latter
       D. None of the above   Ref. p. 1497

SELECT THE MOST APPROPRIATE ANSWER(S):

1425. WHICH OF THE FOLLOWING PATHOLOGICAL ENTITIES BEST EX-
PRESSES THE CAUSE OF PULMONARY COMPLICATIONS WITH
TRACHEO-ESOPHAGEAL FISTULA?:
A. Reflux salivary juice from the blind pouch into the trachea
B. Direct passage of salivary juice into the lower trachea above the
carina
C. No aspiration is involved, however, pulmonary hypoplasia is a com-
mon associated condition
D. Reflux of gastric juice from the stomach into the trachea via a lower
end fistula
E. The frequent association of hyaline membrane disease and T-E
fistula   Ref. p. 1516

1426. IF ON THE FLAT PLATE THERE IS NO AIR IN THE STOMACH OF THE
SUSPECTED NEONATE, ONE MAY:
A. Only observe the child since surgery is not necessary
B. Not be as concerned with a severe chemical peritonitis but still
worry about reflux aspiration
C. Neither   Ref. p. 1517

1427. THE REPAIR OF A T-E FISTULA SHOULD INVOLVE ALL THE
FOLLOWING, EXCEPT:
A. Haight type anastomosis
B. Simple ligature of fistula tract
C. Division of the azygos vein
D. Closure of membraneous tracheal defect
E. All of the above   Ref. p. 1518

1428. PYLORIC STENOSIS IS A DISEASE CHARACTERIZED BY ALL OF THE
FOLLOWING, EXCEPT:
A. Decreased pyloro-muscular ganglion cells
B. First born males
C. Projectile vomiting at 5 to 6 weeks of age
D. Olive shaped mass in the right upper quadrant
E. Surgical mortality rate of 5 per cent
                 Ref. p. 1521

1429. THE CONGENITAL DEFECT MOST FREQUENTLY ASSOCIATED WITH
A PERSISTENT OMPHALOMESENTERIC DUCT IS:
A. Gastroschisis   D. Meckel's diverticulus
B. Omphalocele   E. None of the above
C. Persistent urachus   Ref. p. 1522

1430. WHAT PER CENT OF CHILDREN WITH MECKEL'S DIVERTICULAR
DISEASE PRESENT BEFORE THE AGE OF ONE?:
A. 10 per cent
B. 33 per cent
C. 66 per cent
D. 99 per cent   Ref. p. 1523

1431. THE COVERING OVER AN OMPHALOCELE IS:
A. Skin
B. Amniotic membrane
C. Chorionic membrane
D. None of the above   Ref. p. 1523

1432. WHICH OF THE FOLLOWING MAY BE UTILIZED TO TREAT A LARGE
OMPHALOCELE ?:
   A. Primary closure of skin after amniotic membrane excision
   B. Silver nitrate application to the amniotic membrane
   C. Benzalkonium chloride application to the amniotic membrane
   D. Development of skin flaps
   E. All of the above   Ref. p. 1523-1524

1433. IF IN THE REPAIR OF AN OMPHALOCELE, TENSION IS REQUIRED
TO REPLACE THE ABDOMINAL VISCERA, WHICH OF THE FOLLOW-
ING WILL MOST LIKELY LEAD TO THE PATIENT'S DEMISE ?:
   A. Respiratory embarrassment
   B. Inferior vena cava compression and decreased venous return
   C. Renal shut down
   D. Prolonged paralytic ileus with electrolyte deficiency and starvation
   E. All are equal   Ref. p. 1524

1434. THE LADD PROCEDURE IS FOR WHICH OF THE FOLLOWING CON-
GENITAL ANOMALIES ?:
   A. Persistent urachus
   B. Gastroschisis
   C. Intestinal atresia
   D. Malrotation of cecum and peritoneal bands
   E. Intussusception   Ref. p. 1525-1526

1435. INTESTINAL OBSTRUCTION IS A FREQUENT FINDING ALONG WITH
A MALROTATION. WHICH OF THE FOLLOWING IS USUALLY AF-
FECTED ?:
   A. Duodenal atresia
   B. Jejunal atresia
   C. Ileal atresia
   D. Colonic atresia   Ref. p. 1525

1436. THE MOST FREQUENT CAUSE FOR NEONATAL INTESTINAL OB-
STRUCTION IS:
   A. Meconium ileus   D. Ileal atresia
   B. Malrotation + midgut volvulus   E. Intussusception
   C. Congenital bands   Ref. p. 1526

1437. WHICH OF THE FOLLOWING IS NOT ASSOCIATED WITH A HIGH INCI-
DENCE OF MATERNAL HYDRAMNIOS ?:
   A. Duodenal atresia
   B. Jejunal atresia
   C. Ileal atresia   Ref. p. 1527

1438. WHICH OF THE FOLLOWING IS FREQUENTLY ASSOCIATED WITH
CYSTIC FIBROSIS ?:
   A. Ileal atresia   D. Pulmonary fibrosis
   B. Jejunal atresia   E. None of the above
   C. Malrotation   Ref. p. 1529

1439. THE OPERATIVE TECHNIQUE WHICH DECOMPRESSES AN INTUSSUS-
CEPTION IS DEPENDENT ON:
   A. Constant firm traction on the proximal bowel
   B. Resection of the involved segment without traction
   C. Progressive manual pressure on distal segment to intussusception
                                          Ref. p. 1531

1440. IN HIRSCHSPRUNG'S DISEASE, WHICH OF THE FOLLOWING IS
       ABSENT ?:
       A. Myenteric ganglia
       B. Auerbach's plexus
       C. Neither   Ref. p. 1531

1441. WHICH ORGAN IS MOST OFTEN INVOLVED IN ASSOCIATION WITH A
       COLONIC AGANGLIONOSIS ?:
       A. Pancreas   D. Small intestine
       B. Gall bladder   E. All of the above
       C. Bladder   Ref. p. 1532

1442. THE EASIEST WAY TO DOCUMENT THE DIAGNOSIS OF HIRSCH-
       SPRUNG'S DISEASE IN 90 PER CENT OF THE CASES IS:
       A. Barium enema   D. Sigmoidoscopy
       B. Rectal biopsy (full thickness)   E. None of the above
       C. Intraluminal manometric studies Ref. p. 1532-1533

1443. MANOMETRIC STUDIES OF THE RECTAL SPHINCTER MECHANISM
       IN HIRSCHSPRUNG'S DISEASE INDICATE:
       A. External sphincter contraction and internal sphincter contraction
       B. External sphincter contraction and internal sphincter relaxation
       C. Internal sphincter contraction and external sphincter relaxation
       D. Internal sphincter relaxation and external sphincter relaxation
                                           Ref. p. 1533

1444. RECURRENT RECTAL PROLAPSE IN CHILDREN IS USUALLY TREATED
       BY:
       A. Rectal segment resection
       B. Recurrent digital reduction
       C. Creation of an inflammatory response between rectal wall and sacrum
          by dissection of the area and packing
                                           Ref. p. 1538

1445. IMPERFORATE ANUS OF THE MEMBRANOUS VARIETY SHOULD HAVE:
       A. A sigmoid colostomy
       B. An abdominal perineal pullthrough
       C. A simple digital perforation of the membrane
                                           Ref. p. 1540

SELECT THE MOST APPROPRIATE ANSWER(S):

1446. WHICH OF THE RENAL ARTERIES IS ANATOMICALLY OF GREATER LENGTH?:
A. Right
B. Left
C. Both are equal   Ref. p. 1547

1447. WHICH OF THE FOLLOWING UROLOGIC ORGANS HAS A TRANSITIONAL CELL COVERING:
A. Ureter   D. Bladder
B. Urethra   E. All of the above
C. Renal collecting tubules   Ref. p. 1548

1448. GROSS HEMATURIA IN PATIENTS BETWEEN THE AGES OF 18 AND 40 YEARS IS MOST LIKELY DUE TO:
A. Benign prostatic hypertrophy   D. Leukemia
B. Bladder tumor   E. Renal calculi
C. Cystitis or urethritis   Ref. p. 1549

1449. THE MOST COMMON CAUSE OF ACUTE URINARY RETENTION IN YOUNG MALES IS:
A. Prostatic abscess
B. Urethral stricture due to gonorrhea
C. Bladder calculi
D. Nephrolithiasis with reflux
E. Neurogenic bladder dysfunction   Ref. p. 1550

1450. THE SYMPTOM OF URGENCY IS MOST OFTEN RELATED TO:
A. Obstructing prostatic tumors   D. Vesical outlet inflammation
B. Obstructing bladder tumors   E. Neurogenic bladder
C. Nephrolithiasis   Ref. p. 1550

1451. THE DEVELOPMENT OF A LEFT SIDED VARICOCELE AFTER THE AGE OF 40 YEARS CAN BE AN INDICATION OF:
A. Normal change
B. Renal vein occlusion usually of tumor origin
C. Hernia incarceration
D. Tuberculosis of the prostate
E. None of the above   Ref. p. 1551

1452. MOST URINARY TRACT INFECTIONS ARE:
A. Ascending   D. Present in females
B. Descending   E. Staphylococcal
C. Present in males   Ref. p. 1558

1453. IN WHICH OF THE FOLLOWING PATIENT TYPES IS A SINGLE URINARY TRACT INFECTION AN ABSOLUTE INDICATION FOR A COMPLETE UROLOGIC INVESTIGATION?:
A. Male
B. Female
C. Both A and B
D. Neither   Ref. p. 1558

1454. WHICH OF THE FOLLOWING IS MORE LIKELY DUE TO HEMATOGENOUS ORIGIN?:
A. Escherichia coli
B. Pseudomonas aeruginosa
C. Aerobacter aerogenes
D. Staphylococcus aureus
E. Proteus vulgaris   Ref. p. 1559

1455. URINARY CALCULI ARE RADIOPAQUE IN_____PER CENT OF
CASES:
A. 15   D. 95
B. 30   E. 100
C. 60   Ref. p. 1562

1456. WHICH OF THE FOLLOWING IS NOT AN INDICATION FOR URETHRAL
EXPLORATION?:
A. Nonfunction of kidney on pyelogram with evidence of obstruction on
   retrograde pyelogram
B. Persistent hydronephrosis
C. Obstructing stone associated with infection
D. Frequent episodes of incapacitating colic
E. All of the above   Ref. p. 1563

1457. HYPERKALEMIA IN RENAL SHUTDOWN IS MOST EASILY DOCUMENTED
AND FOLLOWED BY THE ELECTROCARDIOGRAM. WHICH OF THE
FOLLOWING PROVIDES THE BEST CONTROLLING UNIT?:
A. Low voltage QRS complex   D. Spiking P wave
B. Prolonged ST segment   E. Prolonged PQ segment.
C. Spiking T wave   Ref. p. 1565

1458. THE MAIN CONTENDERS IN THE DIFFERENTIAL DIAGNOSIS FOR
WILMS' TUMORS IN THE PEDIATRIC AGE GROUP INCLUDE ALL,
EXCEPT:
A. Neuroblastoma   D. Perinephric abscess
B. Hydronephrosis   E. None of the above
C. Solitary renal cyst   Ref. p. 1567

1459. THE SURVIVAL RATE OF PATIENTS WITH WILMS' TUMORS DIS-
COVERED UNDER THE AGE OF 2 YEARS AND TREATED IS ABOUT:
A. 10 per cent   D. 70 per cent
B. 25 per cent   E. 90 per cent
C. 55 per cent   Ref. p. 1567

1460. CRYPTORCHIDISM IN PREMATURE INFANTS APPEAR IN:
A. 4 per cent   D. 50 per cent
B. 21 per cent   E. 70 per cent
C. 36 per cent   Ref. p. 1570

1461. UNDESCENDED TESTES SHOULD NORMALLY REACH THE SCROTAL
POSITION WITHIN_____AFTER BIRTH:
A. 1 week   D. 12 months
B. 3 weeks   E. 24 months
C. 6 weeks   Ref. p. 1570

FILL IN THE MOST APPROPRIATE ANSWERS: (Questions 1462-1463)

A. Undescended testis in the canal
B. Undescended testis in the abdomen
C. Retractile scrotal testis
D. Eleven
E. Fifty
F. Seventy-five

The incidence of testicular tumors in 1462)_____ carries a higher
incidence of malignant degeneration which is 1463)_____ times
greater.   Ref. p. 1570

SELECT THE MOST APPROPRIATE ANSWER:

1464.   THE SURVIVAL FROM RENAL TUMORS WITHOUT LYMPH NODE
        METASTASES FOLLOWING SURGICAL CORRECTION IS:
        A. 20 per cent   D. 70 per cent
        B. 30 per cent   E. 80 per cent
        C. 50 per cent   Ref. p. 1571

1465.   AN INTRAVENOUS PYELOGRAM IS OFTEN A DIAGNOSTIC TEST FOR
        RENAL CARCINOMA, EXCEPT:
        A. If the BSP is above 25 per cent
        B. In patients with polycythemia
        C. In patients with renal vein occlusion
        D. In cases where renal calcification is noted
        E. All of the above   Ref. p. 1571

1466.   WHICH OF THE FOLLOWING UROLOGIC TUMORS APPEAR TO HAVE
        THE LOWEST INCIDENCE OF METASTATIC SPREAD AND LOCAL
        EXTENSION?:
        A. Renal cell carcinoma
        B. Squamous cell carcinoma of renal pelvis
        C. Prostatic carcinoma
        D. Papillary carcinoma of bladder
        E. Testicular carcinoma   Ref. p. 1573

1467.   WHICH CARRIES A GREATER MORTALITY?:
        A. Transurethral prostatic resection (TUR)
        B. Open prostatectomy
        C. Both are equal   Ref. p. 1577

1468.   WHICH OF THE FOLLOWING IS NOT TRUE WHEN COMPARING A TUR
        TO AN OPEN PROSTATECTOMY?:
        A. TUR has a lower mortality
        B. Postoperative hospitalization with a TUR is shorter
        C. Bleeding problems are greater with a TUR
        D. Sexual potency is preserved with a TUR
        E. Lithotrity can be combined with a TUR
                                        Ref. p. 1577

1469.   THE TREATMENT OF PROSTATIC CARCINOMA INCLUDES ALL OF
        THE FOLLOWING, EXCEPT:
        A. Estrogens
        B. Orchiectomy
        C. TUR
        D. Prostatoseminal vesiculectomy
        E. Corticosteroids   Ref. p. 1578

1470.   IN WHICH DISEASE STATE IS A VIRCHOW'S NODE MOST EXPECTED?:
        A. Hepatic carcinoma   D. Testicular carcinoma
        B. Thyroid carcinoma   E. All of the above
        C. Prostatic carcinoma   Ref. p. 1578

1471.   THE DIFFERENTIAL DIAGNOSIS OF PAGET'S DISEASE FROM
        METASTATIC PROSTATIC CARCINOMA CAN BE MADE MOST EASILY
        WITH:
        A. X-ray
        B. Alkaline phosphatase
        C. Acid phosphatase
        D. Calcium and phosphorus
        E. None of the above   Ref. p. 1578

1472. THE MOST MALIGNANT TESTICULAR TUMOR IS:
   A. Seminoma   D. Choriocarcinoma
   B. Embryonal cell   E. Teratocarcinoma
   C. Teratoma   Ref. p. 1579

1473. WHICH OF THE FOLLOWING IS MOST LIKELY TO HAVE PULMONARY
   METASTASES AT THE TIME OF SURGERY?:
   A. Seminoma   D. Choriocarcinoma
   B. Embryonal cell   E. Teratocarcinoma
   C. Teratoma   Ref. p. 1579

1474. THE THERAPY OF CHORIOCARCINOMA INCLUDES ALL OF THE
   FOLLOWING, EXCEPT:
   A. Orchiectomy   D. 5 fluorouracil
   B. Methotrexate   E. Actinomycin D
   C. Chlorambucil   Ref. p. 1579

1475. IN ABDOMINAL TRAUMA WITH A DIRECT BLOW TO THE PELVIS
   AND NO PELVIC FRACTURE, WHICH HAS A GREATER FREQUENCY?:
   A. Bladder rupture, intraperitoneal
   B. Bladder rupture, extraperitoneal
   C. Both A and B are equal in incidence
                                  Ref. p. 1580

SELECT THE MOST APPROPRIATE ANSWER(S):

1476. THE UTERINE DEVELOPMENT EMBRYOLOGICALLY IS FROM THE:
A. Mullerian duct
B. Wolffian duct
C. Mesonephric duct
D. All of the above fused together   Ref. p. 1590

1477. WHICH OF THE FOLLOWING IS INVOLVED IN GONORRHEA?:
A. Bartholin's glands
B. Skene's glands
C. Both A and B   Ref. p. 1590

1478. IN THE FEMALE, THE STRUCTURE PENETRATING THE INGUINAL
RING IS THE:
A. Ovary   D. Broad ligament
B. Inguinal ligament   E. Cardinal ligament
C. Round ligament   Ref. p. 1591

1479. THE UTERINE ARTERY IS DERIVED FROM THE:
A. Aorta   D. Middle hemorrhoidal artery
B. Common iliac artery   E. Hypogastric artery
C. External iliac artery Ref. p. 1592

1480. THE MOST IMPORTANT STRUCTURES PREVENTING UTERINE
PROLAPSE ARE:
A. Cardinal ligament   D. Uterosacral ligament
B. Round ligament   E. Levator ani muscles
C. Broad ligament   Ref. p. 1592

1481. WEAKNESS OF THE MUSCULAR SUPPORT OF THE FEMALE URO-
GENITAL AREA MAY RESULT IN:
A. Cystocele   D. Uterine prolapse
B. Rectocele   E. All of the above
C. Enterocele   Ref. p. 1592-1593

MATCH THE FOLLOWING. EACH LETTERED ITEM MAY BE USED
MORE THAN ONCE:

1482. Spermatogenesis in the male   A. Luteinizing hormone
1483. Androgen secretion in the male   B. Chorionic gonadotrophic
1484. Maintenance of the corpus luteum   hormone
                                       C. Follicle stimulating hormone
                                       Ref. p. 1593

SELECT THE MOST APPROPRIATE ANSWER(S):

1485. THE GREATEST CONCENTRATIONS OF CHORIONIC GONADOTROPIN
(CHCG) IN THE FEMALE NORMALLY PRESENTS BETWEEN THE
_____OF PREGNANCY:
A. First week and first month
B. Second week and third month
C. Fifth week and fifth month
D. Eighth week and fifth month   Ref. p. 1593

1486. WHICH OF THE FOLLOWING IS <u>NOT</u> TRUE OF ESTROGEN?:
A. Seen in urine as estrone, estradiol and estriol
B. Responsible for "ferning effect"
C. May cause leiomyoma growth
D. Decreases vaginal acidity
E. Increase of myometrium and endometrium
                              Ref. p. 1594-1595

1487. C^{19} COMPOUNDS ARE RESPONSIBLE FOR ELEVATIONS OF WHICH
OF THE FOLLOWING IN A URINE SPECIMEN?:
A. 17 ketosteroids
B. 17 hydroxycorticosteroids
C. Both A and B equally   Ref. p. 1596

1488. THE HORMONE PRIMARILY RESPONSIBLE FOR PUBERTY DEVELOP-
MENT IS:
A. Estrogen   D. FSH
B. Progesterone   E. None of the above
C. LH   Ref. p. 1596

1489. PROGESTERONE IS RESPONSIBLE FOR ALL THE FOLLOWING,
<u>EXCEPT</u>:
A. Endometrial proliferation   D. Coiling of endometrial glands
B. Rise in body temperature   E. All of the above
C. Loss of "ferning effect"   Ref. p. 1597

1490. THE STAINING OF THE CERVIX WITH IODINE IS TERMED THE
SCHILLER TEST. AREAS WHICH DO NOT STAIN:
A. Are usually normal
B. Should be observed
C. Should be biopsied
D. Should have a Pap test
E. Demonstrate an increase in cellular glycogen
                              Ref. p. 1598

1491. A 23 YEAR-OLD FEMALE PRESENTING WITH PRIMARY DYSMENOR-
RHEA SHOULD:
A. Have a D and C   D. Have a conization
B. Have a hysterectomy   E. Have a presacral neurectomy
C. Be treated symptomatically   Ref. p. 1599

1492. WHICH OF THE FOLLOWING MAY RESULT IN SECONDARY
DYSMENORRHEA?:
A. Endometriosis
B. Chronic pelvic inflammatory disease
C. Tight cervical os
D. Intraluminal fibroids
E. All of the above   Ref. p. 1599

1493. IN PATIENTS WITH STRESS INCONTINENCE, THE MOST SIGNIFICANT
DEBILITATING FACTOR IS:
A. Difficulty in walking
B. Loss of posterior urethro-vesical angle
C. Frequency of urination due to development of trigonitis
D. Development of atonic bladder due to neural compression
E. Presence of cystocele   Ref. p. 1600

1494. WHICH OF THE FOLLOWING IS LEAST RESPONSIBLE FOR NON-MENSTRUAL BLEEDING?:
A. Cervical carcinoma
B. Ovarian carcinoma - not hormonally functional
C. Fallopian tube tumor
D. Endometrial carcinoma
E. Early pregnancy   Ref. p. 1602

1495. ALL OF THE FOLLOWING MAY BE RESPONSIBLE FOR PRIMARY AMENORRHEA, EXCEPT:
A. Pituitary chromophobe adenoma   D. Stein-Leventhal syndrome
B. Hypothyroidism   E. All of the above
C. Hyperthyroidism   Ref. p. 1602

1496. THE TREATMENT OF STEIN-LEVENTHAL SYNDROME IS:
A. Bilateral ovarian wedge resection
B. Hydrocortisone administration chronically
C. FSH
D. Clomid (MRL-41) clomiphene citrate
E. All of the above   Ref. p. 1603

1497. THE NORMAL MINIMAL MALE SPERM COUNT IS:
A. 100,000   D. 40,000
B. 80,000   E. 20,000
C. 60,000   Ref. p. 1605

FILL IN THE MOST APPROPRIATE ANSWERS: (Questions 1498-1499)

A. Endometrial carcinoma   A. Methotrexate
B. Cervical carcinoma   B. Prednisone
C. Ovarian carcinoma   C. 5 fluorouracil
D. Choriocarcinoma   D. Vincristine
E. Leiomyosarcoma   E. Azathioprine

Which of the following tumors respond best to chemotherapy?
1498)_____. The chemotherapeutic agent utilized is 1499)_____.
                              Ref. p. 1607

SELECT THE MOST APPROPRIATE ANSWER:

1500. ENDOMETRIOSIS MAY BE DEMONSTRATED IN:
A. Ovary   D. Lung
B. Peritoneum   E. All of the above
C. Colon   Ref. p. 1609

1501. UTERINE LEIOMYOMAS SHOULD UNDERGO SURGICAL CORRECTION BECAUSE OF ALL, EXCEPT:
A. Malignant degeneration (frequent) D. All of the above
B. Associated infertility   E. None of the above
C. Contribution to chronic anemia   Ref. p. 1610

1502. WHICH OF THE FOLLOWING FREQUENTLY UNDERGO MALIGNANT DEGENERATION?:
A. Pseudopolyps of ulcerative colitis
B. Cervical polyps
C. Endometrial polyps
D. Intestinal polyposis of Peutz-Jegher variety
E. None of the above   Ref. p. 1610-1611

1503. THE MOST COMMON MALIGNANT TUMOR IN FEMALES IS:
   A. Breast carcinoma   D. Ovarian carcinoma
   B. Cervical carcinoma   E. Colonic carcinoma
   C. Endometrial carcinoma   Ref. p. 1611

1504. POSTMENOPAUSAL VAGINAL BLEEDING IS MORE COMMONLY:
   A. Cervical carcinoma
   B. Endometrial carcinoma
   C. Equal in incidence   Ref. p. 1611

1505. THE DIAGNOSIS OF CERVICAL CARCINOMA CAN BE MADE
   DEFINITIVELY BY:
   A. Papanicolaou smear
   B. Cervical conization biopsy
   C. Both A and B   Ref. p. 1611

1506. INVASIVE CERVICAL CARCINOMA MAY BE DISTINGUISHED FROM
   CARCINOMA IN SITU BY:
   A. Papanicolaou smear   D. All of the above
   B. Cervical biopsy   E. None of the above
   C. Conization   Ref. p. 1612

1507. CERVICAL CARCINOMA OF STAGE I AND STAGE IIa TYPE SHOULD BE
   TREATED BY:
   A. Radical surgical extirpation
   B. Radiation
   C. Either A or B
   D. Both A and B   Ref. p. 1613

   FILL IN THE MOST APPROPRIATE ANSWERS: (Questions 1508-1509)

   A. 25 per cent
   B. 45 per cent
   C. 65 per cent
   D. 90 per cent
   E. 98 per cent

   The five year survival of Stage I cervical carcinoma without lymph node
   spread is 1508) _____ , and that with lymph node involvement is
   1509) _____ .   Ref. p. 1614

   SELECT THE MOST APPROPRIATE ANSWER(S):

1510. THE MOST COMMON COMPLICATION FOLLOWING RADICAL
   HYSTERECTOMY FOR CERVICAL CARCINOMA IS:
   A. Hemorrhage   D. Urinary tract fistula
   B. Cystitis   E. Claudication intermittents
   C. Rectal stricture   Ref. p. 1615

1511. ENDOMETRIAL CARCINOMA OF THE FUNDUS FOLLOWING TREAT-
   MENT HAS A FIVE YEAR SURVIVAL OF_____PER CENT:
   A. 20   D. 80
   B. 40   E. 90
   C. 60   Ref. p. 1616

1512. RECURRENCE OF ENDOMETRIAL CARCINOMA FOLLOWING SURGERY
   MAY BE TREATED BY:
   A. Radiation   D. Progestational agents
   B. Local excision   E. Estrogens
   C. Diethylstilbestrol   Ref. p. 1616-1617

1513.   PRECANCEROUS STATES OF THE VULVA INCLUDE:
        A. Paget's disease   D. Bowen's disease
        B. Leichen sclerosus et atrophicans   E. All of the above
        C. Leukoplakia   Ref. p. 1617

1514.   CHOCOLATE CYSTS OF THE OVARIES ARISE:
        A. De novo in the ovary
        B. As a product from endometriosus
        C. Have malignant potential
        D. From the corpus luteum
        E. Are enlarged Graafian follicles   Ref. p. 1619

1515.   OVARIAN CARCINOMA IS MORE OFTEN OF WHICH TYPE?:
        A. Pseudomucinous cystadenocarcinoma
        B. Serous cystadenocarcinoma
        C. Endometrial carcinoma
        D. Dysgerminoma
        E. Teratoma   Ref. p. 1620

1516.   WHICH OF THE FOLLOWING TUMORS MAY HAVE MASCULINIZING
        EFFECTS?:
        A. Hilus cell tumor
        B. Arrhenoblastoma
        C. Adrenal rest tumor
        D. Struma ovarii
        E. Choriocarcinoma
        F. Thecoma   Ref. p. 1622

1517.   THE URETER PASSES_____THE UTERINE ARTERY:
        A. Above
        B. Below   Ref. p. 1626

SELECT THE MOST APPROPRIATE ANSWER(S):

1518. THE TRANSMISSION OF SCALP INFECTIONS TO THE INTRACRANIAL
      VAULT IS USUALLY VIA:
      A. Transverse sinus
      B. Sigmoid sinus
      C. Cavernosus sinus
      D. Emissary veins in diploic spaces
      E. Ophthalmic veins   Ref. p. 1633

1519. LACERATION OF THE SCALP OFTEN REQUIRES SUTURE CLOSURE
      WITH LARGE DEEP SUTURES BECAUSE:
      A. The high incidence of subgaleal hematoma development
      B. The blood vessels in the scalp are often held open by the associated
         fibrous tissues adjacent to the vessels
      C. The high incidence of infections in association with galeal lacerations
      D. The increased incidence of cerebral compression if the area is not
         closed   Ref. p. 1633

1520. WHICH OF THE FOLLOWING IS AN INDICATION FOR SURGICAL RE-
      PAIR OF A DURAL LACERATION?:
      A. All dural lacerations must be repaired
      B. All cases with otorrhea
      C. All cases with rhinorrhea
      D. Only those cases with persistent drainage exceeding 10 to 14 days
      E. None of the above   Ref. p. 1633

1521. LOSS OF CONSCIOUSNESS IS FOUND IN WHICH OF THE FOLLOWING
      CONDITIONS?:
      A. Cerebral concussion   D. All of the above
      B. Cerebral contusion   E. None of the above
      C. Cerebral laceration   Ref. p. 1634-1635

1522. WHICH OF THE FOLLOWING STATEMENTS IS CORRECT CONCERN-
      ING SKULL FRACTURES?:
      A. All skull fractures, whether linear or depressed should be hospital-
         ized and observed
      B. Compound fractures of the skull should not be debrided
      C. Depressed fractures of the skull should usually be elevated because
         of the high risk of a tear in the dura
      D. A skull fracture which traverses a paranasal sinus is not considered
         to be a compound fracture   Ref. p. 1634

1523. A PATIENT WITH HEAD TRAUMA PRESENTING WITH A TACHY-
      CARDIA AND HYPOTENSION SHOULD:
      A. Continue to be observed for state of consciousness and slowing of
         pulse rate, which would indicate further progression of cranial dam-
         age before surgery is performed
      B. Should immediately undergo surgery to alleviate cerebral compres-
         sion
      C. Should have a thorough examination of other injured areas since vas-
         cular collapse is rarely caused by head injury alone
      D. None of the above
      E. All of the above   Ref. p. 1635-1636

1524. WHICH OF THE FOLLOWING ARE OF LEAST VALUE IN EVALUATING
      A PATIENT WITH HEAD TRAUMA?:
      A. Lumbar puncture
      B. Skull X-rays
      C. Echo encephalogram
      D. Carotid arteriogram   Ref. p. 1636

1525.   THE MOST IMPORTANT SIGN TO A PHYSICIAN OBSERVING A PATIENT
        WITH HEAD TRAUMA IS:
        A. Pulse rate change, blood pressure change
        B. Change in the state of consciousness
        C. Leakage of cerebral spinal fluid
        D. Change in basal temperature
        E. Sudden elevation of leukocyte count
                                            Ref. p. 1636

1526.   PATIENTS SUSTAINING HEAD TRAUMA SHOULD HAVE ALL OF THE
        FOLLOWING PERFORMED, EXCEPT:
        A. Frequent measurement of the pulse rate and blood pressure
        B. Frequent evaluation of the state of consciousness
        C. Frequent evaluation of the pupil equality
        D. Light sedation for the accompanying agitation
        E. All of the above   Ref. p. 1636

1527.   THE REDUCTION OF CEREBRAL EDEMA AND ITS FORMATION MAY
        BE ACCOMPLISHED WITH THE AID OF:
        A. Mannitol diuretics
        B. Assisted respiration with short positive and long negative phase
        C. Decrease in fluid intake
        D. Slight local hypothermia to the cranial vault
        E. Glucocorticosteroids
        F. All of the above   Ref. p. 1637-1638

1528.   THE MOST COMMON INTRACRANIAL HEMORRHAGE FOLLOWING
        HEAD TRAUMA OCCURS IN THE_____SPACE:
        A. Subdural
        B. Subarachnoid
        C. Epidural   Ref. p. 1638

1529.   WHICH OF THE FOLLOWING PRESENTS WITH EITHER AN ACUTE
        CEREBRAL COMPRESSION AND/OR A CHRONIC, PROGRESSIVE
        CEREBRAL COMPRESSION?:
        A. Subdural hematoma
        B. Subarachnoid hematoma
        C. Epidural hematoma   Ref. p. 1638

1530.   A SUBDURAL HEMATOMA DEVELOPING RAPIDLY AND PRESENTING
        WITH HEMIPARESIS OR OTHER LOCALIZING SYMPTOMS OFTEN:
        A. Is only venous
        B. Is both venous and arterial and is associated with a cerebral lacera-
            tion
        C. Is only arterial
        D. Resolves without treatment   Ref. p. 1638

        MATCH THE FOLLOWING. EACH LETTERED ITEM MAY BE USED
        MORE THAN ONCE:

1531.___ Short state of unconsciousness
1532.___ Lucid interval
1533.___ May be acute, subacute or chronic in development
1534.___ The middle meningeal artery is often lacerated
1535.___ Increases in size because of the osmotic obligation of other fluids
1536.___ Frequently associated third nerve palsy and hemiparesis
                        A. Subdural hematoma
                        B. Subarachnoid hematoma
                        C. Epidural hematoma
                        D. Intracerebral hematoma
                        E. Cerebral concussion
                            Ref. p. 1638-1640

SELECT THE MOST APPROPRIATE ANSWER(S):

1537. SPINAL CORD INJURIES DUE TO FRACTURE-DISLOCATION OF THE
VERTEBRAL COLUMN TEND TO DEVELOP AT THE JUNCTION OF
MOBILE AND FIXED VERTEBRAL AREAS. THESE USUALLY ARE:
A. Upper cervical region   D. Upper lumbar region
B. Lower cervical region   E. Lower lumbar region
C. Mid thoracic region   Ref. p. 1641

1538. WHICH OF THE FOLLOWING IS CONTRAINDICATED BECAUSE OF THE
HIGH RISK OF NEURAL DAMAGE FOLLOWING FRACTURE-DISLOCA-
TION OF THE VERTEBRAL COLUMN?:
A. Skeletal traction
B. Slight extension of the neck
C. Stabilization of the fractured area
D. Closed reduction of the fracture-dislocation
E. None of the above   Ref. p. 1642-1643

1539. A QUECKENSTEDT TEST WHICH DEMONSTRATES A COMPLETE
BLOCK OF THE CEREBROSPINAL FLUID CIRCULATION WOULD BE
INDICATED BY:
A. Rapid rise and fall of the lumbar pressure with compression and
   release of the neck veins
B. Rapid fall and elevation of the lumbar pressure with compression and
   release of the neck veins
C. No change in the lumbar pressure with compression and release of
   the neck veins
D. Rapid rise but no fall of the lumbar pressure with compression and
   release of the neck veins   Ref. p. 1642

FILL IN THE MOST APPROPRIATE ANSWERS: (Questions 1540-1541)

A. 1 week   A. 1 cm
B. 2 weeks   B. 2 cm
C. 3 weeks   C. 3 cm
D. 5 weeks   D. 4 cm
E. 10 weeks   E. 5 cm

Laceration of a peripheral nerve with an immediate neurorrhaphy results
in growth of about 1540)_____to cross the suture line and there-
after 1541)_____ per month.   Ref. p. 1644

SELECT THE MOST APPROPRIATE ANSWER(S):

1542. REINNERVATION OF MUSCLE GROUPS MAY BE EXPECTED TO
FUNCTION IF THE NEURORRHAPHY WAS PERFORMED LESS THAN:
A. 1-3 months   D. 15-20 months
B. 4-10 months   E. 25-30 months
C. 11-14 months   Ref. p. 1644

1543. REINNERVATION OF SENSORY FUNCTION MAY BE EXPECTED IF
THE NEURORRHAPHY WAS PERFORMED:
A. 1-3 months   D. 25-30 months
B. 4-10 months   E. There is no time limit
C. 15-20 months   Ref. p. 1644

1544. EVALUATION OF THE PROGRESSIVE DEVELOPMENT OF A SEVERED
NERVE MAY BE DONE BY UTILIZING:
A. The demonstration of an increase in muscular contractility
B. The demonstration of segmental sensory improvement at the most
distal area
C. The demonstration of a positive Tinel sign by percussing the nerve
in route
D. The demonstration of voluntary motor function of the segment
innervated
E. None of the above   Ref. p. 1645

1545. CAREFUL EVALUATION OF A TRAUMATIZED AREA IS INDICATED TO
ESTABLISH THE CAUSE AND SEVERITY OF PERIPHERAL NERVE
DAMAGE. IF THE DAMAGE PRODUCED IS BY STRETCHING, COM-
PRESSION OR CONTUSION, THE TREATMENT OF CHOICE SHOULD BE:
A. Resect the injured area and perform an end to end neurorrhaphy
B. Close observation of the injured area and no surgical intervention
C. Observe the area for a period not exceeding one month and then
perform an end to end surgical repair
                                        Ref. p. 1645

MATCH THE APPROPRIATE PHRASE AND TYPE OF BRAIN TUMOR:

1546.___ Most common brain tumor   A. Astrocytoma III and IV
1547.___ Most common primary brain tumor B. Astrocytoma I and II
         in the middle-aged and elderly   C. Glioma
1548.___ Most common brain tumor in
         children   Ref. p. 1646

SELECT THE MOST APPROPRIATE ANSWER:

1549. WHICH OF THE FOLLOWING HAS THE GREATER MALIGNANT
POTENTIAL?:
A. Astrocytoma in an adult
B. Astrocytoma in childhood
C. Both are equal   Ref. p. 1646

1550. THE TUMOR WITH A PREDILECTION FOR THE ARACHNOID VILLI
AND ARACHNOID INVAGINATION IS:
A. Astrocytoma III and IV
B. Meningioma
C. Medulloblastoma
D. Astrocytoma I and II   Ref. p. 1646

1551. WHICH OF THE FOLLOWING TENDS TO PRESENT WITH A MORE
LOCALIZED PICTURE OF SYMPTOMS?:
A. Head trauma with subdural hematoma
B. Brain tumor
C. Both are equal   Ref. p. 1646

1552. THE CRANIAL NERVE WHICH HAS THE LONGEST EXTRACEREBRAL
COURSE IN THE CRANIAL VAULT IS THE_____AND IT IS THERE-
FORE LOGICAL THAT AN INCREASE IN CEREBRAL PRESSURE WOULD
PRODUCE A PARALYSIS OF THIS NERVE:
A. Oculomotor nerve   D. Abducens nerve
B. Facial nerve   E. Trochlear nerve
C. Auditory nerve   Ref. p. 1646

FILL IN THE MOST APPROPRIATE ANSWERS: (Questions 1553-1554)

A. Supratentorial
B. Posterior fossa
C. Medulla oblongata

Most adult brain tumors are located 1553)_____and in children the
location is 1554)_____ .   Ref. p. 1646

SELECT THE MOST APPROPRIATE ANSWER:

1555.   THE BRAIN TUMOR(S) FREQUENTLY NOTED TO CONTAIN
        RADIOPAQUE CALCIFICATION IS (ARE):
        A. Craniopharyngioma   D. Oligodendroglioma
        B. Astrocytoma   E. Medulloblastoma
        C. Meningioma   Ref. p. 1648

1556.   WHICH OF THE FOLLOWING HAS LESS MALIGNANT POTENTIAL?:
        A. Primary brain tumors
        B. Primary spinal cord tumors
        C. Both are equal   Ref. p. 1650

1557.   THE METASTATIC TUMORS OF THE SPINAL CORD ARE USUALLY
        (75-85%):
        A. Extradural
        B. Intradural
        C. Intramedullary   Ref. p. 1650

MATCH THE APPROPRIATE PHRASE AND ASSOCIATED TYPE OF
PAIN DUE TO EXTRADURAL TUMORS:

1558.___ Radiated over a dermatome   A. Worse at night and rest
1559.___ Localized to the area of involve- B. Associated with movement
         ment   Ref. p. 1650

SELECT THE MOST APPROPRIATE ANSWER(S):

1560.   INTRAMEDULLARY TUMORS DESTROY_____AND THEREFORE
        PAIN IS NOT A CHARACTERISTIC FINDING:
        A. Radicular elements
        B. Crossing fibers in tracts
        C. Spinal roots   Ref. p. 1651

1561.   MOST INTRADURAL-EXTRAMEDULLARY TUMORS OF THE SPINAL
        CORD ARE (90%):
        A. Metastatic   D. Meningiomas
        B. Neurofibromas   E. Ependymomas
        C. Angiomas   Ref. p. 1651

1562.   PATIENTS WITH ESCHERICHIA COLI MENINGITIS SHOULD BE CARE-
        FULLY EXAMINED FOR_____AS THE POSSIBLE ETIOLOGY OF
        THE DISEASE IN THE LUMBAR REGION:
        A. Spina bifida occulta
        B. Meningocele
        C. Dermal sinus tracts
        D. Neurenteric cysts   Ref. p. 1653

1563. CONGENITAL ANEURYSMS HAVE WHICH OF THE FOLLOWING
CHARACTERISTICS?:
A. Saccular
B. Develop at bifurcation of vessels
C. Increased incidence of rupture when they accompany an aortic
coarctation
D. Correlation to systolic hypertension
E. All of the above   Ref. p. 1660

1564. OSTEOMYELITIS OF THE SKULL APPEARS TO HAVE AS ITS
GREATEST SOURCE:
A. Infection of scalp wounds
B. Hematogenous spread from distant area
C. Paranasal sinus, middle ear and mastoid air cell infections
D. Sepsis with thrombosed cavernous sinus
Ref. p. 1662

1565. EPIDURAL ABSCESS USUALLY DEVELOPS FROM:
A. Infections of the skull   C. Necrotic metastatic tumors
B. Infections of the lung   D. Parasitic infestations Ref. p. 1662

1566. THE MOST COMMON ORGANISM CULTURED IN OSTEOMYELITIS OF
THE SKULL, EPIDURAL ABSCESS AND SUBDURAL EMPYEMA IS:
A. Bacillus proteus   C. Staphylococcus aureus
B. Bacillus pyocyaneus   D. Streptococci viridans Ref. p. 1663

1567. THE SURGICAL MODE OF PAIN RELIEF INCLUDES:
A. Sphlanchnicectomy rhizotomy   D. Sympathectomy
B. Trigeminal tractotomy   E. All of the above
C. Lobotomy and thalomy   Ref. p. 1666

1568. THE PROCEDURE OF CHOICE FOR A YOUNG PATIENT SUFFERING
FROM SEVERE CAUSALGIA INHIBITING HIS ACTIVE MOBILITY AND
REHABILITATION IS:
A. Rhizotomy   D. None of the above
B. Cordotomy   E. All of the above
C. Sympathectomy   Ref. p. 1668

1569. DEGENERATIVE CHANGES IN THE VERTEBRAL COLUMN ARE MOST
OFTEN FOUND IN THE:
A. Upper cervical region   D. Upper lumbar region
B. Lower cervical region   E. Lower lumbar region
C. Mid thoracic region   Ref. p. 1670-1671

1570. THE TERM "SCHMOR'S NODULES" DESCRIBES A DEGENERATIVE
CONDITION OF THE VERTEBRAL COLUMN IN WHICH:
A. The nucleus pulposus herniates through the annulus fibrosis
B. The nucleus pulposus herniates through the vertebral body
C. None of the above
D. Either of the two situations   Ref. p. 1671

1571. NINETY-FIVE PER CENT OF THE HERNIATED DISCS OCCUR IN THE:
A. T_{12} to L_1 level   D. L_4 to L_5 level
B. L_1 to L_2 level   E. L_5 to S_1 level
C. I_2 to L_3 level   Ref. p. 1671

1572. A CLINICAL EVALUATION OF THE POSSIBLE NEUROLOGIC DEFICIT
DUE TO A HERNIATED DISC SHOULD INCLUDE_____(INVOLV-
ING L_4-L_5):
A. Evaluation for foot drop   D. All of these
B. Evaluation for dorsiflexion of the great toe   E. None of these
C. Hypesthesia on the medial aspect of the foot   Ref. p. 1671

186

SECTION XIV -ACQUIRED AND CONGENITAL
MUSCULOSKELETAL DISORDERS: RECONSTRUCTION
AND REHABILITATION

SELECT THE MOST APPROPRIATE ANSWER:

1573. IN WHICH OF THE FOLLOWING IS THERE NO SENSORY END ORGAN?:
A. Muscle
B. Periosteum
C. Synovium
D. Cartilage
E. Capsule
Ref. p. 1677

MATCH THE TYPE OF PAIN WITH THE ETIOLOGIC AGENT:

1574. ___ Deep boring night pain
1575. ___ Sharp piercing pain
1576. ___ Burning pain
A. Fractures
B. Paresthesias
C. Osteoarthritis
Ref. pp. 1677-1678

SELECT THE MOST APPROPRIATE ANSWER(S):

1577. COMPRESSION OF THE NERVE ROOT AT THE INTRAFORAMINAL
LEVEL OF C6 RESULTS IN:
A. Pain and paresthesia over the ulnar side of the forearm, 5th finger
and 4th finger
B. Pain and paresthesia on the radial side of the forearm, thumb and
index finger
C. Pain and paresthesia over the dorsal forearm, wrist and one or all
three middle fingers
D. Chest pain which may be diagnosed as a myocardial infarction
Ref. p. 1680

1578. THE THORACIC INLET SYNDROME (CERVICAL RIB) MAY INVOLVE
THE C8-T1 NERVE ROOTS AND RESULT IN:
A. Motor deficit of radial nerve and sensory deficit in T1 dermatome
B. Motor deficit of median nerve or ulnar nerve and sensory deficit in
T1 dermatome
C. Motor deficit of median nerve or ulnar nerve and sensory deficit in
C8 dermatome
D. None of the above
Ref. p. 1681

1579. WHICH OF THE FOLLOWING ARE CHARACTERISTIC OF THE "LOW
BACK SYNDROME"?:
A. Pain accentuated with movement, cough or sneeze
B. Pain, radicular in nature and not relieved by lying down with flexed
extremities
C. Frequently have higher than normal incidence of spondylolisthesis
and spina bifida
Ref. p. 1682

1580. THE FORWARD SUBLUXATION OF ONE VERTEBRAE OVER ANOTHER
IS COMMONLY KNOWN AS:
A. Spondylolysis
B. Spondylolisthesis
C. Sacroiliac strain
D. Spina bifida
Ref. p. 1684

1581. MOST NEUROLOGIC DEFICIT RESULTING FROM A DISC HERNIATION
IS:
A. Bilateral
B. Unilateral
C. Anterior
D. Posterior
Ref. p. 1686

1582. THE PRINCIPAL CAUSE OF TISSUE LOSS OF THE NUCLEUS
PULPOSUS IS:
A. Necrosis due to vascular compromise
B. Dehydration
C. Both equally   Ref. p. 1687

1583. THE STRAIGHT LEG RAISING TESTING TO (LASEGUE'S SIGN)
DEMONSTRATE THE PRESENCE OF AN INTERVERTEBRAL NUCLEAR
PROTRUSION IS BASED UPON:
A. The free excursion of the spinal roots at L4-L5 and S1-S2 of greater
than 10 mm normally
B. The free excursion of the spinal roots at the L4-L5 and S1-S2 level
of 4 mm which may be increased with flexion of the extremity
C. The lack or excursion of the spinal nerve root at L4-L5 and S1-S2
with extension causing aggravated pain
Ref. p. 1687

1584. THE MOST COMMON PRESENTING SYMPTOM OF PATIENTS WITH A
HERNIATED DISC IS:
A. Radicular sciatic pain
B. Low back pain
C. Limping
D. Motor loss to the involved extremity
E. Sensory loss of the involved extremity
Ref. p. 1687

1585. COMPRESSION OF THE CAUDA EQUINA MAY PRESENT WITH WHICH
OF THE FOLLOWING?:
A. Dysuria   D. Abdominal pain
B. Frequency   E. Fecal incontinence
C. Hematuria   Ref. p. 1687

1586. THE MOST COMMON TUMOR INVOLVING THE VERTEBRAL
COLUMN IS:
A. Fibrosarcoma   D. Giant cell tumor
B. Hodgkin's disease   E. Chondroma
C. Multiple myeloma   Ref. p. 1690

1587. THE METASTATIC LESION MOST OFTEN INVOLVING THE SPINAL
COLUMN IS:
A. Breast   D. Lung
B. Prostate   E. Colon
C. Hypernephroma   Ref. p. 1690

1588. THE MOST COMMON FORM OF MUSCULAR DYSTROPHY IN ADULTS IS:
A. Pseudohypertrophic type (Duchenne)
B. Fascioscapulohumeral type (Landouzy-Degerine)
C. Limb-girdle type (Erb)   Ref. p. 1696

1589. THE DEFINITIVE DIAGNOSIS OF DUCHENNE'S DYSTROPHY USUALLY
IS MADE BY:
A. Muscle biopsy
B. Abnormally low values of aldolase and creatine phosphokinase
C. Abnormally high values of serum aldolase and serum creatine phos-
phokinase in association with clinical findings
D. X-ray examination
E. Chronaxie and rheobase   Ref. p. 1697

SECTION XIV - ACQUIRED AND CONGENITAL
MUSCULOSKELETAL DISORDERS: RECONSTRUCTION
AND REHABILITATION

MATCH THE TYPE OF DEFORMITY WITH THE MUSCLE DEFICIT
WHICH CAUSES IT:

1590. ___ Calcaneus deformity   A. Paralysis of the tibialis anterior
1591. ___ Equinus deformity   B. Paralysis of the calf muscles
1592. ___ Claw hallux deformity   C. Paralysis of the anterior tibial tendon
                                        Ref. p. 1699

MATCH THE DEFINITION WITH THE DISEASE STATE:

1593. ___ An increase in the posterior   A. Scoliosis
          convexity of the thoracic spine   B. Lordosis
1594. ___ A deviation of the spine within   C. Kyphosis
          the frontal plane
1595. ___ A decrease in the posterior con-
          vexity of the thoracic spine   Ref. pp. 1707-1709

SELECT THE MOST APPROPRIATE ANSWER:

1596. THE TYPE OF SCOLIOSIS WHICH APPEARS TO HAVE THE TENDENCY
       TOWARD THE DEVELOPMENT OF PARAPLEGIA IS:
       A. Postural scoliosis   D. Idiopathic scoliosis
       B. Congenital scoliosis   E. Osteopathic scoliosis
       C. Paralytic scoliosis   Ref. p. 1709

1597. THE MAJOR COMPLICATIONS OF SCOLIOSIS INCLUDE ALL OF THE
       FOLLOWING, EXCEPT:
       A. Paraplegia
       B. Cor pulmonale
       C. Back pain which may be confused with renal disease
       D. Reduction of the vital capacity of the lungs
       E. All of the above   Ref. pp. 1707-1711

1598. MUSCLE AND FASCIAL CONTRACTURES INCLUDE:
       A. Congenital torticollis   D. Volkmann's
       B. Club foot   E. All of the above
       C. Dupuytren's   Ref. p. 1716

1599. VOLKMANN'S CONTRACTURE IS FREQUENTLY CAUSED BY:
       A. An autoimmune phenomenon
       B. Supracondylar fracture
       C. Migrating thrombophlebitis
       D. Birth trauma   Ref. p. 1717

IN THE FOLLOWING EPIPHYSEAL DISORDERS, MATCH THE DISEASE
AND THE BONE AFFECTED:

1600. ___ Vertebral body   A. Osgood-Schlatter's disease
1601. ___ Semilunar bone   B. Freiberg's disease
1602. ___ Tarsal navicular   C. Calve's disease
1603. ___ Head of femur   D. Scheuermann's disease
1604. ___ Tubercle of tibia   E. Kienbock's disease
1605. ___ Metatarsals   F. Kohler's disease
1606. ___ Vertebral epiphysis   G. Legg-Calve-Perthe's disease
                                   Ref. p. 1718

SELECT THE MOST APPROPRIATE ANSWER:

1607. TALIPES EQUINOVARUS OR CLUB FOOT HAS ALL OF THE
       FOLLOWING, EXCEPT:
       A. Metatarsus adductus   D. Valgus deformity of femur
       B. Inversion   E. Torsion of the tibia
       C. Equinus at the ankle joint   Ref. p. 1725

1608. CONGENITAL HIP DYSPLASIA IS CLINICALLY DIAGNOSED WITH THE
       HELP OF:
       A. Limitation of hip abduction
       B. Ortolani's sign
       C. Shortening of the thigh with the hip flexed at 90 degrees
       D. Trendelenburg's sign
       E. All of the above   Ref. p. 1726

1609. WHICH OF THE FOLLOWING IS USED IN THE X-RAY DIAGNOSIS OF
       CONGENITAL HIP DYSPLASIA?:
       A. Lengthening of the neck of the femur
       B. Hilgenreiner's lines
       C. Osteochondritis of the femoral head
       D. All of the above
       E. None of the above   Ref. p. 1728

1610. THE TREATMENT OF CHOICE IN PREDISLOCATION, CONGENITAL
       HIP DYSPLASIA IN A CHILD BELOW ONE YEAR OLD IS OFTEN
       ACCOMPLISHED BY:
       A. Surgery
       B. Dennis-Browne splint
       C. Both   Ref. p. 1729

1611. THE MOST COMMON FORM OF CONGENITAL GENU RECURVATUM
       RESULTS FROM:
       A. Developmental type
       B. Embryonic defect
       C. Contracture of extensor muscles due to arthrogryposis
                                         Ref. p. 1732

1612. WHICH OF THE FOLLOWING IS ASSOCIATED WITH NEUROFIBROSIS?:
       A. Metatarsus adductus   D. Talipes equinovarus
       B. Congenital hip dysplasia   E. Pseudoarthrosis of the tibia
       C. Genu recurvatum   Ref. p. 1732

1613. WHICH OF THE DEFECTS IN TALIPIS EQUINOVARUS IS USUALLY
       CORRECTED LAST?:
       A. Adduction deformity
       B. Pes equinus deformity
       C. Both are done together   Ref. p. 1733

1614. COMPLICATIONS OF OVER CORRECTION OF THE ADDUCTUS
       DEFORMITY IN CLUB FOOT INCLUDE:
       A. Osteochronditis
       B. Rocker bottom foot
       C. Inversion of the os calcaneus
       D. None of the above
       E. All of the above   Ref. p. 1734

1615. IN TORTICOLLIS, THE PATIENT'S CHIN POINTS:
A. Down and toward the affected side
B. Up and toward the affected side
C. Down and away from the affected side
D. Up and away from the affected side
Ref. p. 1736

1616. · A MISSED TORTICOLLIS MAY BE PICKED UP IN OLDER CHILDREN AS:
A. Klippelfeil syndrome
B. Atrophy of the face on the affected side
C. Sprengle's deformity
D. Arthrogryposis multiplex congenita
E. Atrophy of the face on the opposite side
F. None of the above
Ref. p. 1737

MATCH THE FOLLOWING:

1617.___ Chondroblast   A. Bone formation
1618.___ Chondroclast   B. Cartilage formation
1619.___ Osteoclast   C. Cartilage destruction
1620.___ Osteoblast   D. Bone destruction
                               Ref. p. 1742

SELECT THE MOST APPROPRIATE ANSWER(S):

1621. WHICH OF THE FOLLOWING ACCOMPANIES THE AGING PROCESS
IN BONE ?:
A. Decrease in crystal size
B. Water displacement by crystals
C. Formation of imperfect crystals   Ref. p. 1742

1622. WHICH OF THE FOLLOWING IS MOST OFTEN ASSOCIATED WITH
HYPERPARATHYROIDISM ?:
A. Increase in serum citrate level
B. Increase in serum potassium level
C. Increase in serum calcium level
D. Increase in serum sodium level
E. All of the above   Ref. p. 1742

1623. ALL OF THE FOLLOWING ARE CHARACTERISTICS OF THE ENZYME
ALKALINE PHOSPHATASE, EXCEPT:
A. Optimal activity at pH 9.0
B. Present in hepatic cells in high concentrations
C. Increased in the serum of patients with rickets and osteomalacia
D. Increased in the serum of patients with scurvy
E. Increased in the serum in patients with healing fractures
Ref. p. 1743

1624. ACID PHOSPHATASE IS FOUND IN HIGHEST CONCENTRATIONS IN:
A. Chondroclasts
B. Chondroblasts
C. Osteoclasts
D. Osteoblasts   Ref. p. 1743

MATCH THE APPROPRIATE CAUSE AND EFFECT. EACH LETTERED
ITEM MAY BE USED MORE THAN ONCE:

1625.___ Osteomalacia   A. Deficit of cartilage differentiation
1626.___ Osteoporosis   B. Deficit of calcium phosphate
1627.___ Achondroplasia   deposition
1628.___ Rickets   C. Deficit in osteogenic-osteolytic
1629.___ Osteitis fibrosis   balance
                                    Ref. p. 1744

MATCH THE APPROPRIATE GROWTH DISTURBANCE WITH THE
MOST FREQUENT SITE OF DAMAGE. EACH LETTERED ITEM MAY
BE USED MORE THAN ONCE:

1630.___ Histiocyte-granulomatosis   A. Epiphysis
1631.___ Neurofibromatosis   B. Metaphysis
1632.___ Multiple enchondromatoma   C. Diaphysis
1633.___ Achondroplasia   D. Marrow
1634.___ Dyschondroplasia   Ref. pp. 1746-1747

SELECT THE MOST APPROPRIATE ANSWER(S):

1635. ACHONDROPLASIA IS CHARACTERIZED BY ALL, EXCEPT:
      A. Normal trunk length
      B. Normal intelligence
      C. Reduced extremity length
      D. Enlarged head
      E. Regular ossification of cartilage   Ref. p. 1747

1636. MULTIPLE ENCHONDROMAS ARE DUE TO PROLIFERATIVE
      CARTILAGINOUS CENTERS AND ARE MOST OFTEN NOTED IN:
      A. Membranous bones
      B. Long bones of the extremities (proximal ends)
      C. Short and long bones of the hands and feet
      D. Ribs   Ref. p. 1748

1637. WHICH OF THE FOLLOWING DISEASES IS CHARACTERIZED BY
      BRITTLE BONES?:
      A. Polyostotic fibrous dysplasia   D. Osteopoikilosis
      B. Osteogenesis imperfecta   E. All of the above
      C. Osteopetrosis   Ref. p. 1750

1638. THE ASSOCIATED DISEASE STATE IN PATIENTS WITH OSTEOGENESIS
      IMPERFECTA IS:
      A. Blindness
      B. Deafness
      C. Congenital cardiac anomalies
      D. Blue sclera   Ref. p. 1750

1639. OSTEOGENESIS IMPERFECTA PRESENTS WITH ALL, EXCEPT:
      A. Blue sclera   D. Osteoporosis
      B. Multiple old fractures   E. All of the above
      C. Wormian bones   Ref. p. 1751

1640. LOCALIZED OSTEOSCLEROSIS MAY BE DUE TO:
      A. Syphilis   D. Neoplasia
      B. Arthritis   E. All of the above
      C. Mechanical stress   Ref. p. 1751

1641. INTESTINAL ABSORPTION OF CALCIUM IS DEPENDENT UPON:
   A. Thyrocalcitonin   D. All of the above
   B. Vitamin D   E. None of the above
   C. Parathormone   Ref. p. 1752

1642. PARATHORMONE INFLUENCES WHICH OF THE FOLLOWING ?:
   A. Intestinal absorption of calcium
   B. Bone absorption of calcium
   C. Urinary excretion of phosphate
   D. Urinary excretion of calcium   Ref. p. 1753

1643. WHICH IS <u>MOST</u> AFFECTED BY PARATHORMONE ?:
   A. Bone absorption
   B. Intestinal absorption of calcium
   C. Soft tissue absorption of calsium
   D. Urinary excretion of phosphate
   E. Urinary excretion of calcium   Ref. p. 1753

1644. THE CLINICAL FINDINGS OF TETANY IN PATIENTS WITH HYPO-
      PARATHYROIDISM RARELY PRESENT WITH VALUES ABOVE:
   A. 5 mg per cent   D. 12 mg per cent
   B. 7 mg per cent   E. 16 mg per cent
   C. 10 mg per cent   Ref. p. 1753

1645. LIST IN ORDER OF OCCURRENCE WHICH SYMPTOMS APPEAR AS THE
      SERUM CALCIUM LEVEL IS DEPRESSED:
   A. ___ Defect in blood coagulation
   B. ___ Positive Chvostek sign
   C. ___ Tingling of the fingers
   D. ___ Tetany

1646. WHICH CELL TYPE IS PRIMARILY RESPONSIBLE FOR THE PRO-
      DUCTION OF ALKALINE PHOSPHATASE ?:
   A. Osteoclast
   B. Osteoblast
   C. Chondroblast   Ref. p. 1754

1647. VITAMIN D ACTS UPON WHICH OF THE FOLLOWING ?:
   A. Intestinal absorption of calcium
   B. Renal tubular phosphate resorption
   C. Calcium absorption from bone
   D. Renal tubular resorption of calcium
   E. Phosphate absorption from bone   Ref. p. 1754

1648. AN ABNORMAL IRREGULAR EPIPHYSEAL LINE AND CALCIFYING
      PEROSTEAL HEMATOMA FORMATION FOUND ON X-RAY EXAMINA-
      TION IS INDICATIVE OF:
   A. Hypoparathyroidism   D. Hypervitaminosis A
   B. Vitamin D insufficiency   E. Infantile rickets
   C. Vitamin C insufficiency   Ref. p. 1756

1649. ENLARGED TENDER EPIPHYSES, BOWING OF LONG BONES AND
      X-RAY EVIDENCE OF DELAYED CARPAL OSSIFICATION SHOULD
      INDICATE THE PRESENCE OF:
   A. Scurvy   D. Hyperparathyroidism
   B. Rickets   E. Hypoparathyroidism
   C. Multiple myeloma   Ref. p. 1757

1650.   HYPOPHOSPHATASIA IS AN "INHERITED RACHITIC DISEASE" WHICH
        IS PRIMARILY AN INABILITY OF THE_____TO SECRETE
        ALKALINE PHOSPHATASE:
        A. Osteoblast
        B. Osteoclast
        C. Chondroblast
        D. Chondroclast   Ref. p. 1759

1651.   OSTEOMALACIA IS CHARACTERIZED BY:
        A. Deficient protein metabolism   D. Slow epiphyseal closure
        B. Deficient collagen deposition   E. X-ray looser's zones
        C. Deficient mineralization   Ref. p. 1759

1652.   OSTEOMALACIA MAY BE DUE TO:
        A. Pregnancy
        B. Starvation
        C. Idiopathic steatorrhea
        D. Increased renal excretion of calcium
        E. All of the above   Ref. p. 1759

1653.   PARATHORMONE PRINCIPALLY ACTS ON AND STIMULATES THE:
        A. Osteoblastic cells   D. Chondroblastic cells
        B. Osteoclastic cells   E. All of the above
        C. Chondroclastic cells   Ref. p. 1760

1654.   OSTEOPOROSIS IS A DEFICIENCY IN:
        A. Calcium metabolism   D. All of the above
        B. Calcium deposition   E. None of the above
        C. Protein supporting tissue   Ref. p. 1761

1655.   CUSHING'S SYNDROME WITH ITS EFFECT ON THE SKELETAL SYSTEM
        IS DUE TO:
        A. Deficit in supporting tissue
        B. An increase in calcium secretion
        C. A demineralization
        D. All of the above
        E. None of the above   Ref. p. 1762

        MATCH THE DISEASE WITH THE MOST APPROPRIATE LABORATORY
        VALUES:

1656. ___ Hyperparathyroidism (primary)
1657. ___ Paget's disease
1658. ___ Multiple myeloma
1659. ___ "Senile" osteoporosis
1660. ___ Osteomalacia

	Calcium	Phosphorus	Alkaline Phosphatase
A.	Normal or low	Low	High
B.	Normal or high	Normal or high	Normal
C.	High	Low	High
D.	Normal	Normal or low	Normal
E.	Normal or high	Normal or high	Very high

                              Ref. p. 1762

SELECT THE MOST APPROPRIATE ANSWER(S):

1661. THE DISEASE STATE WITH INCREASED CIRCULATORY ARTERIO-
VENOUS SHUNTING IS:
A. Congenital hypothyroidism
B. Osteitis deformans (Paget's disease)
C. Acromegaly
D. Hand-Schuller-Christian disease
E. Hodgkin's disease   Ref. p. 1767

1662. THE MOST COMMON MALIGNANT TUMOR PRESENTING BETWEEN
THE AGES OF 15 AND 25 YEARS IS:
A. Wilms'   D. Osteosarcoma
B. Neuroblastoma   E. Seminoma
C. Chondrosarcoma   Ref. p. 1776

MATCH THE FOLLOWING. EACH LETTERED ITEM MAY BE USED
MORE THAN ONCE:

1663.___ Diaphyseal aclasis (10-15%)   A. Osteogenic sarcoma
1664.___ Fibrous dysplasia   B. Chondrosarcoma
1665.___ Irradiated tissues   C. Fibrosarcoma
1666.___ Paget's disease (10-20%)   D. Multiple sarcomas
                                        Ref. p. 1776

SELECT THE MOST APPROPRIATE ANSWER:

1667. OSTEOMA'S ARE MOST FREQUENTLY FOUND:
A. Distal tibia   D. Patella
B. Proximal tibia   E. Humerus
C. Orbit and nasal sinus   Ref. p. 1777

1668. THE DIFFERENTIAL DIAGNOSIS OF OSTEOID OSTEOMA INCLUDES
ALL, EXCEPT:
A. Brodies' abscess   D. Ossifying fibroma
B. Osteogenic carcinoma   E. Metastatic thyroid nodule
C. Ewing's tumor   Ref. p. 1777

1669. THE MOST FREQUENT AREA OF DEVELOPMENT FOR OSTEOGENIC
SARCOMA IS:
A. Proximal tibia   D. Proximal humerus
B. Distal femoral metaphysis E. Iliac crest
C. Distal tibia   Ref. p. 1777

1670. WHICH OF THE FOLLOWING DOES NOT DESCRIBE OSTEOGENIC
SARCOMA:
A. Periosteal "sun ray" effect
B. Frequent lung metastases
C. Anaplastic
D. 25 per cent five year survival
E. Amputation, treatment of choice   Ref. p. 1777

1671. WHICH OF THE FOLLOWING IS THE LESS MALIGNANT FORM OF
OSTEOGENIC SARCOMA ?:
A. Osteoblastic type
B. Osteolytic type
C. Parosteal in juxtacortical position
D. Giant cell tumor
E. Paget's disease   Ref. p. 1779

1672. WHICH OF THE FOLLOWING ARE MOST COMMON IN THE SHORT
BONES OF THE HANDS AND FEET ?:
A. Enchondromas   D. Giant cell tumor
B. Osteoid osteomas   E. Ewing's tumor
C. Osteochondromas   Ref. p. 1779

1673. A TUMOR FOUND IN THE EPIPHYSIS AND OFTEN CONFUSED WITH
OSTEOGENIC SARCOMA BEFORE THE CLOSURE OF THE EPIPHYSIS
IS:
A. Chondrosarcoma   D. Chondroblastoma
B. Ewing's tumor   E. Fibrosarcoma
C. Giant cell tumor   Ref. p. 1780

1674. WHICH OF THE FOLLOWING ARE PRECURSORS FOR
CHONDROSARCOMA ?:
A. Osteochondroma   D. All of the above
B. Ollier's disease   E. None of the above
C. Diaphyseal aclasia   Ref. p. 1780

FILL IN THE MOST APPROPRIATE ANSWERS: (Questions 1675-1677)

A. Flat bones   A. Recur
B. End of long bones   B. Be cured
C. Epiphysis of long bones   C. Hemorrhage
D. Central in metaphysis of long   D. Undergo sarcomatous de-
    bones   generation
E. None of the above   E. Become painful

Osteoclastoma (giant cell tumor) is characteristically found in
1675) _____ and if treated by radiation will most likely 1676) _____
and 1677) _____ .   Ref. p. 1781

SELECT THE MOST APPROPRIATE ANSWER(S):

1678. THE USUAL PRESENTATION OF A UNICAMERAL BONE CYST IS:
A. Humeral pain
B. Pathologic fracture of the humerus
C. Sudden swelling of the upper arm   Ref. p. 1783

1679. EWING'S TUMOR, MOST OFTEN INVADES THE_____OF THE
LONG BONES:
A. Diaphysis
B. Metaphysis
C. Epiphysis   Ref. p. 1784

1680. THE DIFFERENTIAL DIAGNOSIS FOR EWING'S TUMOR SHOULD
INCLUDE:
A. Neuroblastoma   D. Reticulum cell sarcoma
B. Osteogenic sarcoma   E. Fibrosarcoma
C. Chondrosarcoma   Ref. pp. 1784-1785

1681. WHICH OF THE FOLLOWING HAS A MORE FAVORABLE PROGNOSIS ?:
A. Ewing's cell sarcoma
B. Reticulum cell sarcoma
C. Both are equal   Ref. p. 1785

SECTION XIV – ACQUIRED AND CONGENITAL
MUSCULOSKELETAL DISORDERS: RECONSTRUCTION
AND REHABILITATION

1682. THE MOST FREQUENT AREAS OF DEVELOPMENT FOR CHORDOMA
ARE THE:
A. Sphenooccipital region
B. Nucleus pulposus of the vertebral column
C. Sacrococcygeal region
D. Scapulae
E. Symphysis pubis   Ref. p. 1786

1683. THE MOST FREQUENT DISTRIBUTION OF METASTATIC BONE
TUMORS IS: (List in order)
A. Upper end of the femur   D. Scapulae
B. Upper end of the humerus   E. Tibia
C. Spinal column   Ref. p. 1788

1684. METASTATIC TUMORS TO THE BONE ARE MOST OFTEN:
A. Osteolytic
B. Osteoblastic
C. Neither
D. Both A and B in equal incidence   Ref. p. 1788

1685. THE MOST COMMON PRIMARY TUMOR OF THE SPINAL COLUMN IS:
A. Giant cell tumor   D. Fibrosarcoma
B. Hemangioma   E. Multiple myeloma
C. Hodgkin's disease   Ref. p. 1788

1686. THE MODE OF METASTATIC SPREAD FROM THE ABDOMEN AND
THORAX TO BONY TISSUE IS USUALLY IN CONJUNCTION WITH:
A. A system of Batson's veins without veins
B. Direct drainage of lymphatics into the vertebral column
C. Direct extension to the vertebral column
D. The change of intrathoracic and abdominal pressure causing a
reversal of flow into the vertebral venous system
E. All of the above   Ref. p. 1788

1687. THE MOST COMMON METASTATIC BONE LESION WITH OSTEOLYTIC
CAPACITY IS:
A. Prostatic   D. Kidney
B. Breast   E. Ewing's tumor
C. Lung   Ref. p. 1788

1688. HYPERCALCEMIA SECONDARY TO BONE METASTASIS MAY BE AS-
SOCIATED WITH HYPOPHOSPHATEMIA, THE MOST LIKELY CAUSE IS
SECRETION OF VITAMIN D-LIKE AGENT BY THE TUMOR. THE
MOST USEFUL TEST TO ESTABLISH THE PRESENCE OR ABSENCE OF
A PRIMARY TUMOR IN THE PARATHYROIDS IS:
A. Dent test
B. Urinary calcium levels
C. Serum phosphorus levels
D. Serum calcium and phosphorus levels
E. None of the above   Ref. p. 1789

1689. THE TUMOR MOST OFTEN RESPONSIBLE FOR PATHOLOGIC BONE
FRACTURES IS:
A. Lung
B. Kidney
C. Breast
D. Colon
E. Thyroid   Ref. p. 1789

1690. A FRACTURE IN WHICH THERE IS A PARTIAL DISCONTINUITY IN
THE CORTEX IS CALLED A:
A. Greenstick fracture   D. Compression fracture
B. Stress fracture   E. None of the above
C. Torus fracture   Ref. p. 1792

1691. RADIOGRAPHIC EXAMINATION OF A SUSPECTED FRACTURE SITE
SHOULD BE PERFORMED:
A. In two planes 90 degrees from each other
B. In two planes 45 degrees from each other
C. In three planes 45 degrees from each other
D. All of the above
E. None of the above   Ref. p. 1792

1692. WHEN A FRACTURE IS REDUCED AND IMMOBILIZED AND PAIN
PERSISTS, ONE SHOULD SUSPECT:
A. Neural involvement   D. Faulty immobilization
B. Associated vascular involvement   E. None of the above
C. Another fracture   Ref. p. 1795

1693. WHICH OF THE EPIPHYSEAL FRACTURES WILL MOST LIKELY
CAUSE A GROWTH DISTURBANCE ACCORDING TO THE SALTER
HARRIS CLASSIFICATION?:
A. Type I   D. Type IV
B. Type II   E. Type V
C. Type III   Ref. p. 1798

1694. IN WHICH GROUP IS THERE A GREATER FREQUENCY OF BONY
NON-UNION?:
A. Fractures in children
B. Fractures in adults
C. Both are equal   Ref. p. 1799

1695. IN AN INFANT WITH A MIDCLAVICULAR FRACTURE AND BAYONET
OVERRIDING, WHICH OF THE FOLLOWING SHOULD BE PERFORMED?:
A. Reduction of overriding and apposition
B. Figure of eight padding
C. Intramedullary pin
D. Supine bed rest plus interscapular sand bag support
E. None of the above   Ref. p. 1804

1696. WHICH TYPE OF SHOULDER DISLOCATION OCCURS WITH GREATER
FREQUENCY?:
A. Anterior dislocation
B. Posterior dislocation
C. Both occur equally   Ref. p. 1805

1697. THE LEAST TRAUMATIC AND MOST RELIABLE MANEUVER TO RE-
DUCE AN ANTERIOR DISLOCATION OF THE SHOULDER IS:
A. Hippocratic maneuver
B. Kocher maneuver
C. Milch maneuver   Ref. p. 1806

SECTION XIV - ACQUIRED AND CONGENITAL
MUSCULOSKELETAL DISORDERS: RECONSTRUCTION
AND REHABILIATION

1698. A FRACTURE OF_____SHOULD ALERT ONE TO LOOK FOR A
POSTERIOR SHOULDER DISLOCATION:
A. Compression fracture of humeral head, posterior lateral
B. Humeral lesser tuberosity
C. Humeral greater tuberosity
D. Humeral shaft
E. Humeral neck   Ref. p. 1806

1699. HUMERAL SHAFT FRACTURES ARE ROUTINELY TREATED WITH:
A. Open reduction
B. Shoulder spica
C. Coaptation plaster splint plus Velpeau
D. Hanging cast
E. All of the above   Ref. p. 1808

1700. HUMERAL SHAFT FRACTURES DIFFER FROM PROXIMAL HUMERAL
FRACTURES IN THAT:
A. In the former there is often radial nerve involvement
B. Early shoulder motion is indicated in the former
C. Non-union is more frequent in the latter
D. Angulation of the fragments is more common in shaft fractures
E. All of the above   Ref. p. 1808

1701. WHICH NERVE IS MOST OFTEN INJURED AS A RESULT OF A SPIRAL
HUMERAL SHAFT FRACTURE?:
A. Radial nerve
B. Ulnar nerve
C. Median nerve   Ref. p. 1808

1702. THE RADIAL HEAD SHOULD NEVER BE EXCISED DURING CHILDHOOD
FOLLOWING A FRACTURE BECAUSE:
A. It is frequently accompanied by a joint effusion and subsequent loss of
function
B. Shortening develops as a result of epiphyseal loss
C. Associated nerve damage frequently accompanies excision of the
radial head
D. Associated vascular damage is often initiated
                                    Ref. p. 1808

1703. SUSPECTED ELBOW FRACTURES IN THE YOUNG SHOULD HAVE
WHICH OF THE FOLLOWING X-RAYS?:
A. Anterior-posterior; lateral; obliques
B. Anterior-posterior; lateral; obliques of both arms
C. Anterior-posterior view plus lateral view
D. Anterior-posterior view plus oblique views
                                    Ref. p. 1809

1704. VOLKMANN'S ISCHEMIC CONTRACTURE IS A COMPLICATION OF
WHICH OF THE FOLLOWING?:
A. Fracture dislocation of the radial head
B. Fracture dislocation of olecranon process
C. Supracondylar fracture of the humerus
D. Lateral epicondyle fracture of the humerus
E. All of the above   Ref. p. 1810

MATCH THE FOLLOWING. EACH LETTERED ITEM MAY BE USED
ONLY ONCE:

1705.___ Forced abduction of the thumb   A. Subluxation of the radial head
1706.___ Elderly fall with outstretched hand B. Monteggia deformity
1707.___ Hyperextension plus valgus force   C. Lateral epicondyle
1708.___ Forcible pull of arm   D. Smith fracture
1709.___ Kienbock's disease   E. Colles' fracture
1710.___ Direct blow on ulna   F. Navicular fracture
1711.___ Forced flexion of distal phalynx   G. Lunate dislocation
1712.___ Fall on dorsum of wrist   H. Bennett's fracture
1713.___ Young adults fall with outstretched I. Mallet finger
         hand   Ref. pp. 1810-1819

SELECT THE MOST APPROPRIATE ANSWER(S):

1714. A MONTEGGIA DEFORMITY IS:
       A. Dislocation of the radial head plus fracture of proximal 1/3 ulna
       B. Fracture of radial head plus fracture of proximal ulna
       C. Dislocation of the ulna plus fracture of the proximal 1/3 radius
       D. Dislocation of the radial head plus fracture of the coronoid process
       E. Dislocation of the radial head plus fracture of the lateral condyle
                                              Ref. p. 1812

1715. FRACTURES OF THE PROXIMAL 1/3 OF THE ARM USUALLY REQUIRE
       IMMOBILIZATION IN WHICH OF THE FOLLOWING POSITIONS?:
       A. Supination
       B. Pronation
       C. Neutral   Ref. p. 1813

1716. THE PRINCIPLES BEHIND CLOSED REDUCTION INCLUDE ALL OF THE
       FOLLOWING, EXCEPT:
       A. Length regained   D. Reduction of fracture
       B. Angulation increased   E. All of the above
       C. Correct displacement   Ref. p. 1813

1717. A FOREARM FRACTURE IN A CHILD SHOULD BE ACCURATELY RE-
       DUCED AND MAINTAIN LENGTH IN ACCORDANCE WITH THE PRINCI-
       PLES IN THE ABOVE QUESTION. ANGULATION OF THE FRACTURED
       SEGMENTS IS PERMISSIBLE UP TO:
       A. 10 degrees   D. 40 degrees
       B. 20 degrees   E. 50 degrees
       C. 30 degrees   Ref. p. 1813

1718. A COLLES' FRACTURE CONSISTS OF:
       A. Fracture of the distal radius plus ventral angulation and ulna styloid
           fracture
       B. Fracture of the distal radius plus dorsal angulation and ulna styloid
           fracture
       C. Fracture of the distal plus dorsal angulation and radial styloid
           fracture
       D. Fracture of the distal ulna plus ventral angulation and radial styloid
           fracture
       E. None of the above   Ref. p. 1814

1719. THE USUAL TREATMENT OF A NAVICULAR FRACTURE IS A SHORT
ARM CAST INCLUDING THUMB IMMOBILIZATION FOR_____WEEKS:
   A. 4
   B. 8
   C. 16
   D. 20
   E. 24
   F. 28   Ref. p. 1816

1720. POSTOPERATIVE CARE OF THE PATIENT WITH A FEMORAL HEAD
PROSTHESIS SHOULD:
   A. Prevent adduction, flexion and internal rotation
   B. Prevent abduction, flexion and internal rotation
   C. Prevent abduction, extension and external rotation
   D. Prevent adduction, flexion and external rotation
   E. Should always include early mobilization
                                       Ref. p. 1822

1721. WHICH OF THE FOLLOWING FRACTURES MAY BE ACCOMPANIED BY
HEMORRHAGIC SHOCK?:
   A. Subcapital fracture of the femur
   B. Intertrochanteric fracture of the femur
   C. Both are equal   Ref. p. 1823

1722. FEMORAL SHAFT FRACTURES TREATED BY INTRAMEDULLARY
FIXATION HAVE AS A COMPLICATION WOUND SEPSIS AND DELAYED
UNION. THE FREQUENCY OF THE COMBINED COMPLICATIONS IS:
   A. Less than 1 per cent   D. 18 per cent
   B. 6 per cent   E. 24 per cent
   C. 12 per cent   Ref. p. 1824

1723. STEINMAN PIN INSERTION FOR SKELETAL TRACTION OF A DISTAL
FEMORAL SHAFT FRACTURE IS PERFORMED AT THE LEVEL OF THE
TIBIAL TUBERCLE TO PREVENT:
   A. Sepsis   D. Peroneal nerve damage
   B. Popliteal artery damage   E. All of the above
   C. Angulation of the fracture site Ref. p. 1824

1724. THE DISTAL SEGMENT OF A SUPRACONDYLAR FEMORAL FRACTURE
IS:
   A. Shortened and may have a valgus deformity
   B. Is angulated posterior
   C. Is angulated anterior
   D. Has a varus deformity
   E. None of the above   Ref. p. 1825

1725. A LATERAL BLOW AT THE KNEE JOINT LEVEL WILL CAUSE:
   A. Anterior cruciate laceration
   B. Medial collateral ligament laceration
   C. Medial meniscus avulsion
   D. All of the above   Ref. p. 1826

1726.   THE MEDIAL MENISCUS IS ATTACHED TO WHICH OF THE FOLLOW-
ING STRUCTURES?:
A. Anterior cruciate ligament   D. Posterior capsule
B. Medial collateral ligament   E. All of the above
C. Posterior cruciate ligament   Ref. p. 1827

1727.   A SEVERELY COMMINUTED PATELLA FRACTURE IS IDEALLY
TREATED BY:
A. Internal wire fixation
B. Closed reduction cylinder cast
C. Excision of fragments
D. Active mobilization of the knee joint
E. None of the above   Ref. p. 1828

1728.   THE MOST COMMON KNEE INJURY INVOLVES:
A. The lateral collateral ligaments
B. The medial collateral ligaments
C. Both equally   Ref. p. 1832

MATCH THE FOLLOWING:

1729. ___ Bimalleolar fracture   A. External rotation and eversion
1730. ___ Distal tibiofibular diastase   B. External rotation
1731. ___ Lateral malleolus oblique fracture   C. Eversion
                                          Ref. pp. 1832-1834

SELECT THE MOST APPROPRIATE ANSWER:

1732.   A POSTERIOR MALLEOLAR FRACTURE SHOULD UNDERGO OPEN
CORRECTION IF IT EXCEEDS_____PER CENT OF THE ARTICULATE
SURFACE:
A. 5   D. 20
B. 10   E. 30
C. 15   Ref. p. 1833

1733.   THE ANGLE FORMED BY THE AXIS OF THE SUBTALAR JOINT AND
THE TUBEROSITY OF THE CALCANEOUS IS:
A. The most frequent site of calcaneous fracture
B. Delineates Bohler's angle
C. Demonstrates the point of maximum stress on the talus
D. None of the above
E. All of the above   Ref. p. 1834

1734.   THE MOST COMMON TYPE OF HIP DISLOCATION IS:
A. Posterior
B. Anterior
C. Both A and B occur with equal frequency
                                      Ref. p. 1836

1735.   AVASCULAR NECROSIS OF THE FEMORAL HEAD OCCURS MORE
FREQUENTLY IN:
A. Hip dislocation
B. Subcapital fractures
C. Both equally   Ref. p. 1837

SECTION XIV -ACQUIRED AND CONGENITAL
MUSCULOSKELETAL DISORDERS: RECONSTRUCTION
AND REHABILITATION

1736. THE MECHANISM FOR REDUCTION OF A POSTERIOR HIP DISLOCA-
TION IS:
A. External rotation, abduction, flexion
B. Traction adduction, internal rotation, flexion
C. Traction in long axis, gradual abduction, external rotation, extension
Ref. p. 1837

1737. THE MOST COMMON CERVICAL COMPRESSION FRACTURE OCCURS
AT:
A. C1-C4
B. C5-C8
C. Equally at A and B   Ref. p. 1840

MATCH THE FOLLOWING. EACH LETTERED ITEM MAY BE USED
MORE THAN ONCE:

1738.___ Articulation humeri (shoulder joint)   A. Synarthrosis
1739.___ Cranial sutures   B. Syndesmosis
1740.___ Intervertebral joint   C. Diarthrosis
                                                  D. Synchrondrosis
                                                  Ref. p. 1845

SELECT THE MOST APPROPRIATE ANSWER:

1741. WHICH OF THE FOLLOWING ARE COMMON TO ALL JOINTS?:
A. Capsule, two bones, tendons
B. Capsule, two bones, interspace
C. Capsule, two bones, cartilage interface
D. Capsule, two bones interspace with synovial fluid, cartilage
Ref. p. 1846

1742. THE VISCOSITY OF SYNOVIAL FLUID IS MAINLY A RESULT OF:
A. Chondroitin sulfate   D. Albumin
B. Hyaluronate   E. Beta lipoproteins
C. Alpha and beta globulins   Ref. p. 1846

1743. THE NORMAL CELLULAR CONTENT IN SYNOVIAL FLUID IS POLY-
MORPHONUCLEAR NEUTROPHILS, LYMPHOCYTES AND MONOCYTES.
THEY NORMALLY DO NOT EXCEED_____CELLS/MM IN NUMBER:
A. 100   D. 1000
B. 200   E. 2000
C. 500   Ref. p. 1846

1744. THE MOST PAIN SENSITIVE PORTION OF A JOINT INCLUDES:
A. Articular cartilage   D. Bone
B. Meniscus   E. Synovium
C. Capsule   Ref. p. 1847

1745. SYNOVIAL FLUID EXAMINATION IS DIAGNOSTIC IN ALL OF THE
FOLLOWING, EXCEPT:
A. Pyogenic arthritis
B. Gout
C. Tuberculous arthritis
D. Rheumatoid arthritis
E. Pseudogout   Ref. p. 1848

1746. SYNOVIAL FLUID WITH A WEAK MUCINOUS CLOT, DECREASED
VISCOSITY AND INCREASED TURBIDITY IS COMPATIBLE WITH ALL,
EXCEPT:
A. Degenerative arthritis   D. Tuberculous arthritis
B. Septic arthritis   E. Gouty arthritis
C. Rheumatoid arthritis   Ref. p. 1848

1747. THE NORMAL BLOOD-JOINT GLUCOSE DIFFERENCE IS:
A. 100 mg per cent   D. 10 mg per cent
B. 70 mg per cent   E. 0 mg per cent
C. 40 mg per cent   Ref. p. 1848

FOR SYNOVIAL FLUID COLLECTION, MATCH THE COLLECTION
TUBE WITH THE APPROPRIATE TEST. EACH LETTERED ITEM
MAY BE USED MORE THAN ONCE:

1748.___ Urate crystals   A. Culture tube
1749.___ Cell count   B. EDTA
1750.___ Calcium pyrophosphate crystals   C. Empty tube
1751.___ Mucin clot test   D. Acetic acid
                                           Ref. p. 1848

SELECT THE MOST APPROPRIATE ANSWER:

1752. PYOGENIC ARTHRITIS WITH ABSCESS FORMATION DIFFERS FROM
OTHER ABSCESSES BY:
A. A higher concentration of WBC's
B. Its greater sensitivity to systemic antibiotics
C. A thinner capsule
D. Usually is not of staphylococcus origin
E. All are true   Ref. p. 1849

1753. SEPTIC ARTHRITIS IN PREMATURE INFANTS USUALLY AFFECTS
WHICH OF THE FOLLOWING JOINTS?:
A. Shoulder   D. Knee
B. Elbow   E. Wrist
C. Hip   Ref. p. 1849

1754. TO CONFIRM A CLINICAL IMPRESSION OF PYOGENIC ARTHRITIS,
WHICH OF THE FOLLOWING IS CONSIDERED MOST USEFUL?:
A. X-ray
B. Joint aspiration and synovial analysis
C. Clinical findings alone
D. CBC plus sedimentation rate
E. Both A and C   Ref. p. 1849

1755. RHEUMATOID ARTHRITIS PRIMARILY INVOLVES THE JOINT:
A. Capsule   D. Synovium
B. Articular cartilage   E. All simultaneously
C. Bone   Ref. p. 1853

SECTION XIV - ACQUIRED AND CONGENITAL
MUSCULOSKELETAL DISORDERS: RECONSTRUCTION
AND REHABILITATION

1756. CARTILAGE DESTRUCTION IN RHEUMATOID ARTHRITIS APPEARS:
A. Uniformly beneath the pannus
B. Centrally within the joint at the point of maximal pressure
C. At the synovial junction
D. None of the above   Ref. p. 1853

1757. WHICH OF THE FOLLOWING ARTHRITIC STATE PRESENTS WITH THE
GREATEST JOINT FLUID LEUKOCYTOSIS?:
A. Rheumatoid arthritis   D. Tuberculous arthritis
B. Septic arthritis   E. Degenerative osteoarthritis
C. Gonococcal arthritis   Ref. p. 1854

1758. THE X-RAY FINDINGS INDICATIVE OF PERIOSTEAL NEW BONE
GROWTH APPEAR:
A. In the capsular wall
B. In the cartilage
C. At the junction of the bone and capsule wall
                                    Ref. p. 1854

1759. WHICH OF THE FOLLOWING IS (ARE) NOT ASSOCIATED WITH POTTS'
DISEASE?:
A. Intervertebral disc is destroyed early
B. Paraspinal abscess may develop
C. The anterior vertebral border is involved often in the thoracic area
D. Chemotherapy should be continued for at least 1-1/2 years
                                    Ref. p. 1857

1760. THE SURGICAL PROCEDURE CAPABLE OF PREVENTING JOINT
DESTRUCTION IS:
A. McIntosh prosthesis insertion   D. Synovectomy
B. Arthrodesis   E. Arthroplasty
C. Meniscectomy   Ref. p. 1858

1761. WHICH OF THE FOLLOWING ARE NOT COMPLICATIONS OF
RHEUMATOID ARTHRITIS?:
A. Tenosynovitis
B. Rupture of extensor tendons
C. Carpal tunnel syndrome
D. Ulnar deviation at MP joints
E. All are complications   Ref. p. 1859

1762. THE JOINT AREA AFFECTED IN OSTEOARTHRITIS INITIALLY IS:
A. Capsule   D. Bone
B. Synovium   E. Ligaments
C. Articular cartilage   Ref. p. 1860

1763. WHICH OF THE FOLLOWING JOINTS ARE MOST LIKELY TO BE
AFFECTED BY PRIMARY OSTEOARTHRITIS?:
A. Distal interphalangeal joints   D. Shoulder joint
B. Proximal interphalangeal joints   E. Cervial spine
C. Hip joint   Ref. p. 1861

ANSWER THE FOLLOWING QUESTIONS BY USING THE KEY
OUTLINED BELOW:
A. If both statement and reason are correct and related cause and effect
B. If both statement and reason are correct but not related cause and
effect
C. If statement is true but reason is false
D. If statement is false but reason is true
E. If both statement and reason are false

1764.   Primary skeletal tuberculosis is a frequent occurrence BECAUSE of the
declining incidence of pulmonary tuberculosis.
Ref. p. 1850

1765.   The tissue destroyed last in articular tuberculosis is the cartilage
BECAUSE of the developing bony ankylosis.
Ref. p. 1850

1766.   Tuberculous arthritis usually presents in children BECAUSE the
vertebral column is most commonly affected.
Ref. p. 1850

1767.   Osteoarthritis is a degenerative joint disease of diarthrosal joints
BECAUSE of the high incidence of inflammation as a primary mechanism.
Ref. p. 1860

1768.   Heberden's nodes are rheumatic in origin BECAUSE they are found at
the distal interphalangeal joints.   Ref. p. 1861

1769.   Symptomatic arthritis with joint space narrowing, subchondral bone
cysts, subchondral bone sclerosis and osteophyte formation are diagnostic of osteoarthritis BECAUSE these X-ray findings are usually found
in osteoarthritis.   Ref. p. 1861-1862

1770.   Acute episodes of osteoarthritis of the hip may be managed conserva-
tively BECAUSE bed rest, skin traction to the leg and non-weight bear-
ing crutch walking often afford a remission.
Ref. p. 1862

1771.   Chondromalacia of the patella is an early form of osteoarthritis
BECAUSE it frequently is seen in young adults.
Ref. p. 1867

SELECT THE MOST APPROPRIATE ANSWER:

1772.   THE PAIN ASSOCIATED WITH A HALLUX VALGUS DEFORMITY
RESULTS FROM IRRITATION DUE TO:
A. Excessive lateral deviation
B. Osteoarthritis
C. Acute bursitis
D. Callus development over the second and third metatarsal head
Ref. p. 1869

1773. KNEE JOINT ASPIRATION WITH BLOODY OR COFFEE GROUND
SANGUINEOUS FLUID (WITH NO TRAUMATIC ETIOLOGY) MAY
REFLECT:
A. Synovial chondromatosis   D. Charcot's joint
B. Legg-Calve-Perthes disease   E. None of the above
C. Pigmented villinodular synovitis Ref. p. 1872

ANSWER THE FOLLOWING QUESTION BY USING THE KEY
OUTLINED BELOW:
A. If both statement and reason are correct and related cause and effect
B. If both statement and reason are correct but not related cause and
effect
C. If statement is true but reason is false
D. If statement is false but reason is true
E. If both statement and reason are false

1774. The term Charcot's joint refers to joint destruction due to insensitivity
from neurologic disease BECAUSE local trauma may go unnoticed.
                            Ref. p. 1873

SELECT THE MOST APPROPRIATE ANSWER:

1775. ACUTE SHOULDER PAIN WITH AN ONSET AFTER THE THIRD DE-
CADE MAY BE DUE TO:
A. Rotator cuff disruption   D. Pancost's tumor
B. Bicipital tendonitis   E. All of the above
C. Subacromial bursitis   Ref. p. 1874

1776. WHICH OF THE FOLLOWING MAY CONSTITUTE INDICATIONS FOR AN
AMPUTATION?:
A. Infections of an extremity resulting in uncontrolled septicemia
B. Peripheral vascular deficiency
C. Tumors of the extremities
D. Irreversible extremity trauma
E. All of the above   Ref. p. 1879

1777. A GENERAL RULE FOR EXTREMITY AMPUTATIONS IS ALWAYS
PRESERVE LENGTH. EXCEPTIONS TO THIS RULE INCLUDE:
A. Proximal to the knee joint
B. Distal to the elbow joint
C. Proximal to the metatarsophalangeal joint
D. The index digit
E. All of the above   Ref. p. 1880

1778. DISARTICULATION OF A JOINT IS CONSIDERED TO BE AN ADEQUATE
MODE OF TREATMENT IN CHILDREN BECAUSE:
A. Preservation of length takes precedence over ease of application of
the prosthetic appliance
B. The ephyphysis is still functional and should be preserved
C. Disarticulation is a much easier procedure in children
D. Nerve damage above the knee should be avoided at all costs in
children
E. A prosthetic appliance is much easier applied to a disarticulation
area than amputation area in children
                            Ref. p. 1880

MATCH THE FOLLOWING. EACH LETTERED ITEM MAY BE USED
MORE THAN ONCE:

1779. ___ Irreversible below knee trauma in a 4 year-old extending to within
1 inch of the joint
1780. ___ Irreversible below knee trauma in a 30 year-old extending to within
1 inch of the joint
1781. ___ Gangrene of the foot in a patient following popliteal occlusion with a
level of ischemic rubor 2 cm below the knee joint
1782. ___ Gangrene of the foot in a patient following vascular popliteal occlusion
with a histamine flare test positive below the knee by at least 6 inches

    A. Disarticulation
    B. Above knee amputation (A-K)
    C. Below knee amputation (B-K)   Ref. p. 1880

SELECT THE MOST APPROPRIATE ANSWER:

1783. THE MOST RELIABLE INDICATION OF POOR CIRCULATION OF THE
INTENDED AMPUTATION AREA IS:
    A. Histamine flare test
    B. Lack of bleeding at incision level
    C. Lack of pulses at level above incision
    D. Prior history of claudication with minimal exertion
    E. Oscillometry readings above the incision level
                        Ref. p. 1880

1784. FOR BELOW KNEE AMPUTATIONS, WHICH OF THE FOLLOWING
SEEM TO CORRELATE WELL WITH AN EVENTUALLY SUCCESSFUL
RESULT?:
    A. Oscillometry readings of pulsatile circulation
    B. Arteriography
    C. Presence of popliteal pulses
    D. All of the above   Ref. p. 1880

1785. IN A PATIENT SUFFERING FROM DIABETIC KETOACIDOSIS,
GANGRENE OF THE LOWER EXTREMITY AND SHOCK, WHICH OF
THE FOLLOWING PROCEDURES WOULD BE USEFUL TO PERMIT
TIME FOR IMPROVEMENT OF THE PATIENT'S CONDITION?:
    A. Debridment of grossly necrotic tissue
    B. Refrigeration of extremity with ice and application of tourniquet
below the intended amputation site
    C. Switch patient from long acting insulin to crystaline insulin
    D. Wrap extremity in antiseptic impregnated towels
    E. The patient should immediately undergo amputation without attempts
to improve the condition since improvement is dependent on removal
of the infected and necrotic tissue   Ref. p. 1881

1786. WHICH OF THE FOLLOWING AMPUTATION TYPES GIVES THE
POOREST RESULTS?:
    A. Conventional amputation
    B. Osteomyoplastic or myodesis
    C. Guillotine amputation   Ref. p. 1881

SECTION XIV – ACQUIRED AND CONGENITAL
MUSCULOSKELETAL DISORDERS: RECONSTRUCTION
AND REHABILITATION

FILL IN THE MOST APPROPRIATE ANSWERS: (Questions 1787-1788)

A. Cardiac infarction
B. Pulmonary embolism
C. Cerebrovascular accidents
D. Renal shutdown
E. Heparinization

A. Early ambulation
B. High femoral vein ligation
C. Postoperative elevation of
    extremity
D. All of the above

AK amputations for vascular disease frequently carry a mortality rate of
from 30 to 39 per cent due mostly to 1787)_____. The most recent approach to this complication has been 1788)_____.
Ref. p. 1882

MATCH THE FOLLOWING. EACH LETTERED ITEM MAY BE USED
ONLY ONCE:

1789. ___ Necrotic toe with extension to interdigital crease
1790. ___ Necrotic toe distal to PIP joint, no cellulitis or skin edema
1791. ___ Irreversible trauma to third toe with destruction of PIP joint
1792. ___ Irreversible destruction of foot including tarsal bones and metatarsal
        bones

A. Syme amputation
B. Transmetatarsal toe amputation
C. Transmetatarsal foot amputation
D. Transphalangeal amputation   Ref. p. 1883

SELECT THE MOST APPROPRIATE ANSWER(S):

1793. THE TRANSMETATARSAL FOOT AMPUTATION HAS A HEALING RATE
       PROPORTIONAL TO THE VASCULAR SUPPLY AND A_____
       CORRELATION TO THE BLOOD SUPPLY PROVIDED BY THE
       POPLITEAL SYSTEM THAT DOES THE BK OR AK AMPUTATION:
       A. Greater
       B. Lesser
       C. The same   Ref. p. 1883

1794. THE HEALING RATE OF AN AK OR BK AMPUTATION SITE FOR
       PERIPHERAL VASCULAR DISEASE IS_____(INFLUENCED) BY THE
       PRESENCE OF DIABETES MELLITUS:
       A. Greatly
       B. Unaltered   Ref. p. 1885

1795. SACRIFICE OF THE COMPLETE NAIL BED WHEN PARTIALLY
       DESTROYED BY TRAUMATIC DIGITAL AMPUTATION IS INDICATED
       WHEN:
       A. Over 1/4 of the nail bed is removed
       B. Over 1/2 of the nail bed is removed
       C. Over 3/4 of the nail bed is removed
                                       Ref. p. 1890

1796. THE MOST IMPORTANT DIGIT IS THE:
       A. Thumb   D. Ring finger
       B. Index finger   E. All are of equal value
       C. Third finger   Ref. p. 1890

1797. IN CARPOMETACARPAL AMPUTATION THE FUNCTIONAL TENDON
GROUPS WHICH MUST BE PRESERVED AND REINSERTED ARE:
A. Flexor carpi radialis   D. Carpal extensors
B. Digital extensor tendons   E. All are preserved
C. Long flexor tendons   Ref. p. 1891

1798. THE REPAIR OF SYNDACTYLISM INCLUDES WHICH OF THE
FOLLOWING?:
A. Should be performed after 8 years of age
B. Full thickness skin graft is often essential
C. There is no familial tendency
D. Often occurs simultaneously with polydactylism
E. All of the above   Ref. p. 1895

1799. THE TIMING OF SURGICAL INTERVENTION IN SYNDACTYLY IS IMPOR-
TANT. WHEN DIGITS OF DIFFERENT GROWTH RATES ARE INVOLVED,
SEPARATION IS RECOMMENDED PRIOR TO:
A. Age one year   D. Age seven years
B. Age three years   E. Onset of school
C. Age five years   Ref. p. 1895

ASCENDING LYMPHANGITIS WITH SUBSEQUENT NODAL ENLARGE-
MENT MAY BE PREDICTED. MATCH THE FOLLOWING:

1800.___ Little finger and ring finger   A. Axillary nodes
1801.___ Thumb and index finger   B. Deltopectoral nodes
1802.___ Middle finger   C. Epitrochlear nodes
                                           Ref. p. 1897

SELECT THE MOST APPROPRIATE ANSWER(S):

1803. WHICH OF THE FOLLOWING REQUIRE DRAINAGE BECAUSE OF THE
INCREASED INCIDENCE OF OSTEOMYELITIS?:
A. Paronychia   D. Palmar space infection
B. Tenosynovitis   E. All of the above
C. Felon   Ref. p. 1897

1804. OVER 80 PER CENT OF HAND INFECTIONS ARE DUE TO:
A. Escherichia coli   D. Staphylococci
B. Proteus sp.   E. Beta hemolytic streptococci
C. Pseudomonas   Ref. p. 1898

1805. NONSURGICAL INFLAMMATION OF THE HAND OR FINGERS INCLUDES
WHICH OF THE FOLLOWING?:
A. Rheumatoid arthritis   D. Gout
B. Reiter's syndrome   E. Metabolic synovitis
C. Non-specific tenosynovitis   F. All of the above
                                   Ref. p. 1898

1806. OSTEOMYELITIS IS A COMPLICATION OF WHICH OF THE FOLLOWING?:
A. Bacterial tenosynovitis   C. Felon
B. Paronychia   D. Subcutaneous abscess of hand
                                   Ref. p. 1899

SECTION XIV - ACQUIRED AND CONGENITAL
MUSCULOSKELETAL DISORDERS: RECONSTRUCTION
AND REHABILITATION

1807. AN INFECTION OF THE TENDON SHEATH IN THE 5TH DIGIT OF
THE HAND WOULD MOST LIKELY SPREAD TO:
A. The first digit tendon sheath
B. The second digit tendon sheath
C. The third digit tendon sheath
D. The fourth digit tendon sheath
E. All simultaneously   Ref. p. 1901

1808. TO DRAIN A PALMAR SPACE INFECTION ONE MUST:
A. Avoid crossing an area of flexion to prevent a contracture
B. Utilize penicillin, initially as the antibacterial of choice
C. Utilize continuous saline irrigation to prevent sheath-to-tendon ad-
hesions   Ref. p. 1900, 1903

1809. THE USE OF NINHYDRIN WILL INDICATE NERVE DESTRUCTION IN
THE DIGITS. WHICH ARE THE PREDOMINANT NEURAL FIBERS
AFFECTED?:
A. Sensory fibers   D. Autonomic
B. Motor fibers   E. Parasympathetic
C. Sympathetic fibers   Ref. p. 1904

1810. TO TEST THE FLEXOR DIGITORUM SUPERFICIALIS FUNCTION, ONE
MUST:
A. Observe equal flexion of the proximal interphalangeal joints
B. Isolate individual finger placing all others in extension
C. Neither   Ref. p. 1906

1811. WHICH OF THE FOLLOWING MUSCLE GROUPS ARE RESPONSIBLE
FOR MUSCLE DROP AT THE METACARPAL PHALANGEAL LEVEL?:
A. Flexor digitorum profundus
B. Flexor digitorum superficialis
C. Extensor digitorum   Ref. p. 1906

1812. THE ABILITY TO ABDUCT OR ADDUCT ONES FINGERS IS DEPENDENT
UPON THE_____NERVE:
A. Radial
B. Median
C. Ulnar   Ref. p. 1906

1813. WHICH OF THE FOLLOWING NERVE REPAIRS HAS A GREATER
SUCCESS RATE?:
A. Nerve repair per primum
B. Delayed nerve repair at 3 months
C. Both are equally successful   Ref. p. 1908

MATCH THE NERVE DAMAGED WITH THE FUNCTIONAL DEFICIT:

1814. ___ Median nerve palsy   A. Inability to flex M.P. joints of fingers
                                        (pinch)
1815. ___ Ulnar nerve paralysis   B. Inability to position thumb for pulp to
                                        pulp opposition with the fingers
1816. ___ Radial nerve palsy   C. Extensor-supinator group muscle
                                        paralysis
                                                Ref. p. 1910

SELECT THE MOST APPROPRIATE ANSWER(S):

1817. WHICH OF THE FOLLOWING NERVES IS RESPONSIBLE FOR INNER-
VATION OF THE FOLLOWING: THENAR EMINANCE; SUPERFICIAL
HEAD OF THE FLEXOR POLLEXES BREVIS; TWO RADIAL BRANCHES
OF THE LUMBRICLES:
A. Ulnar nerve
B. High median nerve
C. Median nerve (low)
D. Radial nerve   Ref. p. 1911

1818. RADIAL NERVE PARALYSIS IS MOST OFTEN ASSOCIATED WITH:
A. Supracondylar fracture of the humerus
B. Radial head fracture
C. Spiral fracture of the humerus
D. Ulnar mid shaft fracture
E. None of the above   Ref. p. 1911

1819. THE ABILITY TO PINCH IS SEVERELY DIMINISHED IF THE INDEX
FINGER IS AMPUTATED BELOW THE:
A. Distal interphylangeal joint
B. Proximal interphylangeal joint
C. Metacarpophalangeal joint   Ref. p. 1914

1820. THE MOST IMPORTANT DIGITS TO THE FUNCTION OF A HAND ARE:
A. Thumb   D. Index finger
B. Second   E. Fifth
C. Third   Ref. p. 1914

1821. THE BEST WAY TO AVOID POSTOPERATIVE CONTRACTURES OF THE
HAND IS TO AVOID WHICH OF THE FOLLOWING INCISIONS?:
A. Across flexion or extension creases
B. Along flexion or extension creases
C. Neither
D. Both   Ref. p. 1917

MATCH THE FOLLOWING:

1822.___ Donor site heals spontaneously   A. Reverdin graft
1823.___ Vascular supply must be pre-   B. Ollier-Thiersch graft
         served   C. Wolfe graft
1824.___ Represents so-called pinch graft   D. Pedicle flap
1825.___ Results in the most durable and   E. Composite graft
         cosmetically acceptable graft
1826.___ The least reliable graft   Ref. pp. 1923-1924

MATCH THE FOLLOWING. EACH LETTERED ITEM MAY BE USED
MORE THAN ONCE:

1827.___ Eyebrow reconstruction   A. Rotation flap
1828.___ Tip of finger   B. Split thickness graft
1829.___ Burn of axilla   C. Full thickness graft
1830.___ Nasal alae   D. Composite graft
1831.___ Decubitus ulcer   Ref. pp. 1923-1924

SELECT THE MOST APPROPRIATE ANSWER(S):

1832. THE TRANSFER OF A PEDICLE FLAP IS INCONVENIENT BECAUSE OF:
A. Poor cosmetic result
B. Unable to move composite tissues
C. Period of time for tissue transfer
D. It has the least versatility of all grafts
Ref. p. 1925

1833. THE MOST EFFECTIVE TREATMENT OF A WOUND SUSTAINED
FOLLOWING AN EXPLOSION, LEAVING MASSIVE PARTICULATE
MATTER EMBEDDED IN THE SKIN, IS:
A. Excision plus split thickness skin graft
B. Tatooing
C. Microsurgery
D. Dermabrasion
E. Island pedicle flaps   Ref. p. 1934

1834. WHICH OF THE FOLLOWING WOULD MOST LIKELY WARRANT A
TRACHEOTOMY FOR AIRWAY CONTROL?:
A. Zygoma fracture plus nasal fracture
B. Mandibular fracture in two or more places
C. Facial fracture into sinus maxillaris
D. Blowout orbit fracture
E. Basal skull fracture   Ref. p. 1935

1835. WHEN A FACIAL SCAR CROSSES THE NASOLABIAL FOLD, WHICH OF
THE FOLLOWING PROCEDURES WOULD MOST LIKELY BE UTILIZED
TO ADJUST THE BRIDGING DEFECT?:
A. Simple excision of scar and closure
B. Z-plasty
C. Skin graft following simple excision
D. Pedicle flap
E. Bernard procedure   Ref. p. 1935

1836. WITH A TRAUMATIC FACIAL LACERATION, WHICH OF THE FOLLOW-
ING IS OF NO VALUE FOR A GOOD COSMETIC RESULT?:
A. Complete cleansing
B. Debride ragged edges
C. Undermine locally and close without tension
D. Subcutaneous sutures
E. All are essential   Ref. p. 1935

1837. THE NERVE DISTRIBUTION MOST LIKELY INJURED DURING A
MANDIBULAR FRACTURE IS:
A. Trigeminal nerve   D. Facial nerve
B. Mental nerve   E. Lingual nerve
C. Infraorbital nerve   Ref. p. 1936

1838. ORBITAL FLOOR FRACTURES ARE SUGGESTED BY ALL OF THE
FOLLOWING, EXCEPT:
A. Globe depression
B. Diplopia on upward gaze
C. Enophthalmus
D. Paralysis of orbicularis oculi muscle
E. Inferior rectus incarceration with upward gaze
Ref. p. 1938

1839. THE MOST FREQUENTLY FRACTURED BONE OF THE FACE IS:
A. Mandible
B. Maxilla
C. Zygoma
D. Orbital bones   Ref. p. 1938

1840. WHICH OF THE FOLLOWING IS THE CORRECT PROCEDURE PRIOR TO
SUTURING OF A FACIAL LACERATION?:
A. Sensory and motor assessment of the facial nerve before anesthesia
administration
B. Only motor assessment of facial nerve before introduction of local
anesthesia
C. Only sensory assessment of facial nerve before introduction of local
anesthesia   Ref. p. 1940

1841. WHICH OF THE FOLLOWING FRACTURED FACIAL BONES IS MOST
COMMONLY ASSOCIATED WITH A TRIGEMINAL NERVE DEFICIT?:
A. Zygoma   D. Mandible
B. Ethmoid   E. Nasal
C. Maxilla   Ref. p. 1941

1842. LID LACERATIONS ARE EASILY REPAIRED WITHOUT A GREAT
NOTICEABLE DEFECT. THE MOST DIFFICULT PROBLEM ASSOCIATED
WITH LACERATIONS EXTENDING THROUGH THE MEDIAL CANTHUSIS
IS:
A. Entropian   D. Horner's syndrome
B. Lacrimal duct laceration damage E. Lid drop
C. Infraorbital nerve damage   Ref. p. 1943

1843. WHICH OF THE FOLLOWING STATEMENTS ARE TRUE CONCERNING
VERTICAL LACERATIONS OF THE EYELID?:
A. Usually are associated with nasal fracture
B. Usually will develop a contracture if direction is not altered
C. Is associated with prolonged healing because of muscle traction
D. None of the above   Ref. p. 1943

1844. CLEFT LIP REPAIRS ARE ALL VARIATIONS OF WHICH PROCEDURE?:
A. Pedicle flap
B. Composite graft
C. Z-plasty   Ref. p. 1944

1845. IN CLEFT PALATE WITH INVOLVEMENT OF THE "SECONDARY
PALATE" ONE IS CONCERNED WITH WHICH OF THE FOLLOWING?:
A. Lip   D. Soft palate
B. Hard palate   E. All of the above
C. Alveolar ridge   Ref. p. 1944

1846. PATIENTS WITH CLEFT PALATE SHOULD UNDERGO WHICH
SURGICAL REPAIR FIRST?:
A. Soft palate   D. All at once
B. Hard palate   E. None of the above
C. Lip   Ref. p. 1949

1847. THE PALATE REPAIR IS BEST PERFORMED PRIOR TO____YEARS
OF AGE TO ASSURE THE BEST SPEECH RESULTS:
A. 3   D. 24
B. 9   E. 36
C. 12   Ref. p. 1949

1848. THE THYROID ANLAGE OF A THYROGLOSSAL DUCT DEVELOPS FROM:
       A. Foramen cecum   D. First branchial arch
       B. First branchial cleft   E. Second branchial arch
       C. Second branchial cleft   Ref. p. 1952

1849. SINCE THE MOST COMMON COMPLICATION OF THYROGLOSSAL CYST
       SURGERY IS RECURRENCE THE BEST SURGICAL PREVENTION
       SHOULD INCLUDE THE REMOVAL OF:
       A. Thyroid isthmus along the cyst
       B. Thyroid pyramidal lobe along with the cyst
       C. Hyoid bone along with the cyst
       D. The foramen cecum along with the cyst
       E. None of the above   Ref. p. 1952

1850. THE MOST COMMON BRANCHIAL CLEFT ANOMALY INVOLVES:
       A. First branchial arch   D. Third branchial cleft
       B. First branchial cleft   E. Fourth branchial cleft
       C. Second branchial cleft   Ref. p. 1953

       FILL IN THE MOST APPROPRIATE ANSWERS: (Questions 1851-1852)

       A. External auditory canal
       B. Anterior to the sternocleidomastoid muscle
       C. Between the internal and external branch of the carotid artery
       D. Tonsillar fossa
       E. None of the above

       The origin of the most common branchial cleft anomaly is 1851)_____
       and it terminates at 1852)_____ .   Ref. p. 1953-1954

       SELECT THE MOST APPROPRIATE ANSWER:

1853. CENTRAL FACIAL NERVE PALSY MAY BE SUSPECTED BY ALL OF
       THE FOLLOWING, EXCEPT:
       A. Contralateral paralysis of facial muscles except for forehead
       B. Taste loss in anterior 2/3 of tongue
       C. Taste loss of soft palate
       D. Pure motor deficit
       E. All of the above   Ref. p. 1956

1854. THE PERIPHERAL BRANCHES OF THE FACIAL NERVE USUALLY ARE
       FOUND:
       A. At the styloid foramen
       B. Post auricular
       C. Pre-auricular between the superficial and deep lobes of the parotid
           gland
       D. Posterior to the sternocleidomastoid muscle and spreading out
           fan-like beneath the platysma
       E. None of the above   Ref. p. 1956

1855. THE RECONSTRUCTIVE PROCEDURE(S) UTILIZED TO PREVENT
       CORNEAL DAMAGE FOLLOWING FACIAL NERVE PARALYSIS IS:
       A. Tarsorrhaphy
       B. Canthoplasty
       C. Gillie's operation
       D. None of the above
       E. All of the above   Ref. p. 1958

1856. THE PROCEDURE CONSIDERED MOST APPROPRIATE FOR COVERING
DECUBITUS ULCERS IS:
A. Reverdine graft   D. Composite graft
B. Ollier-Thiersh graft   E. Pedicle flap
C. Wolfe graft   Ref. p. 1958

1857. NEONATES WITH HYPOSPADIAS SHOULD:
A. Always have immediate resection of the chordee
B. Undergo a meatotomy with two months
C. Never undergo a circumcision at birth
D. Always have cystoscopy because of associated urethral valves
E. All of the above   Ref. p. 1963

1858. THE GOAL OF REHABILITATION IS BEST DESCRIBED IN TERMS OF:
A. Reestablished active limb mobility
B. Development of both motor and sensory function
C. Reestablishment of functional individual in his environment
D. Return of positive nitrogen balance with full skeletal muscle develop-
ment
E. Reestablishment of anatomic and physiologic function
Ref. p. 1967

1859. FOLLOWING EXTENSIVE SURGERY OR TRAUMA THE PRIMARY LOSS
OF BODY NITROGEN IS_____TISSUE:
A. Adipose   D. Skeletal muscle
B. Connective   E. Bone
C. Hepatic   Ref. p. 1967

1860. VOLKMANN'S CONTRACTURE OF THE ARM IS A_____TYPE OF
DISABILITY:
A. Primary
B. Secondary
C. Neither   Ref. p. 1967

1861. THE PRINCIPLE BEHIND SUCCESS IN EXERCISE AND MUSCLE RE-
EDUCATION IS:
A. Power   D. Speed
B. Coordination   E. Repetition
C. Range of motion   Ref. p. 1968

1862. THE MAJOR PURPOSE OF PASSIVE EXERCISE APPLIED TO A
PATIENT IS:
A. Muscle reeducation
B. To prevent contractures
C. To promote normal range of motion
D. To prevent the development of lymphedema
E. To provide repetition of motion   Ref. p. 1968

1863. WHICH OF THE FOLLOWING TYPES OF EXERCISE REQUIRE
PATIENT COOPERATION?:
A. Active exercise
B. Functional exercise
C. Special exercise
D. Resistive active exercise
E. All of the above   Ref. p. 1968

1864. WHICH OF THE FOLLOWING CAN NOT BE ACCOMPLISHED WITH HEAT?:
A. Pain relief
B. Increase in circulation
C. Relief of non-inflammatory edema
D. Sedation
E. Reduction of muscular tension   Ref. p. 1968

1865. A PATIENT WHO SUSTAINS A 40 PER CENT BURN OVER HIS BODY
WHICH ENCOMPASSED BOTH UPPER EXTREMITIES, WOULD BENEFIT
MOST FROM WHICH OF THE FOLLOWING AFTER INITIAL FLUID
REPLACEMENT?:
A. Whirlpool bath   D. Paraffin application
B. Hubbard tank   E. Infrared radiation
C. Hot packs   Ref. p. 1969

1866. WHICH OF THE FOLLOWING WOULD BE MOST EFFECTIVE IN THE
TREATMENT OF DEEP TISSUES WITH A HIGH WATER CONTENT?:
A. Short wave   D. Infrared radiation
B. Microwave   E. None are effective
C. Ultrasound   Ref. p. 1969

1867. CONTRAINDICATIONS TO THE UTILIZATION OF SHORT WAVE,
MICROWAVE AND ULTRASOUND (i. e. DEEP HEAT) INCLUDE ALL OF
THE FOLLOWING, EXCEPT:
A. Hemorrhagic diathesis
B. Pregnant uterus
C. Fracture site after callus formation
D. All of the above
E. None of the above   Ref. p. 1969

1868. WHICH OF THE FOLLOWING MEDICATIONS MAY CONTRAINDICATE
THE USE OF ULTRAVIOLET THERAPY TO A PATIENT WITH
DECUBITUS ULCERS?:
A. Eclomycin   D. Phenoxybenzamine
B. Thorazine   E. All of the above
C. Amyl nitrate   Ref. p. 1969

1869. ELECTROTHERAPY OR CURRENTS UTILIZED TO STIMULATE MOTOR
AND SENSORY NERVES MOST OFTEN IS THERAPEUTICALLY USED TO:
A. Provide muscular support
B. Prevent edema
C. Reduce muscle tension
D. Maintain denervated muscles is a normal state until nerve regenera-
tion is accomplished
E. Prevent contractures   Ref. p. 1969

1870. WHICH OF THE FOLLOWING WILL NOT BE ACCOMPLISHED BY
MASSAGE?:
A. Increase lymphatic flow
B. Disruption of fibrosis by mechanical stretching
C. Reduce local fat deposition
D. Increase a pain threshold
E. Small vessel vasodilatation   Ref. p. 1969

1871. ALL OF THE FOLLOWING WILL PREVENT MUSCULAR ATROPHY
FOLLOWING INACTIVITY, EXCEPT:
A. Massage   D. Passive exercises
B. Active assistance exercises   E. All will prevent atrophy
C. Functional exercises   Ref. p. 1969

1872. WHICH CONSTITUTES A CONTRAINDICATION TO MASSAGE AS A
THERAPEUTIC MEASURE?:
A. Acute inflammation   D. Skin lesions
B. Malignant tumors   E. All of the above
C. Phlebitis   Ref. p. 1969

1873. COORDINATION OF MOTOR MOVEMENT MAY BEST BE ACCOM-
PLISHED BY WHICH OF THE FOLLOWING THERAPEUTIC MEASURES?:
A. Massage   D. Passive exercise
B. Orthotics   E. All of the above
C. Occupational therapy   Ref. p. 1969

1874. WHICH OF THE FOLLOWING FACTORS SEEMS TO HAVE THE
GREATEST OVERALL INFLUENCE OF SUCCESS OR FAILURE OF
REHABILITATION?:
A. Occupational therapy
B. Physical therapy
C. Psychiatric care of emotional disabilities
D. Application of adequate orthotics   Ref. p. 1970

1875. IN THE FIELD OF ORTHOTICS A DYNAMIC BRACE DEALS WITH:
A. Functional use   D. Provide support
B. Protect an injured area   E. All of the above
C. Prevent contracture   Ref. p. 1971

1876. IN A REHABILITATION PROGRAM THE LOWEST PRIORITY WOULD
BE GIVEN TO:
A. Mobilization of and injured extremity
B. Relief of pain
C. Permit healing
D. Psychiatric support   Ref. p. 1972

1877. IMMOBILIZATION OF A FRACTURE SITE SHOULD INCLUDE:
A. Only the joint involved
B. The joint proximal to the fracture site
C. The joint distal to the fracture site
D. Both the joints proximal and distal to the fracture site
E. None of the above   Ref. p. 1972

1878. AFTER FRACTURE IMMOBILIZATION ACTIVE EXERCISES SHOULD
BE PERFORMED BOTH PROXIMAL AND DISTAL TO THE FRACTURE
SITE. IF SEVERE PAIN PRESENTS DURING EXERCISE ONE SHOULD:
A. Continue with the exercise
B. Reexamine the fracture site because of possible slippage
C. Terminate exercises for two weeks
D. None of the above
E. All of the above   Ref. p. 1972

ANSWER THE FOLLOWING QUESTION BY USING THE KEY
OUTLINED BELOW:
A. If both statement and reason are correct and related cause and effect
B. If both statement and reason are correct but not related cause and
effect
C. If statement is true but reason is false
D. If statement is false but reason is true
E. If both statement and reason are false

1879. Most patients who undergo extremity amputations who are over the age of
60 years are successfully rehabilitated BECAUSE the cause of the disease
state is simultaneously cured.   Ref. p. 1972

SECTION XIV – ACQUIRED AND CONGENITAL MUSCULOSKELETAL DISORDERS: RECONSTRUCTION AND REHABILITATION

SELECT THE MOST APPROPRIATE ANSWER:

1880. THE SUCCESS OF AN AMPUTEE IN ADJUSTING TO A PROSTHESIS DEPENDS ON:
A. The amputation stump
B. Patient motivation
C. Patient cardiovascular stability
D. Type of prosthesis
E. All of the above
Ref. p. 1973

1881. THE IDEAL AMPUTATION STUMP FOR PROSTHETIC FITTING:
A. Tapers from above downward
B. Tapers from side to side
C. Tapers from right upper to left lower
D. Permits the bony end to be covered by only skin
E. All are correct   Ref. p. 1973

ANSWER THE FOLLOWING QUESTIONS BY USING THE KEY OUTLINED BELOW:
A. If both statement and reason are correct and related cause and effect
B. If both statement and reason are correct but not related cause and effect
C. If statement is true but reason is false
D. If statement is false but reason is true
E. If both statement and reason are false

1882. To complete the closure of an amputation site a myofascial bridge is considered an excellent cover over the bone BECAUSE it permits the skin flaps to maintain mobility over the end of the stump.
                                        Ref. p. 1973

1883. Amputations below the knee are always desirable when possible BECAUSE the presence of less than two inches below the knee joint provides adequate support and prosthetic function with short levers.
                                        Ref. p. 1973

1884. Above the knee amputations should always preserve the length of the femur to but not including the joint space BECAUSE the prosthesis applied on a stump with four inches of the joint results in asymmetry of the two extremities.   Ref. p. 1973

SELECT THE MOST APPROPRIATE ANSWER:

1885. WHICH OF THE FOLLOWING SHOULD BE CONSIDERED WHEN PERFORMING AN AMPUTATION?:
A. Knee disarticulation is a poor procedure
B. Amputations within 2 inches above or below the knee are undesirable
C. Above knee amputations are best performed 4 inches above the knee joint
D. Short stumps of 2 inches or less are not desirable
E. All of the above   Ref. p. 1973

1886. THE STAGING OF AMPUTEES ACCORDING TO THE INTENDED END RESULT AFTER PROSTHETIC APPLICATION IS IMPORTANT AS A MEANS OF COMMUNICATION AMONG PHYSICIANS. A CLASS 5 REPRESENTS:
A. Full restoration
B. Self-care minus
C. Partial restoration
D. Self-care plus
E. Cosmetic plus
F. Not feasible

Ref. p. 1974

1887. THE USE OF NEW TECHNIQUES FOR EARLY PROSTHETIC APPLICA-
TION PERMIT A PATIENT TO WEAR A PERMANENT PROSTHESIS
WITHIN:
   A. 1-2 weeks   D. 6-8 weeks
   B. 2-4 weeks   E. 8-10 weeks
   C. 4-6 weeks   Ref. p. 1975

1888. THE MINIMAL TIME PERIOD OF IMMOBILIZATION FOLLOWING AN
EARLY OR DELAYED TENDON REPAIR IS:
   A. 3 weeks   D. 12 weeks
   B. 6 weeks   E. 15 weeks
   C. 9 weeks   Ref. p. 1975

1889. NERVE REGENERATION FROM THE PROXIMAL SECTION FOLLOWING
TRAUMA PROGRESSES AT_____PER DAY:
   A. 1.5 mm   D. 4.5 mm
   B. 2.5 mm   E. 5.5 mm
   C. 3.5 mm   Ref. p. 1977

1890. DURING THE PHASE OF NERVE REGENERATION WHICH OF THE
FOLLOWING EXERCISES IS MOST USEFUL?:
   A. Active assisted exercises
   B. Active exercises
   C. Passive exercises
   D. Functional exercises   Ref. p. 1977

1891. ELASTIC EXTENSIONS FROM THE FINGERS EXTENDING ON THE
EXTENSIOR SURFACE OF THE HANDS AND AFFIXED TO A SOLID
SUPPORT IS UTILIZED IN WHICH OF THE FOLLOWING?:
   A. Median nerve injury   D. Long thoracic nerve injury
   B. Axillary nerve injury   E. Ulnar nerve injury
   C. Radial nerve injury   Ref. p. 1977

1892. THE MOST USEFUL INITIAL THERAPEUTIC MEASURE FOLLOWING A
PERONEAL NERVE INJURY IS:
   A. Splint with negator springs
   B. Posterior splint
   C. Short leg cast
   D. None of the above   Ref. p. 1977

1893. THE MOST FREQUENT CAUSE OF DEATH IN PATIENTS WITH LESIONS
AT C6 OR C7 ARE OF_____ORIGIN:
   A. Respiratory
   B. Cardiac
   C. Urogenic
   D. Hepatic   Ref. p. 1979

1894. THE NEUROGENIC BLADDER RESULTING IN A LARGE RESIDUAL
VOLUME OFTEN REQUIRES WHICH OF THE FOLLOWING FOR LOWER
MOTOR NEURON LESIONS?:
   A. Pudendal neurectomy
   B. Transurethral resection
   C. Anterior and posterior sacral rhizotomy
   D. Cordectomy
   E. Intrathecal alcohol injection   Ref. p. 1979

The author has made every effort to thoroughly verify the answers to the questions which appear on the preceding pages. However, as in any text, some inaccuracies and ambiguities may occur. Therefore, if in doubt, please consult your reference: Schwartz, S.I., Lillehei, R.C., Shires, G.T., Spencer, F.C. and Storer, E.H.: Principles of Surgery, 2nd Edition, McGraw-Hill, 1974.

1. B✓	57. C	113. B	168. B	224. C	280. C	336. F
2. C✓	58. E	114. D	169. C	225. BD	281. B	337. D
3. C✓	59. B	115. D	170. C	226. C	282. AD	338. C
4. C✓	60. AC	116. B	171. C	227. A	283. A	339. C
5. B	61. A	117. C	172. A	228. A	284. AC	340. B
6. D✓	62. F	118. E	173. B	229. C	285. B	341. C
7. D	63. B	119. D	174. D	230. E	286. CB	342. C
8. AC	64. C	120. T	175. B	231. T	287. E	343. E
9. A	65. D	121. C	176. A	232. AC	288. A	344. B
10. D	66. E	122. D	177. E	233. BD	289. DE	345. C
11. A	67. E	123. D	178. D	234. ABC	290. E	346. E
12. B	68. A	124. B	179. D	235. B	291. D	347. B
13. E	69. AC	125. C	180. DB	236. B	292. A	348. C
14. A	70. AD	126. A	181. D	237. E	293. C	349. B
15. E	71. B	127. D	182. D	238. B	294. B	350. C
16. C	72. B	128. E	183. D	239. A	295. A	351. C
17. D	73. D	129. B	184. A	240. E	296. B	352. C
18. B	74. A	130. C	185. AC	241. C	297. C	353. D
19. F	75. A	131. A	186. C	242. D	298. C	354. AD
20. E	76. A	132. E	187. A	243. A	299. E	355. D
21. A	77. D	133. D	188. F	244. C	300. F	356. B
22. C	78. A	134. A	189. T	245. CA	301. B	357. C
23. A	79. B	135. T	190. T	246. D	302. BDE	358. A
24. T	80. B	136. T	191. A	247. B	303. C	359. D
25. B	81. A	137. A	192. F	248. B	304. D	360. B
26. A	82. D	138. A	193. D	249. B	305. ACD	361. E
27. B	83. E	139. A	194. A	250. T	306. A	362. B
28. A	84. B	140. A	195. B	251. A	307. AED	363. A
29. C	85. D	141. C	196. F	252. F	308. B	364. A
30. A	86. A	142. B	197. T	253. A	309. A	365. C
31. A	87. C	143. C	198. F	254. T	310. D	366. B
32. A	88. A	144. D	199. T	255. B	311. D	367. B
33. C	89. D	145. A	200. E	256. CE	312. B	368. D
34. B	90. C	146. D	201. D	257. D	313. D	369. D
35. AD	91. B	147. C	202. D	258. BA	314. C	370. A
36. A	92. C	148. B	203. E	259. D	315. E	371. B
37. E	93. C	149. D	204. C	260. BA	316. B	372. C
38. A	94. B	150. C	205. A	261. A	317. B	373. E
39. C	95. C	151. C	206. AC	262. A	318. C	374. C
40. A	96. B	152. AD	207. C	263. E	319. D	375. B
41. C	97. AC	153. C	208. F	264. A	320. B	376. E
42. A	98. D	154. E	209. D	265. F	321. B	377. C
43. E	99. B	155. C	210. C	266. T	322. AD	378. T
44. D	100. E	156. ACB DE	211. A	267. B	323. D	379. B
45. A	101. AC		212. AD	268. C	324. T	380. T
46. B	102. D	157. C	213. ABC	269. B	325. F	381. A
47. A	103. C	158. B	214. F	270. A	326. B	382. D
48. D	104. AD	159. C	215. D	271. D	327. E	383. AC
49. E	105. AC	160. BD	216. AC	272. BD	328. A	384. T
50. C	106. A	161. T	217. A	273. D	329. A	385. D
51. A	107. B	162. E	218. A	274. B	330. A	386. B
52. E	108. A	163. B	219. AC	275. A	331. C	387. E
53. B	109. BD	164. C	220. D	276. D	332. B	388. D
54. C	110. T	165. A	221. D	277. E	333. D	389. D
55. E	111. A	166. C	222. BC	278. B	334. A	390. D
56. A	112. C	167. D	223. ABC	279. B	335. D	391. C

ANSWER KEY221

392. A
393. E
394. A
395. C
396. B
397. B
398. A
399. A
400. D
401. B
402. C
403. A
404. C
405. C
406. A
407. B
408. T
409. D
410. T
411. C
412. A
413. B
414. B
415. B
416. B
417. CE
418. C
419. C
420. B
421. A
422. A
423. C
424. A
425. B
426. A
427. C
428. A
429. D
430. D
431. E
432. A
433. AD
434. E
435. C
436. B
437. A
438. F
439. G
440. D
441. E
442. D
443. A
444. C
445. B
446. B
447. C (70%)
448. A
449. B
450. B
451. A
452. T

453. A (immune lymphocytes and macrophages)
454. F
455. F
456. A
457. B
458. C
459. C
460. C
461. F
462. A
463. B
464. T
465. A
466. C
467. E
468. D
469. C
470. E
471. E (2%)
472. B
473. C
474. B
475. B
476. B
477. D
478. CA
479. A
480. C
481. (1) A (2) B
482. T
483. A
484. D
485. A
486. AC
487. E
488. C
489. A
490. C
491. A
492. A
493. B
494. E
495. A
496. A
497. E
498. E
499. B
500. C
501. A
502. D
503. A
504. BD
505. A
506. AD
507. E
508. C
509. E
510. BD

511. C
512. A
513. A
514. C
515. A
516. AC
517. D
518. E
519. A
520. D
521. D
522. C
523. C
524. D
525. A
526. A
527. C
528. C
529. D
530. A
531. A
532. C
533. B
534. E
535. C
536. E
537. E
538. C
539. F
540. A
541. C
542. F
543. A
544. E
545. D
546. A
547. BE
548. CA
549. E
550. AD
551. C
552. D
553. D
554. A
555. C
556. C
557. D
558. B
559. A
560. B
561. D
562. C
563. B
564. C
565. A
566. A
567. BD
568. C
569. D
570. D
571. A
572. E

573. B
574. B
575. A
576. A
577. AD
578. ABC
579. B
580. E
581. C
582. D
583. A
584. D
585. A
586. C
587. B
588. C
589. E
590. AD
591. A
592. D
593. D
594. A
595. B
596. B
597. T
598. A
599. AC
600. C
601. AC
602. B
603. C
604. D
605. C
606. D
607. C
608. D
609. E
610. B
611. D
612. A
613. D
614. C
615. A
616. AD
617. B
618. D
619. B
620. A
621. C
622. E
623. C
624. ABC
625. B
626. C
627. E
628. B
629. B
630. D
631. D
632. B
633. C
634. D

635. E
636. D
637. B
638. E
639. C
640. C
641. B
642. B
643. A
644. B
645. D
646. C
647. D
648. D
649. B
650. E
651. E
652. B
653. D
654. A
655. D
656. D
657. B
658. D
659. C
660. A
661. B
662. ABE
663. C
664. A
665. D
666. C
667. A
668. F
669. E
670. D
671. B
672. C
673. D
674. C
675. D
676. B
677. D
678. C
679. A
680. B
681. C
682. D
683. A
684. B
685. B
686. B
687. D
688. C
689. F
690. B
691. H
692. G
693. D
694. T
695. T
696. F

697. C
698. B
699. E
700. C
701. C
702. C
703. B
704. E
705. A
706. E
707. A
708. A
709. C
710. A
711. E
712. C
713. E
714. A
715. D
716. A
717. E
718. A
719. C
720. A
721. D
722. D
723. B
724. A
725. B
726. B
727. ABC
728. A
729. D
730. A
731. D
732. E
733. D
734. D
735. A
736. C
737. AD
738. D
739. D
740. A
741. BD
742. D
743. A
744. B
745. AC
746. B
747. A
748. C
749. D
750. D
751. A
752. C
753. E
754. A
755. BD
756. D
757. B
758. B

759. A	817. D	879. C	940. B	998. A	1060. C	1122. A
760. ABC	818. E	880. E	941. B	999. B	1061. AD	1123. A
761. ABC	819. B	881. D	942. E	1000. C	1062. B	1124. B
762. B	820. E	882. D	943. C	1001. A	1063. D	1125. C
763. B	821. C	883. B	944. A	1002. A	1064. B	1126. AD
764. D	822. B	884. B	945. A	1003. C	1065. A	1127. C
765. T	823. B	885. B	946. C	1004. D	1066. C	1128. B
766. A	824. D	886. A	947. E	1005. D	1067. D	1129. C
767. B	825. C	887. B	948. B	1006. C	1068. E	1130. A
768. E	826. A	888. B	949. A	1007. F	1069. A	1131. C
769. C	827. A	889. B	950. D	1008. A	1070. C	1132. A
770. B	828. D	890. D	951. C	1009. AD	1071. BD	1133. D
(20%)	829. A	891. B	952. B	1010. C	1072. B	1134. AD
771. D	830. C	892. E	953. A	1011. D	1073. E	1135. A
772. A	831. B	893. D	954. C	1012. A	1074. B	1136. E
773. A	832. B	894. E	955. D	1013. C	1075. B	1137. B
774. BD	833. E	895. D	956. B	1014. E	1076. B	1138. D
775. D	834. C	896. BD	(60 to	1015. B	1077. B	1139. C
776. D	835. C	897. E	70%)	1016. C	1078. B	1140. B
777. ABC	836. E	898. C	957. AD	1017. A	1079. D	1141. E
778. T	837. B	899. C	958. C	1018. C	1080. E	1142. B
779. A	838. C	900. B	959. A	1019. C	1081. A	1143. C
780. A	839. T	901. F	(60 to	1020. D	1082. C	1144. B
781. E	840. D	902. B	70%)	1021. B	1083. B	1145. B
782. C	841. D	903. D	960. C	1022. D	1084. D	1146. A
783. B	842. B	904. B	961. B	1023. A	1085. D	1147. C
784. D	843. C	905. AD	962. B	1024. B	1086. C	1148. C
785. A	844. C	906. B	963. D	1025. E	1087. A	1149. C
786. D	845. E	907. A	964. C	1026. B	1088. C	1150. B
(50%)	846. D	908. D	965. B	1027. AD	1089. C	1151. B
787. F	847. B	909. E	966. D	1028. ABC	1090. D	1152. C
788. ABC	848. B	910. C	967. A	1029. E	1091. B	1153. D
789. A	849. C	911. A	968. C	1030. B	1092. D	1154. E
790. C	850. E	912. B	969. D	1031. D	1093. E	1155. A
(42%)	851. B	913. C	970. E	1032. C	1094. E	1156. C
791. B	852. T	914. B	971. A	1033. B	1095. B	1157. B
792. E	853. AD	915. B	972. B	1034. C	1096. BD	1158. B
793. E	854. C	916. A	973. B	1035. D	1097. E	1159. C
794. C	855. E	917. B	974. D	1036. A	1098. C	1160. C
(right)	856. D	918. C	975. A	1037. BD	1099. D	1161. A
795. AD	857. D	919. D	976. C	1038. D	1100. A	1162. D
796. D	858. D	920. C	977. B	1039. B	1101. A	1163. B
797. B	859. C	921. C	978. A	1040. C	1102. B	1164. A
798. B	860. B	922. B	979. E	1041. C	1103. C	1165. B
799. ABC	861. C	923. E	980. C	1042. E	1104. C	1166. B
800. A	862. B	924. A	981. B	1043. C	1105. E	1167. B
801. B	863. C	925. ABC	982. C	1044. D	1106. A	1168. E
802. B	864. D	926. BD	983. B	1045. E	1107. ABC	1169. E
803. A	865. B	927. B	984. D	1046. B	1108. A	1170. C
804. A	866. B	928. A	985. B	1047. C	1109. E	1171. C
805. B	867. A	929. D	986. E	1048. E	1110. F	1172. F
806. AD	868. D	930. E	987. A	1049. A	1111. D	1173. D
807. D	869. B	931. B	988. C	1050. B	1112. D	1174. A
808. AD	870. E	932. A	989. A	1051. D	1113. F	1175. T
809. D	871. D	933. A	990. A	1052. C	1114. B	1176. C
810. A	872. D	934. C	991. A	1053. D	1115. C	1177. C
811. C	873. A	935. A	992. D	1054. C	1116. C	1178. AC
812. B	874. E	(10%)	993. D	1055. B	1117. AD	1179. AC
813. C	875. B	936. A	994. A	1056. B	1118. A	1180. E
814. D	876. C	937. C	995. C	1057. A	1119. B	1181. T
815. A	877. A	938. C	996. E	1058. D	1120. B	1182. ABC
816. B	878. B	939. D	997. B	1059. A	1121. B	1183. E

1184. AC	1245. AB	1307. D	1366. BD	1426. B	1488. A
1185. BD	1246. BC	1308. D	1367. A	1427. B	1489. A
1186. D	1247. C	1309. D	1368. AD	1428. E	1490. C
1187. E	1248. E	1310. B	1369. AD	1429. D	1491. C
1188. B	1249. C	1311. A	1370. C	1430. B	1492. E
1189. A	1250. A	1312. E	1371. T	1431. B	1493. B
1190. B (50%)	1251. D	1313. B	1372. E	1432. E	1494. B
1191. C	1252. B	1314. A	1373. B	1433. A	1495. E
1192. C	1253. D	1315. C	1374. B	1434. D	1496. AD
1193. C	1254. AC	1316. B	1375. A	1435. A	1497. E
1194. A	1255. A	1317. A	1376. A	1436. D	1498. D
1195. D	1256. E	1318. C	1377. C	1437. C	1499. A
1196. A	1257. BD	1319. B	1378. A	1438. D	1500. E
1197. D	1258. A	1320. D	1379. D	1439. C	1501. A
1198. T	1259. C	1321. C	1380. A	1440. A	1502. E
1199. T	1260. C	1322. B	1381. D	1441. C	1503. A
1200. D	1261. B	1323. B	1382. D	1442. B	1504. B
1201. T	1262. C	1324. D	1383. F	1443. C	1505. B
1202. AC	1263. C	1325. B	1384. B	1444. B	1506. C
1203. ABC	1264. A	1326. C	1385. A (2%)	1445. C	1507. C
1204. B	1265. B	1327. A	1386. A	1446. A	1508. D
1205. C	1266. C	1328. AD	1387. C	1447. AD	1509. A
1206. C	1267. D	1329. D	1388. E	1448. C	1510. D
1207. B	1268. B	1330. B	1389. A	1449. A	1511. D
1208. B	1269. C	1331. C	1390. C	1450. D	1512. AD
1209. A	1270. E	1332. A	1391. D	1451. B	1513. AD
1210. E	1271. BCE	1333. A	1392. B	1452. AD	1514. B
1211. B	1272. B	1334. C	1393. B	1453. A	1515. B
1212. A	1273. C	1335. AD	1394. B	1454. D	1516. ABC
1213. B	1274. E	1336. B	1395. C	1455. D	1517. B
1214. A	1275. B	1337. B	1396. ABC	1456. E	1518. C
1215. A	1276. C	1338. B	1397. A	1457. C	1519. B
1216. C	1277. A	1339. B	1398. B	1458. D	1520. D
1217. D	1278. D	1340. D	1399. E	1459. D	1521. D
1218. ABC	1279. A	1341. C	1400. D	1460. E	1522. ACD
1219. C	1280. D	1342. E	1401. C	1461. C	1523. C
1220. C	1281. B	1343. AD	1402. A	1462. B	1524. A
1221. D	1282. B	1344. B	1403. B	1463. E	1525. B
1222. B	1283. B	1345. B	1404. F	1464. C	1526. D
1223. D	1284. D	1346. B	1405. C	1465. C	1527. F
1224. B	1285. C	1347. D	1406. F	1466. D	1528. B
1225. D	1286. B	1348. AD	1407. F	1467. B	1529. A
1226. E	1287. F	1349. A (24%)	1408. T	1468. C	1530. B
1227. D	1288. A	1350. B	1409. B	1469. E	1531. E
1228. BD	1289. C	1351. A	1410. B	1470. C	1532. C
1229. D	1290. C	1352. A	1411. A (78%)	1471. A	1533. C
1230. C	1291. B	1353. B	1412. C	1472. D	1534. A
1231. A	1292. B	1354. E	1413. B	1473. D	1535. C
1232. C	1293. B	1355. E	1414. B	1474. D	1536. A
1233. D	1294. B	1356. AD	1415. B	1475. A	1537. BD
1234. C	1295. A	1357. T	1416. B	1476. A	1538. D
1235. B	1296. B	1358. C	1417. B	1477. B	1539. C
1236. A	1297. B	1359. A	1418. D	1478. C	1540. C
1237. E	1298. C	1360. B	1419. B	1479. E	1541. A
1238. B	1299. C	1361. D	1420. D	1480. AD	1542. D
1239. AD	1300. A	1362. A	1421. D	1481. ABC	1543. E
1240. B	1301. B	1363. B	1422. A	1482. C	1544. C
1241. B	1302. D	1364. D	1423. C	1483. A	1545. B
1242. C	1303. C	1365. D (2-3 days)	1424. B	1484. A	1546. C
1243. C	1304. A		1425. AD	1485. B	1547. A
1244. B	1305. B			1486. D	1548. B
	1306. CDAB			1487. A	1549. A

1550. B	1612. E	1674. D	1735. C	1797. AD	1859. D
1551. B	1613. B	1675. B	1736. C	1798. B	1860. B
1552. D	1614. B	1676. A	1737. B	1799. A	1861. E
1553. A	1615. D	1677. D	1738. C	1800. C	1862. B
1554. B	1616. B	1678. B	1739. AB	1801. A	1863. E
1555. ACD	1617. B	1679. A	1740. AD	1802. B	1864. C
1556. B	1618. C	1680. AD	1741. B	1803. C	1865. B
1557. A	1619. D	1681. B	1742. B	1804. D	1866. B
1558. AB	1620. A	1682. C	1743. B	1805. F	1867. C
1559. B	1621. B	(60%)	1744. C	1806. C	1868. A
1560. B	1622. AC	1683. ABC	1745. D	1807. A	1869. D
1561. BD	1623. E	1684. A	1746. A	1808. A	1870. C
1562. C	1624. D	1685. E	1747. D	1809. C	1871. A
1563. E	1625. B	1686. AD	1748. C	1810. B	1872. E
1564. C	1626. C	1687. B	1749. B	1811. C	1873. C
1565. A	1627. A	1688. A	1750. C	1812. C	1874. C
1566. C	1628. B	1689. C	1751. D	1813. C	1875. A
1567. E	1629. C	1690. C	1752. B	1814. B	1876. A
1568. C	1630. D	1691. A	1753. C	1815. A	1877. D
1569. BE	1631. B	1692. B	1754. B	1816. C	1878. B
1570. B	1632. B	1693. DE	1755. D	1817. C	1879. C
1571. DE	1633. A	1694. B	1756. C	1818. C	1880. E
1572. D	1634. C	1695. B	1757. A	1819. B	1881. A
1573. D	1635. E	1696. A	1758. C	1820. AD	1882. A
1574. C	1636. C	1697. C	1759. A	1821. A	1883. C
1575. A	1637. B	1698. B	1760. D	1822. B	1884. D
1576. B	1638. B	1699. C	1761. E	1823. D	1885. E
1577. B	1639. D	1700. AD	1762. C	1824. A	1886. E
1578. D	1640. E	1701. A	1763. C	1825. C	1887. D
1579. A	1641. B	1702. B	1764. E	1826. E	1888. A
1580. B	1642. BC	1703. B	1765. C	1827. D	1889. A
1581. BC	1643. AD	1704. C	1766. B	1828. C	1890. C
1582. B	1644. B	1705. H	1767. C	1829. B	1891. C
1583. C	1645. BCDA	1706. E	1768. D	1830. D	1892. B
1584. B	1646. B	1707. C	1769. D	1831. A	1893. C
1585. B	1647. AB	1708. A	1770. A	1832. C	1894. B
1586. C	1648. C	1709. G	1771. B	1833. D	
1587. A	1649. B	1710. B	1772. C	1834. B	
1588. B	1650. A	1711. I	1773. C	1835. B	
1589. C	1651. CE	1712. D	1774. A	1836. E	
1590. B	1652. E	1713. F	1775. E	1837. B	
1591. C	1653. B	1714. A	1776. E	1838. D	
1592. A	1654. C	1715. A	1777. A	1839. A	
1593. C	1655. A	1716. E	1778. B	1840. B	
1594. A	1656. C	1717. C	1779. A	1841. D	
1595. B	1657. E	1718. B	1780. B	1842. B	
1596. B	1658. B	1719. C	1781. B	1843. B	
1597. E	1659. D	1720. A	1782. C	1844. C	
1598. E	1660. A	1721. B	1783. B	1845. BD	
1599. B	1661. B	1722. B	1784. D	1846. C	
1600. C	1662. D	1723. B	1785. B	1847. D	
1601. E	1663. B	1724. D	1786. C	1848. A	
1602. F	1664. C	1725. D	1787. B	1849. C	
1603. G	1665. A	1726. BD	1788. B	1850. C	
1604. A	1666. DAB	1727. C	1789. C	1851. D	
1605. B	1667. C	1728. A	1790. D	1852. B	
1606. D	1668. D	1729. A	1791. B	1853. D	
1607. D	1669. B	1730. C	1792. A	1854. C	
1608. E	1670. D	1731. B	1793. A	1855. E	
1609. B	1671. C	1732. E	1794. B	1856. E	
1610. B	1672. A	1733. B	1795. B	1857. C	
1611. A	1673. D	1734. A	1796. A	1858. C	

Other Books Available

MEDICAL EXAM REVIEW BOOKS

101	Vol. 1	Comprehensive................	$12.00
102	Vol. 2	Clinical Medicine.............	7.50
123	Vol. 2A	Txtbk. Study Guide Int. Med......	7.50
130	Vol. 2B	Txtbk. Study Guide Int. Med......	7.50
153	Vol. 2C	Textbook Study Guide of Cardiology.	7.50
103	Vol. 3	Basic Sciences	7.50
104	Vol. 4	Obstetrics - Gynecology	7.50
152	Vol. 4A	Textbook Study Guide of Gynecology	7.50
105	Vol. 5	Surgery...................	7.50
150	Vol. 5A	Textbook Study Guide of Surgery ...	7.50
106	Vol. 6	Public Health & Preventive Medicine	7.50
156	Vol. 7A	Textbook Study Guide of Psychiatry.	7.50
108	Vol. 8	Psychiatry & Neurology.........	7.50
111	Vol. 11	Pediatrics..................	7.50
112	Vol. 12	Anesthesiology	7.50
113	Vol. 13	Orthopaedics................	12.00
114	Vol. 14	Urology	12.00
115	Vol. 15	Ophthalmology..............	12.00
116	Vol. 16	Otolaryngology..............	12.00
117	Vol. 17	Radiology.................	12.00
118	Vol. 18	Thoracic Surgery	12.00
119	Vol. 19	Neurological Surgery..........	15.00
128	Vol. 20	Physical Medicine	12.00
127	Vol. 21	Dermatology	12.00
141	Vol. 22	Gastroenterology	12.00
126	Vol. 23	Child Psychiatry	12.00
143	Vol. 24	Pulmonary Diseases	12.00
133	Vol. 25	Nuclear Medicine	12.00
132	Vol. 26	Allergy...................	12.00
129	Vol. 27	Plastic Surgery	12.00
138	Vol. 28	Cardiovascular Diseases	12.00
146	Vol. 29	Oncology	12.00
147	Vol. 30	Infectious Diseases	12.00
144	Vol. 31	Rheumatology	12.00
148	Vol. 32	Hematology................	12.00
131	Vol. 33	Endocrinology	12.00
120	ECFMG Exam Review — Part One........		7.50
121	ECFMG Exam Review — Part Two		7.50

BASIC SCIENCE REVIEW BOOKS

201	Anatomy Review....................	$ 7.00
202	Biochemistry Review................	7.00
215	Digestive System Basic Sciences.........	7.00
207	Embryology Review.................	7.00
212	Heart & Vascular Systems Basic Sciences ...	7.00
203	Microbiology Review................	7.00
210	Nervous System Basic Sciences..........	7.00
204	Pathology Review..................	7.00
205	Pharmacology Review	7.00
206	Physiology Review	7.00
213	Respiratory System Basic Sciences........	7.00
214	Urinary System Basic Sciences	7.00
151	Histology Textbook Study Guide......	7.00
155	Medical Physiology Textbook Study Guide ..	7.00

STATE BOARD REVIEW BOOKS

411	Medical State Board Review – Basic Sciences .	$10.00
412	Medical State Board Review – Clinic. Sciences	10.00

SPECIALTY BOARD REVIEW BOOKS

314	Cardiology Specialty Board Review.......	$12.00
311	Dermatology Specialty Board Review.......	12.00
309	Family Practice Specialty Board Review	12.00
303	Internal Medicine Specialty Board Review ...	12.00
306	Neurology Specialty Board Review	12.00
304	Obstetrics - Gynecology Specialty Board Review	12.00
305	Pathology Specialty Board Review	12.00
301	Pediatrics Specialty Board Review........	12.00
312	Psychiatry Specialty Board Review........	12.00
302	Surgery Specialty Board Review..........	12.00
313	The Otolaryngology Boards.............	10.00
307	The Psychiatry Boards................	8.00

CASE STUDY BOOKS

027	Allergy Case Studies.................	$10.00
001	Cardiology Case Studies..............	10.00
012	Chest Diseases Case Studies	10.00
029	Child Psychiatry Case Studies..........	10.00
014	Cutaneous Medicine Case Studies........	7.50
003	ECG Case Studies	7.50
040	Echocardiography Case Studies	12.00
008	Endocrinology Case Studies	12.00
020	Hematology Case Studies..............	10.00
011	Infectious Diseases Case Studies.........	10.00
022	Kidney Disease Case Studies	12.00
006	Neurology Case Studies	10.00
030	Orthopedic Surgery Case Studies	10.00
021	Otolaryngology Case Studies............	10.00
018	Pediatric Hematology Case Studies........	10.00
023	Pediatric Oculo-Neural Diseases Case Studies	10.00
019	Respiratory Care Case Studies...........	7.50
038	Thyroid Case Studies.................	10.00
017	Urology Case Studies.................	10.00
026	X-Ray Case Studies..................	10.00

PRACTITIONERS GUIDES

705	E.N.T. Disorders	$10.00
709	Hypertension	10.00
704	OB-Gynecology Disorders.............	10.00
703	Ophthalmologic Disorders.............	10.00

JOURNAL ARTICLE COMPILATIONS

795	Emergency Room Journal Articles.........	$ 8.00
799	Hospital Pharmacy Journal Articles	10.00
530	Medical Psychiatry Journal Articles.......	12.00
797	Outpatient Services Journal Articles, 2nd Ed..	10.00
524	Rec. Adv. Myocard. Infarc. Shock Jrnl. Art. ..	24.00
523	Selected Papers in Inhalation Therapy......	10.00

Prices subject to change.

M

Other Books Available